Fundamentals of Medical Management

Second Edition

Edited by Jerry L. Hammon, MD, FACPE

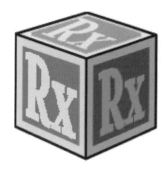

American College of Physician Executives
4890 W. Kennedy Boulevard
Suite 200
Tampa, Florida 33609

ISBN: 0-924674-66-0
Library of Congress Card Number: 99-63142
Printed in the United States of America by Hillsboro Printing Company, Tampa, Florida

Preface

For several years now, the American College of Physician Executives has conducted a group of special educational programs intended for physicians who are just entering the first stages of medical management. Aimed at medical staff leaders, department and section chiefs, and physicians becoming involved in the governance of medical group practices, these courses introduce the fundamentals of management to help these individuals understand the nature of the task that they have undertaken. These courses are different from the College's Physician in Management seminar series, in that they provide only a few critical survival skills. They are not intended to build a solid foundation in management.

Many of the graduates of these courses indicated both an interest in and a need for a reference that would remind them of the content of courses after they return to their organizations. And so the first edition of this book from the College was produced in 1993. Members of the College's Society on Hospitals undertook the project, many of them serving as authors of chapters. Dr. Jerry Hammon, the editor, was Chair of the Society during the book project and volunteered to oversee its design and production. He carefully read every manuscript, offering guidance for revisions as necessary.

Many of the authors of chapters in the first edition of the book are back again in this new edition, but their chapters have been expanded and revised to acknowledge the phenomenal changes that have occurred in the health care field over the past seven or so years. Much of the most basic elements of medical management are immutable, but the technical content has undergone sometimes cataclysmic transformations over the past decade. The new physician executive may not find comfort in this book, but he or she will certainly find knowledge that will guide him or her more effectively into a medical management career.

Combined with *New Leadership in Health Care Management: The Physician Executive,* another hardcover book in the College's catalog of publications, this book not only assists the physician new to medical management to deal effectively with his or her new responsibilities but also further defines and refines the medical management profession itself. There are all manner of environments and levels of responsibility in the medical management profession. *Fundamentals of Medical Management: A Guide for the New Physician Executive* is where it all begins.

Wesley Curry
American College of Physician Executives
Tampa, Florida
November 2000

Foreword

I am assuming that you have taken or are contemplating taking a plunge into the mysterious waters of medical management. And I am also assuming that, in preparation for that plunge, you acquired this book about medical management, hoping that it would be your life preserver and keep you afloat until you could become proficient in the many life-saving strokes needed in the swirling waters of medical management.

Each of the chapters of this book has been written, reviewed, and/or edited by members of the American College of Physician Executives who are very actively engaged in some form of medical management. The subjects involve specific directions for acquiring the skills needed to begin the handling of basic problems you may encounter in medical management. Each chapter is, in itself, a mini-life-saver. Of course, how you handle each of these "life-savers" will depend upon you and upon the circumstances that you encounter when you need the skills.

Review and application of the many helpful basics found in this volume will be as necessary as review and practice of any life-saving technique. If, after review and practice, there is a need for more help, you will find that not only will the authors be willing to respond to your call of, "help, I'm over my head," but also other experienced members of the College will rush to your aid if they hear your call. Just make the request.

A final word of warning. This treatise is intended to get you started in this administrative ocean. If used correctly, it can keep you afloat. But please be aware that, just as in all other endeavors, there are the unseen dangers. You should be able to survive these dangers and gain even more expertise in the pursuit of a very successful career in medical management. However, be forewarned that there will be some "sharks" in this pool. As always, your best defense is a good offense. That offense can best be developed from the many superb and readily available educational experiences offered through ACPE. Take advantage of these opportunities as frequently as possible. The rewards are immense.

Since the first edition of this book in 1993, there have been many more changes in the fields of medicine and medical management. These changes are usually quick, but many seem to have been at warp speed. Therefore, in warning you above of the "swirling waters" and the "sharks," I should also have cautioned you to be aware of the tidal waves, octopi, electric eels, and multiple other lethal pitfalls that may suddenly seem to overwhelm you or even eliminate many medical managers (downsizing seems to be the fashion at times). The beautiful Portuguese man of war is colorful and fascinating to watch, but, like it, so many management cost containment and insurance and government intrusions can entangle and painfully neutralize a medical manager before he or she knows it. Beware, but be prepared.

The best of everything for a satisfying and successful new career.

Jerry L. Hammon, MD, FACPE
West Milton, Ohio
November 2000

Contents

Chapter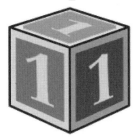

Clinical Practice to Medical Management: A Case Study

by Frank J. Volpe, MD, FACPE

The road to medical management and to success in this newly chosen career is a personal journey. Like all journeys, it requires considerable planning. In this lead chapter to the book, a veteran physician executive shares the story of his transition into and travels through a medical management career. He provides some sage advice, based on personal experiences, on how to navigate the sometimes turbulent waters of medical management.

"Let's sit by the pool."

"Great! I'd like that."

Pool side was their favorite retreat, a quiet place to have their cocktails, to unwind after a busy day, to enjoy each other's company. He missed that closeness when he got home too late. He was too late too often in the two years since being in his first full-time medical directorship.

They sat, sipped. He felt relaxation taking over.

"We have to talk. Serious," she gently said.

Tension displaced relaxation. He feared he knew the topic. They had often discussed his job and what the stress was doing to him, to them, to their marriage. It was easy to discuss things with her; she was always calm, reasonable, caring, never demanding or threatening, and, above all, loving. He could not blame her if she brought it up again. He realized he was making a major investment of energy and time to learn his job, management, and how to deal with the multiple problems that came his way, an investment he felt was necessary to be successful, not only for himself, but for them. He had to admit that, despite his earlier intentions, assurances, and promises, little had changed. But, as he often told her, once over the initial learning-hump, things would get better, a lot better.

They started talking. His fear was justified. Their conversation followed the familiar pattern; the dynamics were the same until she said something totally out of character.

Calmly, deliberately, she said, "I know, and believe, you meant it before when you told me things would change. So far, nothing has. It's tearing me up inside." After a brief silence, she added, "My bags are upstairs. Packed. If you're not committed to change, committed to start that change right now, I'm leaving."

In this chapter, I share my thoughts on, and experiences in, medical management, especially on the transition from practice to management, with the hope that a physician who is contemplating, or has just made, such a move will find something to make the transition easier. We physicians are used to increasing our clinical knowledge and skills through case studies, so I will share my case to illustrate what I think is important to know on the journey into medical management—what knowledge and skills are needed, and how I acquired them. I do so realizing I risk exposing my biases, weaknesses, and failures; perhaps there are lessons in those too.

My first action outside the doctor-patient interchange occurred in the mid-1950s, in the year after internship, my first of two years in the United States Public Health Service (USPHS) to satisfy my draft obligation. The federal prison system was my assignment. The routine for all new inmates included a medical evaluation and a smallpox immunization, but there was nothing concerning tetanus. My prison, located in the Southwest, had an inmate population of over 90 percent Mexican nationals serving time for illegal entry into the United States. I was concerned. I called my superior officer, the medical director of the prison system who was located in Washington, D.C., told him of my concern, and recommended that we change our routine to include updating tetanus immunization. He said no one had ever raised the question—the existing routine had been established with the assumption that all federal prisoners had spent time in the U.S. military and, hence, had tetanus immunizations. He thought my idea had merit. I expected him to change the systemwide protocols. He did not. He asked me to run a pilot project in my prison and report to him with numbers and cost. I did. The routine then was changed.

I include this small incident to bring us to the definition of medical management, a definition I find difficult, as difficult as that for the practice of medicine. Diagnosing and treating an acute otitis media is medical practice, as is doing an organ transplant; yet, there is a world of difference in the knowledge and skills needed for the two treatments. So, too, is there a wide difference in knowledge and skills needs for the physician whose only responsibility outside the doctor-patient interchange is chair of a department and for the physician who has become the president of a multimillion dollar health care entity. To me, any responsibility or action taken by a physician to affect some or all of the environment in which the doctor-patient interchange takes place can be called medical management. The scope of focus, the range of responsibilities, and the knowledge and skills needed vary greatly as one travels deeper and deeper into medical management.

It can be helpful when planning a journey to know something of your route and destination so you can know what to take with you, what you will need. Of all your possessions, only some will be appropriate; others have to be left behind lest they make the trip more difficult. Some new things you will need to start your journey; some will have to be acquired along the way. This holds true for the journey from practice to management. Let us consider some of the nonmaterial possessions a clinician already has, things I will call traits.

- Physicians are intelligent and knowledgeable. Their having completed schooling and training evidence this. A good physician recognizes his or her knowledge is never complete; changing medical knowledge and technology dictate the need for lifelong learning.

- Physicians are diagnosticians. They have the training and skill to look beyond the obvious to determine causes. A good physician is not just a symptom treater, but a medical detective, always searching for root causes and always aware that new information may dictate a change in diagnosis or treatment plan.

- Physicians need to be right. Great pains are taken to be sure that a diagnosis or a treatment is right for a patient. Making an error, especially a serious error, is abhorred.

- Physicians have power. Their unique knowledge and skills have given them power, both physical and emotional, over patients' lives. The good physician recognizes this power and uses it judiciously lest he or she harm the patient, or even him- or herself.

- Physicians are independent, decisive decision makers. The practice of medicine demands this trait. A physician's training has strongly emphasized the need to be able to act independently and be comfortable doing so.

- Physicians expect to be obeyed. Orders, instructions, and advice to patients are expected to be followed exactly. Patients who refuse are termed noncompliant, a term that implies an error on the patient's part.

- Physicians need approval and appreciation. These are part of the non-monetary compensation in medicine. They are received by the occasional spoken thank you, the established patient continuing to return for care, and new patients seeking care. These direct and indirect manifestations are powerful ego builders; they can be addicting.

- Physicians are patient advocates. Their training has fostered this trait. They want the best for their patients. Anything that interferes is seen as a negative, an obstacle to be overcome.

The last trait, I believe, is the one that has propelled many physicians into medical management. Some have looked beyond the doctor-patient interchange to the environment in which it occurs and have seen problems they felt they could solve. I felt a drive, a force, result from combining this trait with my natural tendency to ask my four favorite questions:

- What are we doing?

- Why are we doing it?

- Is it accomplishing what it should?

- Is there a better way?

That force led me down the road to medical management without my fully realizing it, until I faced the decision to make a career change. The going was not always easy. My lack of management knowledge and skills made the journey more complicated than it could have been. With that ignorance, I packed up all my traits and took them, unmodified, with me. Let me share some experiences.

My pediatric residency was in a county hospital that had its maternity and neonatal units in a separate, one-story, wood-frame building. On hot summer days, its interior became stifling. Some neonates would show fever, requiring a work-up that almost always was negative. My predecessors had argued the need for air conditioning to no avail. I had to try. I met with the administrator with data from the previous three years showing the number of affected infants and the diagnostic studies done and made a strong plea for air conditioning. My answer was an acknowledgment that there was a problem, brief lessons on hospital budgeting, and a promise to consider a change during the next year's budget process. I left, unsatisfied.

The head nurse also was disappointed when I told her the news. She, however, supported an idea I had. She gathered up large pans and fans while I purchased 50-pound blocks of ice. We arranged them throughout the nursery and let the breeze blow over the ice. The room temperature dropped. I phoned the administrator, told him of the drop, and invited him to come see how we did it. He came, looked, said little, and left. Three days later, a crew was at work installing window air conditioners in the nursery.

Some months later, I had an "Ah-Ha!" experience. Suddenly, I saw a change that would solve multiple problems. My vision was to establish an all-day, five-days-a-week pediatric clinic that would function much like a pediatrician's office, including the ability to speak with patients by telephone. All children would be seen by pediatrics personnel, instead of those with acute illnesses being seen in an acute clinic for all ages staffed by only an intern who was at liberty to call a resident in any specialty for help. The new clinic would eliminate the erroneous diagnoses and treatments we had seen resulting from the existing arrangement. Mothers would be given appointment times rather than all coming at eight a.m. for morning visits or one p.m. for afternoon visits, thus improving access and the appointment failure rate. Pediatric training would be improved by a stronger involvement in ambulatory care, the kind of care most common in practice.

The first step was to enlist the support of the house staff. While they thought the idea had merit, the attitude was it would never happen, administration would never buy it, etc. Surprised and discouraged, I did not quit but pushed on. With the support and help of the head nurses of the pediatric ward and of the ambulatory clinics, a plan was developed. We went to administration. It was approved, and we were made responsible for it.

Within a few months, we were operational. It was a success; it worked smoothly. The naysayers were at first surprised, then supportive. It was not a short-term success; 14 years later when I left town, the clinic was still operating as started.

Those two experiences during residency, along with a few others that effected environmental changes, led me to believe I had a knack. I could see a problem, diagnose it, and treat it. I had confidence in this ability, a confidence that bordered on, if not crossed over into, arrogance, a confidence born out of a few successes within a narrow scope. Lessons lay in wait. Humility had to be learned.

Twelve years in private practice, entered into without management or business training, provided on-the-job learning and experience in many areas, including staffing and its management, patient relations, medical record design, budgeting, purchasing, accounting, and systems design and redesign. My accountant and physicians with office experience were great sources of helpful ideas. Regular discussions with office staff also helped my learning process. Our approach to office management was to ask my favorite four questions. The answers resulted in many small changes that improved our operation, medical records, and patient satisfaction. In office matters, successes were easy; outside the office was another matter.

The county medical society formed an ad hoc committee of 18 physicians to review its bylaws and make recommendations for changes. I was asked to be chair. I had served on other committees and had been frustrated by our meetings. They were in the evening; business was conducted after a light dinner with wine, which followed a cocktail hour. Too often, a few attendees became quite verbose and hogged a meeting, a happening I felt was fueled by alcohol. I vowed my committee would be different. My treatment for these sick meetings was two actions I took without consulting anyone: No alcohol would be served until business was completed, and no physician could speak again until all others had a chance to have their say.

After a series of meetings, our task was done. Committee members had participated actively and expressed pride in our product. The executive director also was pleased with our recommendations and expressed surprise that we had completed our task in such a short time. The society membership voted acceptance of all our recommendations as written. I felt proud; my treatment worked.

Gradually, my pride was displaced by distress. I heard directly from a few committee members and indirectly from other sources that rather than being appreciated, which I assumed would be the case, for focusing on the business at hand and guiding us to complete it in record time, I was being criticized for my two actions. I felt hurt, felt they did not understand, felt they were wrong.

Obviously I failed, for I was never again asked to chair or to serve on a committee for the society. It was not my only failure; another happened a few years later.

Repeated small talk over coffee among a dozen of us practicing pediatricians gave birth to the idea of establishing a large group practice. Innovative office design and operation could reduce facility costs and overhead expenses we experienced in our one- to four-doctor practices. As we became more serious, my peers asked me to lead the group. I accepted.

Recognizing I knew too little about group function and how to go about the task, I sought the help of the medical society's executive director, who knew of, and supported, our idea, help that was freely given. He assisted by guiding me throughout our work.

Meetings were regularly held, subcommittees were formed and did their work. Though we discussed many issues and made what appeared to be reasonable decisions on how the new office should work, I felt something was missing, felt that we were not dealing with basic issues, felt perhaps we were avoiding them. With the group's approval, and the support of the executive director, I contacted a pediatrician known to all of us from his articles in the literature on practice management. My feeling was justified. He quickly focused on our failure to fully explore and articulate what the project would mean to each of us, focused on our planning an operation based on assumptions of compatibility and like values. At the next meeting, I reported my conversation with the pediatrician. There was unanimous agreement to seek the first step he had to offer, a step without charge. Each of us filled out and returned the survey instrument he sent. After review, he said that he saw no major incompatibilities and that the next step should be personal interviews with each of us. These he would do for a fee and reimbursed travel expenses; the total cost averaged a little over one hundred dollars per physician. I thought it was a bargain.

At our next meeting, I reported on his findings and recommendations, The group voted two less than unanimously not to seek his services, despite my strong argument that his advice was sound, that we needed help. I was deeply disappointed and feared for the project. Meetings did continue, various issues were discussed, but the basic requirements for a successful plan were ignored. Within a few more months, the group and our vision died.

Only later did I see how I contributed to these failures, that blaming only others for them was not honest or accurate. In the first instance, I made my diagnosis and started treatment independently. While my objectives for the task were correct and met, I failed to consider how the other members would feel about my prescriptions. I failed to understand their values and expectations and to address them. In the second instance, I failed because I could not clearly communicate how I saw our vision, because I failed to determine or understand how others saw the vision, and because I was unable to influence them to deal with basic issues. Though the executive director was helpful to me, I had inadequate knowledge and skills in communication to improve the chances for success. After this second failure, I swore that, henceforth, all my efforts would be directed to my practice only, an area in which I was successful and comfortable.

In 1972, after 12 years in private practice, I made a change having nothing to do with medical management. During the last few years of that time, my observations on what was happening in medicine, its problems, and of the growth of prepaid medicine led me to change. I left to join a prepaid group practice (PPGP), the predecessors to HMOs, as a full-time, salaried practicing pediatrician. Little did I realize, or expect, that in this new setting I would hear the siren's call of medical management.

I was the third pediatrician in the not-for-profit, 18-physician PPGP that practiced in four ambulatory clinics. I was assigned to the largest of the clinics. Practice was fun, I thoroughly enjoyed it in this new medical financing environment. I felt I was doing very well until, a few months after being on board, the boss called me in to see him.

The boss was the physician who started the PPGP some years earlier. I had met with him four times during our interview process before joining the group. I admired him for his starting the group, managing its growth and its success. At the time, he was the PPGP's president and medical director. I had noted he often made reference to the need to learn management and to manage well to be successful. I had also noted he was a lecturer in the school of business of a local college.

Our meeting was brief. He immediately got to the point by saying, "Frank, I know you are a good pediatrician. I hear good things about you from the other doctors and staff. But, for the life of me, I can't figure out why, of all our physicians, your productivity is the worst."

Stunned, after a moment to collect my thoughts, I calmly asked to see the figures. He handed me the report. He was right. I was dead last. He explained the figures were the dollar values of services rendered, the fee-for-service (FFS) equivalent. I asked how they were derived; he said I should speak to the finance department for the details. I said I would and be back in two weeks with my answer.

After considerable research I had my answers. The following summarizes my report to him at our next meeting, one that had me apprehensive, because I had to tell him his methods had errors:

- The finance department staff members assigning the relative value codes, units, and dollar amounts for inpatient services performed did so incorrectly. They had helpfully processed inpatient service slips for five hypothetical cases I supplied them. The result was that the FFS equivalent was 60 percent below what it should have been.

- After reviewing medical records and speaking with the other physicians, I found that patients were having unnecessary visits. For example, a child with acute otitis media would be seen every other day after treatment was started until healed. I saw such a patient once for diagnosis and treatment and a second time after the completion of therapy. Physicians freely admitted they did this to make their productivity numbers look better.

- Each physician's productivity figures included the FFS equivalent of all laboratory and radiology work done in our centers ordered by him.This meant that overutilization was rewarded rather than discovered and dealt with, an approach not in keeping with the financial principles of a PPGP.

He listened; I knew from his expression and behavior that he had heard me. He thanked me for my report and added that he would have to get with finance. He changed the subject and said, "Frank, we are growing fast. Soon we will have our fourth pediatrician. I think it is time we have a department chair. Will you accept the job?" Feeling that would better position me to effect change, I accepted on the spot. I was on the road to medical management –willingly, eagerly.

The chair position was easy and fun. As we grew to six pediatricians plus two nurse practitioners, we were able to introduce many changes that improved our care, access to it, and costs. During our monthly meetings, I remembered my past errors and did not assume others' views were the same as mine or that they understood my views; clear, thorough communication and understanding among us was the objective. Without realizing it, I was developing credibility. One challenge arose that involved more than my department.

The physician in charge of utilization management asked for my help with requests for referrals to outside otolaryngologists (ENT), especially from our family practitioners; he felt there were too many, resulting in too many tonsillectomies and adenoidectomies (T&A). After reviewing the data and some of the authorization requests, I agreed with him. I was sure I knew the problem and had the answer: establish a common set of indications in my department and have the family practitioners refer all children for pediatric consultations when the question of a T&A arose. While I had the authority to issue a memorandum changing our routine to fit my solution, I would not do it. I told him I would have our department discuss the issue. I felt I had to listen to my peers, find out how they saw the problem, and seek their input on possible solutions. I chose a two-step process.

At our next pediatrics meeting, I told of my discussion with the utilization physician and my findings on review of the data. I then asked if anyone had any ideas on how to address the issue. A lively discussion followed. Most comments were outwardly directed; faults of the family physicians and their need for education were the focus. One member suggested that all the children in question should be referred to us; the others thought that a good idea. I asked whether all of us agreed on the indications for a T&A. Another lively discussion followed revealing we did not and seemingly never would. I suggested having a professor of ENT from a local medical school assist us in developing an up-to-date set of indications. There was unanimous agreement to do so. At our next meeting, the professor was instrumental in our quickly developing an agreed-upon set of indications. That done, my peers turned to me and asked what we would do about the family physicians. I was honest. I said I was not sure but would meet with their chair.

Before that meeting, I carefully thought about what to say. I felt that my objective, if stated bluntly, could have two negative effects. First, it could be seen as an accusation that his physicians were not doing things right. Second, it could be interpreted as a step to take patients away from his physicians. I thought of an approach to use if needed.

The family practice department was much larger than mine; its physicians provided routine care to many children in our program and referred to pediatricians when they thought it necessary. I met with the chair, informed him of the problem, and told him of my department's development of indications. I asked if he had any ideas about how we could address the issue of ENT referrals. He spoke of education need, of obtaining our new set of indications, and of having his department adhere to them. I felt we lacked significant progress, so I used my backup approach. I said I understood the pressure brought by parents on physicians for tonsillectomies and added that my department was willing to see all such children by referral, thus relieving his physicians of the burden of demanding parents. He thought that would be welcome and invited me to his department's next meeting. I accepted. There my proposal received enthusiastic endorsement.

The changes were made. Our referrals to ENT specialists and T&As dropped markedly. We had achieved better medicine at less cost. The success felt good.

I did not realize then that my behavioral changes were in keeping with good management. I kept my diagnosis of and treatment for the problem to myself until I had elicited the views of those involved or affected. By judicious use of questions, I was able to guide others to an acceptable resolution, one acceptable to members of both departments. Further, physicians' input was listened to and discussed; as a result, they developed a sense of ownership in the resolution. I felt my credibility rise in their eyes, also in mine.

Some months later, a second role was added to my chair duties; I was made the area clinic chief, the one responsible for the physicians in my ambulatory center. Responsibilities included interviewing all physician candidates, ensuring coverage was appropriate, monitoring and evaluating physician behavior and performance, and interfacing with those to whom nursing and other staff reported to ensure a smoothly running center. Shortly before my first anniversary with the group, I was given a third hat, chair of our quality assurance (QA) committee, of which I had been a member for five months.

QA meetings were monthly over lunch. We five physicians would eat while reviewing a large stack of charts gathered from our now six centers. Our routine was to look at the last entry for appropriateness. If a problem was noted, a message was sent to the area clinic chief to counsel the physician who made the entry. I began to ask myself my favorite four questions. Other than producing good-looking numbers for QA activity that were impressive to state regulators, I felt we were not grappling with issues of quality. I thought the process was ailing, but I was not sure. One Sunday, I let myself into my center, went to the record room, and started reviewing charts from the patient's first visit through the last. I had planned to do 50 to 100 charts to see if my suspicions were correct. It took only 20 for me to identify quality issues, some serious, and to see the pattern of how we practiced. Of interest, most of the problems had our systems as a major contributor; while one could focus on the last physician who saw the patient and blame him or her, it was really the way we did things that provided the fertile ground for these errors. Our QA program was not well, but I had no firm idea how to treat it.

At our next PPGP's physician meeting, I objectively presented my findings with specifics on what I found, without revealing patient or physician names. Discussion followed. Consensus quickly developed that we had to do something. I thanked the group for their attention and support for change and said the committee would work on it and keep them informed.

With input and concurrence of the committee members, we changed how we reviewed charts. Findings revealed the need for system changes. Each member contributed new ideas. Quite often, I had no, or a poor, idea for change. I was not trying to influence others to my way, only attempting to elicit others' ideas for effective change. It worked. Over the months, we made many changes, including medical records forms, how reports were filed into records, appointment scheduling, having the physician review the record of those who missed an appointment, etc.—all of which changed our environment so that it helped practicing physicians provide good care. The changes were welcomed. I was proud. My credibility went higher.

Eighteen months after I joined the PPGP, the president asked if I was interested in being the group's medical director. I was surprised and concerned. Six months earlier, he had given up that role and appointed a family practitioner who had been with the group for years as our first full-time medical director. Before I could express my concern, he quickly added that the family practitioner was unhappy being in administration and wanted to return to practice. That did not surprise me for, unfortunately, he was not doing well in the position; fortunately, he recognized it. I expressed interest, but said I had to think about it. He encouraged me to do so and ended our meeting with a comment I never forgot. He said with a grin, "The problem with making a competent doctor a medical director is that you lose a good clinician and gain a lousy administrator."

The decision was not an easy one. The president and I met three times to discuss his expectations, define the job, and consider my ideas. During those sessions, he made clear that, while I had done many good things, the first task I faced was learning how to manage. Further, he expected a commitment to management, a commitment that meant I had to quit practice, for he was of the strong opinion that the job was full-time. My wife and I discussed this opportunity at length, sharing our thoughts and feelings on what it would mean to us for me to quit what I was doing and start over in a new career. We agreed on the decision. I accepted. Three months later, I took over the job, vowing to myself to learn management, to be a good medical director, and to prove my boss's comment wrong.

Enrolling in management seminars was immediate. None yet had been developed for physicians, so I attended general management seminars put on by local colleges and national management associations. Initially, I was on a fast track, attending short seminars on topics such as personnel evaluation, communication, conflict management, time management, priority setting, planning, negotiation, etc. A great new vista lay before me, one in which I had little knowledge. Learning was easy, turning the new knowledge into skills was not. It was similar to one's trying to improve one's tennis serve; no matter how much one reads, how many tapes one watches, how many lessons one takes, serving skills will not improve without practice, and more practice.

Management education was not limited to seminars. Serving on committees—management, finance, planning, member grievance—was fertile ground for learning. Discussions with other department managers also were of great help. Within the company, the greatest day-to-day help I had was from my boss. He was always available to serve as a tutor, a function I found very helpful and reassuring, a function I feel can be of equal value to any physician new in management, whether the tutor is in the company or outside it. I had other help. Our PPGP belonged to Group Health Association of America, the national trade organization of PPGPs. By regularly attending its meetings, I met many other medical directors who also struggled in their jobs. We often discussed our problems and offered one another advice. Outside the meetings, we felt free to call on one another to continue mutual assistance.

After a year in the new job, I became a charter member of the American Academy of Medical Directors (AAMD), the predecessor organization to the American College of Physician Executives (ACPE). While its management courses would come later, the meetings provided additional contacts with physicians in management with whom to share problems and solutions.

While education had to be sought over time, I had a job to do. My highest priority outside physician staff matters was our benefit contract language, which defined what services were covered, partially covered, or not covered and our responsibilities to our members. It contained ambiguities, a few inaccuracies, and language not in keeping with changing medical knowledge and technology and was the cause of numerous misunderstandings by members and sometimes by our physicians. One simple, noncontroversial item was the benefit of an annual complete examination for all members of any age, clearly a benefit that was not necessary as stated. In my second month, I created an ad hoc committee composed of those responsible for marketing, finance, operations, legal, member relations, utilization management, and myself to revise the language. The president approved the changes and implemented them.

This was my first attempt to work closely with other than health professionals, a valuable experience. Quickly I learned that others had views that differed from mine, including how they perceived the role of physicians; learned that others saw problems where I did not; learned they had suggestions for change that never would have occurred to me. This experience also reinforced my belief that actions in one department can affect other departments; we existed to benefit the company as a whole and had to communicate well to ensure its health, not just that of our own department. I had learned to listen, to ensure that each participant had full input into the issues and proposed changes, to ensure that there was consensus for each change.

As the months sped by, other lessons were learned, lessons about the differences between medicine and management:

- Management is accomplishing things through others. The effective manager is not a Lone Ranger who single-handedly solves problems.

- Problems keep coming no matter how many you have. There is no appointment schedule as in practice, a schedule that prompts prospective patients to seek care elsewhere when it is full.

- Problems are your responsibility; there is no way to refer them. Even if others can be enlisted in the effort, permitting you to delegate, your responsibility remains intact.

- Other managers respected me as a physician, but not as a manager. I had to earn that respect through consistent performance.

- To the physicians, I was now one of "them." Before, I was seen as a peer who was working to change administration. Now I was part of administration. The credibility I had was put on hold until I could demonstrate that I still understood the practice of medicine and would continue to work to improve the environment in which they practiced. Further, there were subtle changes in my personal relationship with many physicians. Now I was their boss and had power over their fate; established friendships tended to become more distant.

- I had underestimated my dependence on the steady flow of appreciation and ego strokes I experienced in medicine. In their place was a void that I had to fill by developing my own appreciation when a job was well done, by developing faith in my abilities based on my successes.

Work was demanding, long, but fun. Many changes were made to improve our physician recruiting, evaluations, and compensation. Other changes improved access to care and its quality, improved our members' perception of us, and kept the costs of care in control. Some things I could have done better or more easily, but successes outweighed failures. Challenges were plentiful, challenges I accepted willingly until I hit a bump in my road.

This chapter started with a true story; my wife and I were the characters. It happened just as I finished a five-month executive management course at a local university, a course I found excellent, but one that fostered a growing discomfort; I began to see that how we managed our company was not always the best. My wife's loving ultimatum that evening, added to that growing discomfort, precipitated an epiphany. I suddenly saw how I was failing. My energies had been focused on my company and my profession; I had been neglecting myself; I was failing to manage myself as a person, a husband, a father.

Change did come over time. I had to learn to ask my favorite four questions about my own behavior. Hard at first, it became easier with time and practice. It developed into a skill, one I think most important for the physician manager. Slowly, I began to see how I was changing and in that change had to find the best balance possible among my company's, my profession's, and my personal values and priorities. I gradually saw that I had ignored, even denied, certain problems at work, problems I was powerless to change or have changed. One example will suffice.

In the first month as medical director, I was given the task to go to the state capitol and continue my boss' long-standing argument that our laboratory did not need certification; it should be considered as any private doctor's office laboratory. I succeeded; the issue was put off for another year, yet I was not proud. Our physician staff had low confidence in our lab and often would repeat tests. While practicing, I had noted a problem with our selective media for strep cultures. The local hospital helped me document the problem, and I was able to effect a change of media suppliers. Our laboratory studies were done by our x-ray technicians, who were trained in-house to do lab work; we had no certified laboratory technicians. I finally convinced the boss that we should hire a certified technician. I collaborated with the operations director, the one to whom laboratory and x-ray reported, for the hiring. I was able to delegate the cooperative working relationship with operations to an interested physician who agreed to work with the laboratory technician in developing an improved department. The physician also agreed with my objective to obtain state certification. Short of a year after my trip to the capitol, we had our inspection. We achieved certification.

As our plan continued to grow, I saw the need to have a second certified laboratory technician, to have one in each of the two largest of our six centers. I approached the operations director with the request and reasons. It would be considered. A few weeks later my boss met with me, asked if I was seeking a second technician. I said yes and explained why. His response was clear and forceful. He said, "We are not hiring another—ever! Forget you even thought of it and don't bring it up again!"

This and other issues I found as I got deeper and deeper into the company, including a seat on the board of directors, were fertile ground for my newly developed skill of self-evaluation. I finally decided I had only four options:

- Quit management and return to practice.

- Remain in the job and suppress my growing frustration.

- Change my values and principles and be comfortable remaining on the job.

- Leave.

The first was not an option; I enjoyed having an impact on the environment of medical practice, an impact that far exceeded what I could do in practice. I was living the second option, except for being able to suppress frustration; even if I could, I felt it would not be conducive to good physical and mental health, or the health of my marriage. The third was not possible; I would not, could not, change my basic principles. I left.

The next five years were spent back on active duty in the USPHS, where most of my work was with HMOs. Technical assistance and consultation was provided to developing HMOs and to those seeking federal qualification. Toward the end of the five years, while I was Director, Division of Qualification, I was contacted by a physician who had started an HMO that was acquired by a large insurance company for which he then became national medical director. He offered me a medical director position in one of three HMOs in his company's developing national network of HMOs. The opportunity to return to line management prompted me to accept. I became a regional medical director in a large staff-model HMO, one with more than 300,000 members, that had been purchased by the insurance company. The first 20 months in this company, I served as one of five regional medical directors; then I was promoted to the medical directorship of the plan, which continued to grow to an enrollment of about 400,000 with 30 ambulatory centers with a staff of 400 physicians plus support staff, a plan 10 times larger than my previous HMO. Another difference for me was that all of health care operations were under my direction—physicians, nurses, medical assistants, medical records, laboratory, x-ray, pharmacy, optometry, and dentistry. This position brought me to my largest scope of responsibilities.

AAMD had developed management seminars for physicians that I started to attend on joining this new company. They were a breath of fresh air. I found them highly helpful, informative, and well directed to physicians interested in medical management. They were far superior to the general management seminars I had attended; they were more practical. AAMD had grown considerably and offered a large number of new contacts with whom to share problems and solutions. I continued attending its various seminars over my subsequent years in medical management and always found something new, something to help further development of management knowledge and skills.

While one must be a lifelong student in management as in medicine, there is a difference. Increasing clinical knowledge and skills can result in a narrower scope of medicine; specialization and subspecialization are evidence of this. In management, however, the more one learns, the more skills one develops, the more prepared one is to broaden one's scope and focus, the more prepared for new opportunities.

If you are about to, or recently did, start your journey into medical management, what physician traits should you take, change, or leave behind; what new knowledge and skills will you need? Perhaps you already saw some answers in my case. Permit me to be more specific by sharing my thoughts, first on physician traits.

Intelligence and Knowledge

These you will need. There will be much to learn about management. It will help to view every event as a possible learning experience. Further, your knowledge of medicine, not only clinical facts but also how medicine is practiced and its nuances, can enhance your credibility with physicians. Board certification in a clinical discipline will also increase your credibility. While you have extensive clinical knowledge, it is of little use in management by itself.

Diagnostic Ability

Take this with you into management. The skill to look behind the obvious to discover basic issues will be needed; you may have to adapt this skill to management, but it is an important one to keep. Beware of assumptions. It is important to recognize when behavior is based on assumption. Use your diagnostic skills to discover when this is the case and dig deeper to check the assumption. An example:

There was no physician policy manual in the large HMO when I arrived as a regional medical director. One of my physicians, in my first month on the job, had a question about a leave benefit for which I did not know the answer. I called our plan's medical director, who had been on the job a little over a year; he advised me to check with one of the other regional medical directors for the answer, as they had been with the company for years. I did, but did not stop there. I called each one of the other four with the question and received definite answers, all of which varied significantly. The assumption that the medical directors knew policy was wrong. This experience prompted us to review our physicians' benefit policies and to create a written physicians' manual.

The Need to Be Right

This trait is best left behind, or at least severely modified. Often, in management, there is no one right answer, but a choice of a number of options, each with advantages and disadvantages. Often decisions cannot, or should not, be delayed until all the facts are known. You will make mistakes. We all have and will continue to make them. No reasonable person expects perfection in a medical manager. If you recognize, admit, and learn from your mistakes, you will stand a greater chance of being perceived as human and increasing your credibility.

Power

In a management position you probably will have power. Usually different from power in clinical practice, it will come because of your position, not necessarily because of your knowledge. It is wise to keep this power in reserve for things that are both urgent and important; for most matters, use your other skills.

Independent Decision Making

As with power, this needs to be kept, but used with caution. Much of management is better accomplished through involving others unless circumstances dictate otherwise. One of the most valuable things I learned about decision making was its different levels:

- I independently decide and tell those involved what my decision is.

- I ask for information from others and make the decision.

- I ask for information and recommendations from others and then make the decision.

- I surrender my decision-making authority to the group, participate in the group's deliberations, and implement the group's decision.

This chapter is not appropriate for a full explanation of decision making. It is important to learn when each method is appropriate and to be sure those involved understand how a decision will be made. There will be times when the first approach is appropriate because of importance or urgency. However, the more you involve others in the decision-making process, the greater their sense of participation and acceptance of decisions, and the greater the chance of improving the quality of decisions.

Expecting to Be Obeyed

This is best left behind. While it may be a reasonable trait in practice, having this attitude in management can be deadly to the morale of those you manage and, in the long run, can prevent your advancing in management. Only in rare circumstances is it appropriate to have this expectation.

Approval Need

The need for a steady flow of approval from others is best left behind. Instead, develop and substitute self-approval for a job well done. While it may be intellectually easy to do, emotionally it can be difficult. Management does not provide a steady stream of ego strokes. This should not be surprising, for in medicine a patient comes seeking your help to relieve distress; in management those you lead have not always sought your services, nor are your actions always perceived as beneficial to them. If you expect to be an instrument of change, it is wise to recognize that most people do not like change and are often distressed during the process, an outcome not prone to bring you immediate plaudits.

Being a Patient Advocate

I think this trait is important to keep, although it needs to be transformed. A medical manager has to develop the skill to be an advocate not only for an individual patient, but also for groups of patients. Effecting environmental changes that support and improve the doctor-patient interchange is a form of this advocacy. Further, part of that environment is the expectations and attitudes that the physician and patient each bring to their interchange. Hence, efforts to affect those expectations and attitudes can be very appropriate forms of this advocacy. At times, you may encounter a conflict between advocacy and your company's behavior, as the following example illustrates.

The plan medical director of the large HMO called an urgent telephone conference with the plan's regional medial directors near the end of the year. He instructed us to cancel immediately all elective surgery because our financial performance against budget was not looking good. When pressed, he admitted he was doing so at the instruction of the plan's president, who was not a physician. Protests filled the air; however, he persisted and ended the call. Calls among the regional medical directors to discuss this directive quickly followed. We all were suspicious that the reason was not solely our financial performance. The fact that the president's annual bonus was based on that performance made us suspect he wanted to maximize what he would get, a suspicion we could not prove nor expect anyone to admit. I gained the support of the others for my immediately speaking with our director. I saw him that afternoon and made the following points:

- Canceling elective surgeries would not save money; it would increase our costs. Hospital contracts were to be renewed at the end of the year and rates were to rise, meaning that cases postponed until after the end of the year would cost us more.

- Our surgeons all were on salary; canceling surgery would leave them unproductive while their pay would continue. Further, moving cases would cause a bulge in the amount of their work in the first few months of the new year.

- Many patients had their surgery scheduled around the holidays and had made arrangements with employers and families; cancellation would be the source of many complaints by patients and employers.

He listened, saw the light, and went to our president. The following day, there was a conference call to announce that the directive was changed; all scheduled surgery would be done as planned, but no new elective surgery could be scheduled before the end of the year. This we found acceptable.

I felt that, in this instance, our plan's medical director succumbed to the influence of the president and lost sight of what medicine was about, lost sight of his role as patient advocate. I must add this was only one incident, not a pattern of our medical director's behavior, but it is illustrative of how the values of medicine can be subverted by those of a company, illustrative of how one must consider all possible results of a planned action.

New traits will be needed in management, traits that will require new knowledge and repeated practice in its application so you can become skillful. Those I think most important at any level of management are noted below, with comments from my experiences.

Communication Skills

Both clinical practice and management require good communication skills, but there are significant differences between the two. In practice, a patient usually comes to a physician without broad knowledge of medicine with the purpose of seeking a resolution to a problem. The physician uses his or her skills to elicit a good history; measures the patient's responses against a fund of medical knowledge; makes a judgment concerning further work up, diagnosis, or treatment; and then communicates recommendations to the patient. In this exchange, the physician has a position of power, somewhat like that of a professor with a student.

In management, the physician no longer has the advantage of this kind of power. His or her vast clinical knowledge is of little use, and knowledge of management is rudimentary in the early years. Often, others do not seek the physician's wisdom, but come with the objective of convincing him or her their perceptions and judgments on issues are correct. Most of the communication in practice is one on one; in management, much is not. Different skills in communication will be needed and must be learned.

Reading is of vital importance. Not only will one need to keep up with changes in medicine, but one may need to learn more about other specialties if the management role includes them. The job of management itself will bring much to read in the performance of the job. Further, it will be necessary to read and study management to become more effective. I found that a speed reading course I took in my private practice years was of great help.

Writing skills may seem elementary, but, much to my dismay, I have too often seen writing that was ambiguous or incomplete, and even writing that delivered a message that was not intended. I found two steps helped me greatly. First, I would write my message and then reread it for completeness and clarity, making necessary revisions. Second, as is possible with almost all writing, I put it aside for a day and then reread it; often additional changes were needed.

Speaking skills are needed. You will be speaking with individuals and groups in and outside your entity. In conversations, there is no time for preparation, but taking a few seconds to think about what you will say and how you will say it can be of great help. You will probably be called upon to do public speaking, a task that requires preparation similar to that for writing. I found public speaking a difficult skill to develop and improve, one with which I struggled without reaching the level I desired.

Active listening is an essential skill for the manager. Through its use, it is much easier to learn and understand the perspectives of others, their values and priorities; to learn what others see as problems and options; and to gain feedback on how you are perceived. Becoming a skilled listener early in your management involvement is advisable.

Conflict Management Skills

You will need these skills. Conflict cannot be avoided; you will meet it at any level of involvement in management. If you find yourself without conflict, you are either denying it or not doing your job. Most important is to avoid personalization in dealing with conflict. You will need to separate the person from an issue; you will also need to separate yourself emotionally from an issue to be able to be effective. I strongly recommend learning the techniques of conflict management early in your management education.

Meeting Skills

While the object of many jokes and derogatory remarks, meetings are needed and can be pertinent, productive, and an excellent forum for communication, especially among parties with varied interests. They are vital to the health of a company. Learning about meetings and various techniques is not a subject for this chapter, but permit me to share a few thoughts about them:

- The agenda should be in writing and distributed in advance.

- Starting and ending times should be on the agenda.

- The nature of the meeting elements should be noted—reports, informational items, discussion items, decision items.

- To respect others' time, they should start and end on time.

- Tangential discussions should be kept to a minimum.

- When asking if anyone has further comments, wait quietly for 30 seconds for input before proceeding.

- Decisions need to be clearly articulated, and each attendee should understand a decision has been made and what it is.

- Minutes should be brief and pertinent, include all decisions, and be distributed as soon as possible after the meeting.

Time Management, Priority Setting, Delegation Skills

Practicing physicians are used to seeing and treating patients as they come, one at a time in sequence. Using this approach with problems and issues that come your way will spell disaster for your management career. In a sense, the first step in dealing with them is triage, followed by deciding what you will do, when, and in what order. To do so effectively requires these three skills. While seminars on these skills were very helpful in my early days of management, I always welcomed periodic, continuing education addressing them.

A technique I found helpful was to daily, in the quiet of my home or office before the day started, write a list of all that had to be done. Often, the list was very long and represented many days work. Then I determined the urgency and importance of each item. The next step was to determine what I could delegate and what required only my attention. Finally, I selected six to eight of the most important and most urgent things that required my doing and those were my work for the day. It took great discipline to avoid giving an item a higher priority because it was something easier to do or because I liked to do it; it was harder, but necessary, to set priorities on the needs for action, not my personal likes and dislikes.

Delegation is a special skill. It requires knowing who is suitable for the task; having clear communication on what is to be done and by when; establishing how progress will be communicated; and, while you retain responsibility for what is done, being sure the person has the resources and freedom to complete the task.

I kept my daily lists of things to do. I used the previous day's list when making out a new day's list. I carried over undone items. I found some items that I had carried forward for many days that were not of great importance or urgency often no longer had to be done; some that appeared important but not of great urgency also disappeared from the list. This daily review helped me learn the mistakes I made in prioritizing items. It also helped me see patterns of problems that prompted my diagnostic skills to find the underlying cause. An example:

There were recurring issues with various hospitals with which we contracted. I saw that there was no scheduled communication except at contract renewal time. Only when problems became intolerable was there communication at other times. After consulting with finance and legal departments, we included in our next contract with each hospital the requirement of quarterly meetings of key personnel from the hospital and our company concerned with finance, claims, and medical operations. These regular meetings were usually brief and permitted a review of our business relationship and early identification and resolution of problems before they became major; they also improved our relationships with key persons at the hospitals and eased communication.

Admission of Ignorance Skills

Physicians do not enter practice until they have achieved a high level of clinical knowledge and have developed some practice skills during their training. Physicians commonly enter management roles with two levels of ignorance: incomplete knowledge of management and ignorance of many of the aspects of the entity in which they will manage. There is not the leisure to gain all the necessary knowledge about management or the entity before starting. It is important to know when you do not know something and to learn to feel free to ask. Most important is to avoid assuming you know. I found that nonphysicians appreciated my admitting I did not know something and were pleased to help me learn. My best example concerns finance.

While I successfully managed my own finances and books in private practice, I was the proverbial babe-in-the-woods at my first finance committee meetings in the first PPGP. Only by asking questions over time was I able to learn how our books were kept, how to read financial statements, how we budgeted, what our reports reported, how reserves were established for claims incurred but not yet received, etc. Gradually, it became possible for me to be a fully participating member of the committee. Once my knowledge had grown, I felt comfortable addressing how physician productivity was measured and reported and making recommendations for changes. Incidentally, although my boss still felt it appropriate to include the FFS equivalent of lab and x-ray ordered and performed within our company, I was able to have the other measures subtotaled and then below that put the FFS for lab and X-ray. I had my measure, the boss had his on the same report.

Self-Evaluation Skill

This, I believe, is a vital skill, especially to the physician who progresses deeper into management. Simply put, it is the ability to evaluate as objectively as possible your own behavior to see if it is compatible with the values and priorities of the company, the medical profession, and your personal values and priorities. I found the lure of management initially so consumed me that I became dysfunctional as a whole person. I started by weekly taking my daily lists of things to do and reviewing what I had done and what I had neglected, and asked my favorite four questions of myself in the light of those three sets of values and priorities. The objective was to find balance among them. I found my company and I were both undergoing change, even my profession had some changes; ongoing evaluation was needed to be sure I had achieved the best balance possible in light of those ongoing changes. I strongly recommend that all physicians in management become skillful at self-evaluation.

There are many other skills to be developed, depending on your level of involvement. More accurately stated, there is more knowledge that may be necessary that you have to apply in a skillful way. A skill is not really a thing, it is the effective, facile manner in which you apply your knowledge, be it in the above topics or in negotiation, budgeting, finance, legal matters, marketing, etc. If you expect to advance in a medical management career, you must be prepared to learn throughout your career and constantly improve the skills you have and develop new ones. Other skills that can stand you in good stead include how to honestly admit your mistakes, how to graciously deal with criticism and disappointment without personalizing them, how to find and share humor on the job, and how and when to say no when inappropriate demands are placed on your energy or time.

I have shared some of my experiences with you. What follows is from my recent experience but is really about another person. A physician I had known became a medical director of an large IPA HMO in the mid-1990s and found himself pulled in many directions. He was concerned about the demands on him and also about how the HMO was managed. Over time, we had conversed by telephone about his frustrations. He asked me to provide consultation on the HMO and his job. After his president agreed, I visited the operation. While there were a number of issues about the HMO operation in general, I will share only what I observed of him in his job.

He had taken a number of management courses, some from the ACPE. However, watching his behavior, one would never guess it. Simply put, he was using the same behavior pattern that was appropriate to clinical practice and behaved as if he missed practice. He insisted on answering all his telephone calls, no matter how many interruptions. It appeared he felt lonely and, hence, pined for personal contact with the person presenting a problem and eagerly wanted to take charge to fix it. He dealt with problems as they came much as one sees patients. He worked with things that were comfortable, putting off tasks that were difficult or that made him uneasy. Needless to say, he was harried. While he had the ultimate responsibility for utilization management and its authorizations, he had never read the benefit contract to understand what it said and, thereby, missed the opportunity to discover wording that needed improvement to minimize problems. While he was responsible for interfacing with the various medical groups with which the HMO contracted, he had not read the contracts that were in force. While he dealt with many patient complaints, he had never reviewed the marketing brochures or what the marketing representatives were telling employers and potential enrollees. I could go on.

What I sadly saw was a physician working hard and long, but getting nowhere. He had not developed the necessary skills, despite his courses, to manage his job or himself. It remains to be seen whether he has that ability. Not all physicians can be good managers; he may be one. My recommendations to him included the need to manage his time, set priorities, delegate, read all the contracts, read all the literature produced by the company that can have an impact on health care delivery and its costs, and recognize the interdependence of departments within the HMO. Whether he changes remains to be seen. If he continues as he is, I suspect he will remain miserable until he quits, or is fired.

Let us return to the definition of medical management I used. It is obvious that persons other than physicians can, and do, affect the environment in which the doctor-patient interchange takes place. Why, then, have physicians take time from practice, or leave it, to work in a management role? Physicians have unique knowledge and experience that they can bring to management, specifically how medicine is practiced and all the nuances therein, and they have a greater understanding of how physicians think and behave. The physician manager stands a greater chance to achieve early credibility among physicians, especially if he or she has impeccable credentials, including clinical specialty board certification and significant practice experience. Most important, physicians can bring to the decision-making process for change the values and priorities of the profession, a need I am not sure is being fully met.

While I can never be sure of another's motives, I have seen behavior of some physicians in management that leads me to suspect that their focus has been on the priorities and values of the company at the expense of those of the profession. I have noted others who appear to have placed their personal priorities above their company's and their profession's. These observations have caused me to question whether all physicians in management are still medical managers. Some appear to have left behind their profession and its values while progressing down the management road; they appear to be physicians who happen to be managers rather than physicians devoted to medical management as I have defined it.

I believe physicians in medical management must consistently remember our medical profession's obligation to be of service to others. The challenge is to remember that obligation while working to effect positive changes. The need for medical managers has grown and will continue to do so. Opportunities are there to work for order in the present confusing, changing, distressing arena of health care service delivery and its financing. Opportunities are there to remain true to our first chosen profession, and possibly to rescue it.

Physicians entering medical management today are fortunate to have a variety of educational opportunities for their new line of work that did not exist for many of us who preceded them. Take advantage of them. Develop management skills from that knowledge. Work for change. You are needed, especially if you will remember the mission, values, and responsibilities of the medical profession.

Bon voyage!

Frank J. Volpe, MD, FACPE, is a retired physician executive living in Lake Havasu City, Arizona.

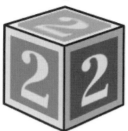

Chapter

Life as a Medical Manager

by Laurence G. Roth, MD, FACPE

Experience is a necessary but insufficient generator of the skills that are needed for success in medical management. The serious student of medical management will seek a variety of educational opportunities to acquire the credentials that can lead to lasting success.

What does it mean to be a medical director, a vice president of medical affairs, or a physician executive with a related title that says you are involved in the business side of medicine? Within every group of physicians or other health care provider large enough to require leadership and management, there is a potential position for a physician executive. Opportunities are found in group practices, hospital and medical staff administration, and larger institutions providing managed care at multiple sites, and in sections within these organizations. There are medical managers in industries producing equipment, supplies, and pharmaceuticals; in research programs; and in the many agencies of local, state, and federal government. In recognition of the need for medical management, the military has been sending its personnel for training and experience so that they can qualify for assignments with managerial responsibilities. There is also increasing awareness of the appropriateness of medical management in academia.

Although the titles of these positions vary widely in relation to the spectrum of opportunities, all of them involve managing people and programs as contrasted with treating patients in clinical situations. There are more meetings to attend and much more paper work for managers than for pure clinicians. Managing people, however, is the keystone of management. In the evolving scheme of things, there are more team leadership responsibilities and the possibility of the need to negotiate with employers who pay for the health care of their employees and dependents. This chapter is an introduction to the general aspects of medical management as the profession is now constituted. For the most part, this chapter will be based on the provision of hospital-based health care but with indications of other possibilities covered more fully in the other chapters.

New York State revised its hospital code in 1988 to require medical management in every hospital in the state. The new code said, "The governing board shall appoint a physician, referred to as the medical director, who shall be responsible for directing the medical staff organization."[1] As a result, medical directors began to do things that had not been done previously. Now, hospitals no longer are willing to do without them, because the benefits have been significant. It has also become evident that the role of medical management is not for the casual participant. It is an important function best undertaken by those who have the essential qualifications to be medical managers in addition to expertise in clinical practice.

The definition of responsibility in the New York code establishes the hospital medical director as the focus of attention in medical matters for the medical staff, administration, and the governing board. The definition serves as a useful beginning for understanding what it means to be a medical director or a physician executive generally. It emphasizes the interesting and challenging role that the medical director assumes in being an advocate for each one of the three entities to the other two in a hospital environment, but the medical manager role is similar regardless of the environment in which the person serves.

The liaison and advocacy role of the medical director is essential in any operation in which successfully getting and giving information on medical matters is of paramount importance. For example, the medical manager's role in quality assurance and risk management will demand constant emphasis on adequate communication and documentation. In this, as in other aspects of medical management, the medical director should expect to set an example of how to communicate with everyone and of how to properly document findings, recommendations, and actions.

In the transition from clinical practice to medical management, most of the characteristics of the clinician must give way to those of the manager, but there is one feature of clinical practice that is retained without loss of significance. It is most important for the medical manager to continue to be an advocate for the patient. In evaluating medical care and reviewing medical staff practices, there is a unique opportunity for the medical manager to facilitate achievement of what is best for the patient. Other actors in the organization may have concerns about cost containment, avoidance of liability, or personal preferences that affect their actions and subsequent decisions. This is especially true in the present-day proliferation of capitated, hospital-centered, vertically integrated systems. A medical manager is usually not encumbered to the same degree by these considerations and can speak to what is in the best interests of the patient.

Planning products, services, and programs and devising innovations to make improvements in an organization's operations are among the ways in which the medical manager contributes to the successful outcome of the work of the organization. Much of this will require leadership of teams to provide the combination of managerial and medical expertise necessary to bring together all of the elements needed for solutions. Generally, the activities of the medical manager, especially in a provider setting, are still tied, even if indirectly, to health care delivery. Modern medical management gives attention to what is termed "continuous quality improvement" or "total quality management." This approach represents adaptation of principles established in industry that are proving to be of great value in health care.[2-4] (Medical quality management concepts are discussed in detail in Chapter 15 of this book.) Crosby[5] has written about the concept, "Do it right the first time." This is a goal for every patient-physician encounter and a great guideline for every medical manager.

In order to play a leading role in the design and implementation of programs that address medical quality and other issues of current concern, the medical manager must learn a wide variety of new and very different concepts and skills. The learning that must take place is especially intense for the newly recruited medical manager who is just beginning to gain experience. In a review of the dynamics of the "revolution in our midst," Goldener[6] lists many of the physician manager's tasks—having a customer focus, developing a strong technological push, learning business and its language, learning negotiation skills, avoiding risk, practicing team work, acquiring listening skills, and practicing stress management. This list can be expanded by adding such things as being aware of local, state, and federal regulations and of how to cope or coexist with them. Knowing the players who operate in this area can be a valuable asset in solving some problems expeditiously. To enhance understanding and appreciation of community needs and expectations, participation in such activities as the local chamber of commerce and service clubs will provide opportunities to better serve in the role of patient and community advocate.

The manager is an important support person. Vested with central responsibility and authority, the medical manager works with and for many people who come for advice and direction. The manager assists others in carrying out tasks that they might not otherwise be able to accomplish. This helps others to overcome their reluctance to follow through on programs and projects and helps them to avoid or overcome obstacles to progress.

The medical manager operates out of what becomes a central command post. Information comes from administration, the governing board, the medical staff and its committees, and regulatory and certifying agencies. With knowledge of the resources available, pertinent data, and what has to be done, the position becomes akin to the President's Chief of Staff in relation to the leaders of the U.S. Senate and House of Representatives. There is the need and the opportunity to assist in devising policy and then seeing that it is carried out, all the while being responsible to those whom he or she serves. The guidance of the medical manager is especially important for members of the medical staff who have leadership responsibilities but who perhaps lack the knowledge, the motivation, or the time to carry out those responsibilities, just one example of team leadership responsibilities.

A manager also serves as a counselor to the many individuals who come to be listened to, to be encouraged, and to be guided to solutions they find acceptable. The availability of the medical manager leads to the solution of many problems that might otherwise persist and cause trouble. Existence of the position is a signal to practitioners and others that help is available from a person who understands their concerns.

There is a significant relationship between the medical manager and new members of the medical staff. The indoctrination that is essential starts each physician off in harmony with the way things are done locally. This opens communication that can be used in other matters. There are always problems for the new physician with the various regulatory agencies, and guidance here can eliminate a lot of grief later. If the medical manager has an effective open door policy, physicians feel free to come in and discuss potential as well as real problems that pertain to them as individuals or to their relationships with committees and departments. Many of these encounters are unscheduled. The medical manager's just being available is most helpful to everyone concerned.

The typical hospital-based physician executive has had an active clinical practice in the specialty for which she or he is board certified. It is a full-time position, reporting to the chief executive officer. The major responsibilities are for quality assurance, credentialing, risk management, and utilization review. Compensation is adequate and includes not only salary but also the schedule of working hours, vacations, and continuing education. It may afford a different lifestyle that is attractive in comparison to some clinical practices that are so busy that they limit satisfaction of personal goals.

The medical manager has a position of influence, derived to a large extent from the organizational authority necessary to be an effective leader with major responsibilities. But it is also the result of the manager's effectiveness in processing information, such as external regulations and internal policies that affect the personnel and the work of the organization. Interpretation and application of these regulations and policies are an important part of the medical manager's job and have a significant impact on the operations of the organization. The busy practitioner does not have time to investigate all the information that is available. By attending meetings at which in-depth discussions are conducted and having time to read materials that are circulated, the medical manager becomes a resource who permits pragmatic application of the information through reliable advice to busy practitioners.

The opportunity to be the one to receive information and to give advice allows the medical manager to greatly affect the smoothness of the organization's work and the satisfaction of everyone's work life. Much of this is accomplished in the role of educator, both directly and indirectly. In many situations, the medical manager is in charge of continuing education programs. The medical staff is consulted on its special needs, programs are arranged locally where feasible, and other sources of education are developed. The medical manager is also an educator by example and through counseling of both individuals and groups with whom he or she comes in contact.

The medical manager faces the paradox of being the "good guy," with responsibilities for medical quality management, but may also be perceived as the "bad guy" when dealing with inappropriate or disruptive physician behavior. The former achievements will often be taken for granted by the organization, and the latter will consume both time and energy with little in the way of positive recognition. Self-confidence and the ability to evaluate performance objectively are essential in both cases. The ultimate achievement for the manager is self-management, dealing with the responsibilities that are part of the management package with fairness and forthrightness. The manager is a large visible target for anyone with an ax to grind and is infrequently rewarded with praise. The job requires a well-honed ability to cope with these facts of management life.

Management skills are not an inherent part of any person's abilities. They have to be acquired. As the skills are used and mistakes are made, the skills become increasingly effective. The necessary skills have to be actively identified and then aggressively sought and polished. A major purpose of the American College of Physician Executives (ACPE) is to provide opportunities for management education.[7] Its goal is to introduce physicians interested in pursuing a management career to the full range of knowledge and skills that they will need for success. Of course, an allied purpose is to provide these educational opportunities in a setting and at a pace that are least disruptive to physicians' professional and personal lives. For some, however, there are programs leading to master's level degrees. There are now several university programs specifically oriented to medical management. ACPE has struck arrangements with several universities by which College educational programs may lead to master's degrees in medical management.

The field of medical management is growing rapidly, with future opportunities for both those in the profession and those considering a move in this direction. It is always a good idea to talk with someone who is a practicing medical manager and to learn how he or she came to be in that position. The educational programs and conferences of ACPE are excellent experiences that allow exploration of the career of medical management with its great variety of opportunities. They are also an opportunity to meet many individuals with similar interests and varying degrees of experience.

The management career will not have universal appeal for physicians. For those who are interested, the opportunities are good and the work is satisfying. This book is intended to help practicing physicians with some curiosity about such a career to determine if it fits their needs and to help them understand the road that will have to be traveled.

References

1. *New York State Public Health Law* Part 405, Subchapter A of Chapter V, Title 10, Sections 405.2(e)(2), and 405.4.

2. Scherkenbach, W. *The Deming Route to Quality and Productivity: Road Maps and Road Blocks.* Washington, D.C.: George Washington University, Cee Press Books, 1988.

3. Juran, J. *Juran on Planning for Quality.* New York, N.Y.: Free Press, 1988.

4. Berwick, D., and others. *Curing Health Care: New Strategies for Quality Improvement.* San Francisco, Calif.: Jossey-Bass Publishers, 1990.

5. Crosby, P. *Quality without Tears:* The Art of Hassle-Free Management. New York, N.Y.: McGraw Hill, 1984.

6. Goldener, J. "After the Revolution: The Physician Executive of the Future." *Physician Executive* 24(4):40-4, July-Aug. 1998.

7. *New Leadership in Health Care Management:* The Physician Executive, Second Edition. Curry, W., Editor. Tampa, Fla.: American College of Physician Executives, 1994.

Laurence G. Roth, MD, FACS, FACOG, FACPE, is retired from service as Executive Vice President for Medical Affairs, Genesee Memorial Hospital, Batavia, N.Y.

Chapter

Getting Oriented for Success as a New Physician Executive

by Marilyn Szymialis Radke, MD, MPH, MA, FACPM, CPE, FACPE

The first month a new physician executive is on the job presents a critical opportunity for integration into the corporate culture of an organization. The corporate leadership should use this time to make sure the new physician executive is set up to succeed in the position by implementing a strategic orientation program to help the new person become part of the team and aligned with the organization's mission and vision. Responsibility for orienting the new employee should be shared by the corporate leadership, including the CEO or supervisor, the physician executive's peers, and even the recruiter. When the new employer does not orient new employees, new physician executives should do it themselves.

Although health care organizations are spending more and more time and money on physician executive searches, experts say that corporate leadership is not always making sure the new hire is set up to succeed in the position. Responsibility for orienting the new employee should be shared by the corporate leadership, including the CEO or supervisor, the physician executive's peers, and even the recruiter, because executive recruiters are often familiar with the organization's corporate culture.[1] When the new employer does not orient new employees, new physician executives should do it themselves. The new physician executive who takes the initiative in his or her orientation at an organization can be successful if restraint and care are exercised and if the emphasis is placed on listening and taking in information rather than sending out information.

Corporate culture has been described as the informal organization, with its values, norms, mores, and unwritten expectations and assumptions.[2] The issue of fitting into the corporate culture is so important that it deserves formal attention.[3] Discuss mission, vision, values, goals, and how the strategic plan is implemented and reviewed with your supervisor and the CEO if possible.[1] Investigate corporate taboos or known failure paths, myths and honored traditions, and the level of initiative and assertiveness you may use regarding different responsibilities.[4] Discover unwritten reporting relationships, which are even more significant than the organizational chart.[5] It is important to be sure that there is buy-in from the various critical parts of the organization, especially if the position is new and will affect the power of other individuals in the organization.[6]

Identify available resources, including human, technical, and organizational. Structural and systemic arrangements and processes regarding information, communication, and training should be understood.[7] Obtain an organizational chart, with names, titles, and phone numbers of key individuals, and a list of professional contacts.[8] Find out about things such as business cards and office supplies, computer and phone access, where to buy stamps or lunch, and where to park the first day.[1] Prepare a press release with biosketch and announcement for publication internally for the organization and externally as appropriate.[8]

Seek a mentor or advisor to help you to assess difficult situations that may be encountered in the start-up phase and to generate strategies that can show your progress as early as possible.[9] Establish collegial relationships with your peers in the organization during the orientation period by having lunch and discussing their projects with them. Persuade your supervisor or CEO to facilitate the use of staff time for such team building.[1]

Most important, however, carve out some time to spend with your supervisor, an investment that will pay future dividends. New employees need good communication and clear expectations from the very beginning. Know the status of your work, especially during the orientation period. Feedback on your performance during the first weeks is vital.[10]

The following is practical, expert advice for newly hired physician executives who take the initiative in their own orientation at an organization:

- Observe how people interact and note whether they use memos or communicate face-to-face.

- Review the organization's publications to see what is being highlighted.

- Learn about the corporate culture by joining a lunch group.

- Find a mentor, an experienced person from a noncompetitive area of the organization, to discover how things are done.

- Explore the entire organization by visiting every area from clinic to kitchen and laboratory to library.[1]

The rule for orientation is: The more time you spend up front with your supervisor, the less time is required later. If the learning function is neglected, you may be oriented in unfavorable ways that will take months to change by retraining. One expert suggests the following five-day orientation plan for a new physician executive:

Day One.

Spend almost the entire day with the person to whom you report directly.[11] Review the job description in detail, including level of responsibility, reporting hierarchy, and sources of positional power.[5] Make sure you meet everyone in the immediate work unit. Request that others join you and the supervisor on coffee breaks. Make a tour of the entire organization, and begin exploring politics, policies, and procedures. Find a mentor.

Day Two.

Ask questions that you may have as a result of the first day. Complete three to four hours of substantive work, then meet with your supervisor to obtain feedback and ask more questions.

Day Three.

Arrange to meet with all those with whom you will interact to learn their expectations. Ask for feedback on the meetings.

Day Four.

Have lunch with your supervisor and top management if possible. Review the telephone directory and discover who does what, how supplies are requisitioned, etc.

Day Five.

Spend an hour with your supervisor discussing the job as a whole. On day six you will be doing it all solo, with your supervisor being available but not standing by. Ask all the questions you can think of now.[12]

Often, a physician executive is hired to fill a newly created position and must blaze a new trail in an organization. The profession is new enough that health care organizations may not have many preconceived notions about the role, and the new physician executive can become an architect of the position. In this case, the new hire does not have to wade through a lot of history concerning the job, but still has to learn the organization's culture.[13]

The physician executive can never escape the title of "Doctor" and will always be perceived as a physician and one of "them" by nonphysician executives and staff of the organization. Historically, "they" have always been an adversarial group; therefore, allegiances, commitment, and dedication of the physician executive will always be questioned.[14] At the same time, physician executives enjoy a certain mystique and respect among corporation executives because of the awesome responsibility and basic intelligence credited to physicians. Even if the CEO and others in top management are physicians, however, the corporate culture is that of business and not medicine.[15]

It may be a major challenge to resist the avalanche of problems that beset the new physician executive upon arrival in an organization. It is natural to react to whatever demands attention and to do whatever is more enjoyable or less stressful, whether or not it is what needs to be done. Discrimination is an important managerial skill to cultivate.[13] When asked how they viewed the performance of physician executives under their direct supervision, non-physician managers in one company reported that concerns often focused around time and task management and communication.[16] New physician executives may need to switch from a time schedule totally driven by the clinical needs of patients to a schedule mostly driven by the administrative needs of an organization. The focus shifts more toward important and not urgent activities in order to build relationships and avoid crisis situations. This requires being more active than reactive, emphasizing prevention over cure, and delegating more activities.[17]

When the new physician executive is the CEO of an organization, he or she alone is responsible for learning all he or she can about the corporate culture of the organization as fast as possible. It is common for a new CEO to become caught up immediately in a few obvious problems and to find out later that he or she does not know the organization when long-range changes need to be made.[1] The corporate culture must be defined before it can be influenced. A perspective on organizational history may be gained by knowing the expectations created by predecessors, learning the impacts of legal ordinances, appraising key personalities, and assessing existing organizational commitments and anticipated alliances. Learning something as abstract as the corporate culture by oneself can be an uncomfortable task. This may be especially true for physicians who are accustomed to personal mastery over health care problems and to relying on consultants and referral sources.[18] Finding a mentor among the network of professional colleagues outside the organization can help.

Corporate culture has been described as an ecosystem of independent relationships that must be balanced synergistically.[19] No matter how brilliant or charismatic, no one in an organization succeeds alone, and organizations are only as successful as their personnel. The gold standard for a new leadership team is to integrate people with new ideas and different organizational experiences with those who have knowledge of the organization and its clients or constituents. Unfortunately, the corporate leadership of many health care organizations focuses little attention on orientation and training of their new physician executives. It is a fallacy to assume that a skilled and experienced physician, researcher, scientist, clinician, or academician will evolve automatically into an accomplished executive administrator. Physician executives will not be respected or effective leaders merely because of their titles or their status; their success will be more a function of process than of structure. Individual initiatives as a technical or professional expert may gain entry into the executive suite, but these qualities will not suffice in the leadership of contemporary health care organizations. The new physician executive must be skillful in becoming acclimated, oriented, and integrated into the corporate culture in order to succeed in an executive role in a health care organization.[20]

References

1. Eubanks, P. "Acclimating the New Exec Should Be First Goal." *Hospitals* 65(9):50, May 5, 1991.

2. Covey, S. *Principal Centered Leadership.* New York, N. Y.: Simon and Schuster, 1992, pp. 227-8.

3. Linney, G., and Linney, B. *Medical Directors: What, Why, How.* Tampa, Fla.: American College of Physician Executives, 1992, p. 20.

4. Covey, S., *op cit.,* pp. 192-3.

5. Hammon, J., Editor. *Fundamentals of Medical Management: A Guide for the New Physician Executive.* Tampa, Fla.: American College of Physician Executives, 1993, p. 63.

6. Linney, G., and Linney, B., *op. cit.,* p. 16.

7. Covey, S., *op. cit.,* p. 193.

8. Simmons, S. "Orientation: The Bridge from Recruitment to Retention." *Association of Staff Physician Recruiters* 2(1):6, Spring 1995.

9. Aluise, J. *The Art of Leadership the Science of Management.* Durham, N. C.: Wellness Publishing, 1995, p. 212.

10. Aluise, J., *op. cit.,* p. 159.

11. Curry, W., Editor. *New Leadership in Health Care Management: The Physician Executive.* Tampa, Fla.: American College of Physician Executives, 1994, p. 295.

12. Curry, W., *op. cit.,* pp. 295-6.

13. *Ibid.,* p. 98.

14. *Ibid.,* p. 86.

15. *Ibid.,* pp. 145-6.

16. *Ibid.,* p. 149.

17. Hammon, J., *op. cit.,* pp. 75-81.

18. Curry, W., *op. cit.,* p. 147.

19. Covey, S., *op. cit.,* p. 254.

20. Aluise, J., *op. cit.,* p. 212-214.

Marilyn Szymialis Radke, MD, MPH, MA, FACPM, CPE, FACPE, was Medical Officer, Drug Enforcement Administration, Arlington, Virginia, when this chapter was written. She is now an occupational medicine physician at Mankato Clinic, Ltd., Mankato, Minnesota.

Chapter

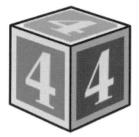

Organization Theory

by Robert J. Inguagiato, MBA

Organizations are complex, ever-changing entities. While it is rarely possible to have a perfect handle on every aspect of organizational dynamics, the simple model described in this chapter can lead to better understanding of the meaning behind organizational behavior. The ultimate secret of success is for the leader's expectations to be congruent with the phase at which the organization operates.

Today's health care world finds few organizations that have not been touched by mergers, acquisitions, strategic partnerships, and alliances. These shifting organizational foundations have created even greater challenges for the new leaders in medical management. A physician making the entry into management used to focus on an organization known as a hospital, a clinic, or some other single-unit entity. Now, the hospital is part of a chain or health care system and has probably formed a strategic alliance with other health care providers as well. The dynamics of organizations are exhilarating, challenging, confusing, and sometimes contradictory. And, with the advent of new organizational relationships, organizations certainly are not dull. For many physicians who have been nonmanagerial participants in organizations, the organization was a place to apply professional competencies, and the intricacies of how the organization operated generally were not of much concern. The changing landscape in health care organizations has changed that attitude, and, for those who are making the transition to leadership roles, an understanding of the organizational landscape can be of critical importance.

Your clinical training, skills, and talents were crucial precursors to entering the leadership world. However, you will quickly find that your new role requires something much more of you if you are to be a successful leader in today's health care landscape. You will need managerial and leadership competencies, particularly in areas such as consensus building, team building, networking, and understanding the consequences of change in the dynamic systems you are working in. In some cases, these leadership competencies will be applied in uncharted organizational waters and, in most cases, with systems that are under stress.

Pursuit of these managerial and leadership competencies can seem chaotic. Organizational leadership and managerial theories abound in today's literature. A theory is adopted, tried for a few years, and then abandoned for another new theory. Which ones should you choose, which ones should you believe, and which ones are accurate? The answer is all of them and none of them. You should choose the ones that will allow you to add value to your stakeholders, patients, staff, CEO, board members, investors, and the community at large. If you are flexible in your approach and are willing to select what seems to make most sense for you and your stakeholders at the time, and then are willing to fine tune and continually modify your approach based on observations and feedback, you will do well. If you select one theory, hang on to it regardless of the changing landscape, you will find yourself frustrated and dissatisfied, both with the results and with the organizational system in which you are operating.

Organization theory places meaning and understanding on the dynamics operating in organizations. You will find it helpful to have one, if not several, paradigms available to interpret the forces at play. My bias is to provide you with a simple model that explains the complexities of organization life, rather than a complex model that explains the simplicities of life in an organization.

This chapter has four objectives:

- To explain the three phases of organizational evolution.

- To discuss the behavioral characteristics associated with these phases.

- To take an exploratory look at the variables creating this dynamic ebb and flow.

- To put all this information together through the eyes of the health care leader.

The Three Phases of Organizational Evolution

Most health care organizations will undergo three distinct phases of evolution. In the first edition of this book, I used the phrase organization growth rather than evolution to describe these three phases. I have changed the term to evolution, because I think the term growth implies moving to something more effective. I now believe that one phase of development is no better or worse than another, just different. These three phases will often be characterized by how an organization is structured, as if these phases were landmarks to recognize what phase the organization is in at the moment. Out of these structures will flow behaviors that people exhibit in these organizations. For most leaders, it is the behaviors that can cause confusion and frustration. It is the behaviors that drive performance and the bottom line. What causes confusion is when the behaviors do not match what you expected the organization to accomplish. It is as if the behaviors are being exhibited in defiance of the organization structure. Yet, it is quite the opposite. Most people behave the way the organizational system encourages them to behave. These phases of evolution can be observed at the macro level (the entire organization or system) or at the micro level (department or section). Observing the structure of an organization will tell you much about how decisions are made, the level of trust, the level of maturity, the leadership styles that are likely to prevail, and the behavioral expectations placed on staff.

Organizational evolution implies that an organization moves from one phase to another. That does happen, but organizations can and will move back and forth from one phase to another. This can happen because they are not happy with the results of the present structure, because they have just merged with another organization and are adopting the structure of the parent organization, or for any number of other reasons. The point is that these structures will change like the tides in the ocean. An effective leader will do well to learn how to read these changing tides, or to change the tides themselves, to get the organization to perform differently.

Dependency is the first phase of organizational evolution. This type of organization produces highly dependent behavior in its staff. A dependent organization is analogous to a child who is dependent on parents for most major life-support systems. Decision making is highly centralized. At times, this phase will be characterized by a large headquarters staff. The working environment is highly control-oriented, and decision making is in the hands of a relative few. The dependency phase can be seen in start-up ventures where maturity and experience are low, in departments that are either new or in trouble, and in organizations that must follow exacting detail in their daily performance. The level of trust in highly dependent organizations is low. People are expected to do as they are told, and behaviors that cause waves are quickly extinguished. This type of organization generally rewards autocratic leadership behavior for those who are among the chosen few. It is rare to see participative leadership styles used with any success in a department or organization of this nature.

Independence is the second phase of organizational evolution. It is common to have an organization evolve from a highly dependent structure to one of independence. This phase of organizational evolution is analogous to a young adult who strikes off on his or her own. On an organizational level, this independence would be characterized by departments and functions being very independent of each other. Each unit makes decisions with its own immediate world in mind. Decision making is decentralized, departments and functions operate in an autonomous manner, and individual performance is highly cherished and rewarded. Little emphasis is placed on interdepartmental relationships, and at times staff members will wonder if they are all working for the same institution. This type of organizational structure can breed a high level of internal competition that, if not carefully monitored, can cause counterproductive outcomes. The level of trust in an independent organization is generally high, and the level of control, evidenced by organizational systems, is considerably lower than in a dependent organization. An independent organization generally expresses confidence in its staff members' abilities and encourages them to maximize their potential.

The first two phases of organizational evolution, dependency and independence, are used often in heath care systems and can be successful under the right conditions. However, each phase has a major drawback. The dependent organization does not fully utilize the talents of its staff members and runs the risk of not treating them with dignity. The independent organization, on the other hand, uses and recognizes the talents of individual staff members but often loses the synergy available through cross-functional cooperation and collaboration.

The third phase of evolution, interdependence, has become more popular in the past decade and is particularly popular in contemporary organizations, both for better and for worse. An interdependent organization takes the best of the dependent and independent organization phases and adds one additional element, synergy. An interdependent organization has a decentralized decision-making process; however, there is a strong emphasis on not making decisions in a vacuum. Departments and functions are encouraged, if not required, to consult with one another to discuss the ramifications of their decisions, and, in most cases a collaborative approach is emphasized. A strong emphasis is placed on the need for staff from different organizational teams to come together in the decision-making process. Again, the collaborative approach is evident in the day-to-day life of the organization. A strong emphasis is placed on interdepartmental cooperation rather than competition. Although individual contributors are considered important, a higher value is placed on teamwork. Occasionally, organizational achievement will occur more slowly, but with much more commitment by the staff. The synergy of cross-functional cooperation and collaboration is an expected outcome of organizations that have an interdependent structure.

Behavioral Characteristics of the Three Phases of Evolution

Why is it necessary to identify the key behavioral characteristics for each of these evolutionary phases? The answer is congruency and understanding. If, as the leader, you expect your staff to behave in certain ways, you must have an understanding of what behaviors your organizational structure is shaping and reinforcing. For example, it is particularly frustrating for a leader to expect his or her staff to exhibit collaborative behaviors when the organizational structure is causing and reinforcing people to behave independently of each other. It is not uncommon, in the example above, to diagnose this behavioral problem as one caused by lack of appropriate training. A word of advice, before you jump on the training bandwagon; first look at what your organization's structure and systems are asking for in terms of behavior. In instances such as those above, people will behave according to what the systems and structure are reinforcing them to do, regardless of the espoused desire. As a leader, if there is congruency among your organizational structure, systems, and leadership behavior, there is a higher likelihood that your staff will behave in ways that will meet your expectations. Naturally, your expectations should be based on realistic outcomes of these forces or you will be disappointed. The following discussion is designed to help you identify realistic behavioral expectations based on these three phases of organizational evolution.

A dependent organization produces staff behaviors that are hinged on a few people providing direction for the entire staff. Consequently, if you expect your staff to be self-directional, a dependent organizational structure will not produce such behaviors. The staff will not have a feeling of empowerment. As a result, you should not expect staff members to take matters into their own hands if a situation calls for action outside of their specific job description. Individual discretionary effort would not be reinforced in a dependent organization.

Dependent organizations tend to produce consistent but rarely superior performance. If you need consistently average performance, a dependent organization may well help you achieve that goal. Dependent organizations produce a low level of innovation. This is particularly important if you expect staff members to be innovators. What innovation is developed must come from the few decision makers in the organization. If the organization has exacting work systems and procedures in place that reduce the need for individual judgment, the level of efficiency in the organization can be high. The emphasis is on the phrase "exacting detail." If you have covered every possible contingency, and have it documented, this form of organization structure can work well. This structure does not work well in environments that are experiencing rapid change. Professional work standards must be articulated in fine detail if you expect the staff to meet the organization's goals. As you have observed, a dependent organization produces and reinforces a host of staff behaviors. What is crucial for you to be aware of is what you are asking for when you develop a dependent organization. If your leadership expectations are congruent with the outcomes of a dependent organization, you will not be disappointed.

An independent organization produces and reinforces a different set of staff behaviors. Staff members will be encouraged to be more self-directive in their day-to-day work. It is not unusual to have reward systems in an independent organization that reinforce individual initiative. Staff members will often use discretionary effort to accomplish their work. If a situation calls for an individual to do more than his or her job description states, it is not unusual for that staff member to go beyond the call of duty. Independent organizations tend to produce a higher level of overall individual performance. A dependent organization will produce a consistent average performance and very little, if any, superior performance. An independent organization will produce more variability in performance, but a higher likelihood of more superior staff performance. If you are looking for strict adherence to deeply documented procedures, policies, etc. an independent organizational structure will probably not meet your expectations. An independent organization will adapt well to a changing landscape and can be very effective in stimulating the maximum potential of individuals.

The level of innovation by individual staff members in an independent organization could be high, if the organization's reward systems encourage such behavior. The independent organization is very individual oriented; thus, staff members are encouraged and expected to have their own internal standards of quality, in addition to what may be formally spelled out by the organization. An independent organization places a great deal of emphasis on individual and departmental autonomy, which, in turn, produces behavior that is congruent with this structure and phase. If your expectations as a leader of a department or function are congruent with the type of organization you create, the likelihood of your being confused or frustrated by staff behaviors are lessened considerably.

An interdependent organization encourages collaborative and cooperative staff behaviors. As in an independent organization, staff members are likely to express self-direction. However, the interdependent organization will encourage and reinforce self-directive behaviors that take into account other people and other departments, rather than behavior that is self-oriented. Staff members will generally behave in ways that reflect a sense of empowerment and also will demonstrate a sense of responsibility for other staff members' work. They not only will perform their jobs but often will go beyond them if the situation calls for more latitude. Staff members of an interdependent organization tend to behave in ways that demonstrate a concern for the global good of the organization, rather than focusing on themselves.

An interdependent organization, similar to an independent organization, is likely to produce superior performance, particularly in a changing landscape. However, this superior performance will be more observable on a systemwide basis, rather than on an individual level. The amount of discretionary effort individual staff members may exhibit can be quite high, especially when they see the ramifications of their actions on the entire organizational system. The level of innovation in an interdependent organization can be even higher than in an independent organization. The synergistic effect of collaboration between individuals and departments stimulates the level of innovation. The organization will not need to spell out individual work standards in exacting detail, but can paint a vision of the expected outcomes of the team. An interdependent organization emphasizes team performance and collaboration rather than individual performance. Individual performance is valued in an interdependent organization. However, relationships and their impact on the overall performance of the organization are valued even more.

Understanding the behavioral characteristics of the different stages of organizational evolution will often explain why individuals, departments, and organizational systems behave the way they do. The main issue is congruency. If your expectations are congruent with the behavioral outcomes of the organizational structure, the likelihood of these outcomes being what you want are high. However, additional variables also affect performance. These variables, in combination with the stage of organizational evolution, will have a major impact on the behavioral performance of individuals and, subsequently, on the organization.

Dynamic Variables of Organizational Life

The stage of organizational life, i.e., dependent, independent, or interdependent, and its corresponding behavioral characteristics are major factors in shaping organizational life. However, they are not the only variables at play in this dynamic ebb and flow. There are five other components that help shape life in organizations: espoused organizational values, mission/goals, systems (psychological and technical), external competition, and leadership behavior.

The espoused values of an organization, and, on a micro level, of a department, help create behavioral expectations. If a health care system states that one of its fundamental values is to provide a working environment that encourages individual initiative, it is stating a behavioral expectation that it has of its staff. Concurrently, this value statement is also saying that staff can expect the organization to behave in a manner that will support and encourage such behavior. The adage, "Be careful of what you ask for because you are likely to get it," is a critical factor in organizational values. Organizational values help create the rules of the game for organizational life. The real values, as opposed to the espoused values, of an organization are evidenced in what stories are printed in the internal newsletters, the types of behaviors that are rewarded through promotions, the internal role models for success, and dozens of other actions that occur on a daily basis. If a significant difference occurs between espoused values and actual values, incongruence develops. Once this occurs, it is difficult to understand and shape behavior, and the impact of other variables becomes less predictable as well.

The mission and goals of the organization help create a sense of purpose and direction that tell staff what game they are participating in. If a health care organization states that one of its goals is to provide the highest quality of patient care, its staff will use this goal to provide direction for day-to-day behavior. However, if staff members observe the organization continually making exceptions to this goal, they can only interpret these changes as the new goal. Inevitably, inconsistencies such as this are what create new organizational goals, much to the surprise of the organization.

Organizational systems, both psychological and technical, have a major impact on organizational life. Psychological systems, such as performance appraisals, internal newsletters, compensation plans, career progression systems, and organizational role models, will shape the behavior and the performance of staff members in powerful ways. For example, if a health care system has an espoused value of only hiring the best professionals in the field and then develops a performance appraisal system that forces the majority of staff to be evaluated as adequate, staff members will soon get the message that adequate behavior is all that is really wanted in the organization. Inevitably, this outcome will become the new norm and will come as a surprise to the organization and its leadership.

Technical systems, such as management information reports, the budget process, and resource acquisition systems, also will have an impact on the life and behavior of staff members. For example, if an organization is in its independent phase and has a resource acquisition system that requires CEO approval for the most insignificant of purchases, a staff member will become confused about the message the organization is attempting to deliver.

External competition, mergers, acquisitions, and strategic alliances can all have an impact on the stress an organization experiences. This stress, like stress to a physiological system, can cause behavioral reaction that may be different from those expected. Under these circumstances, it is particularly important to examine the variables at play, to ensure that your organizational structure is congruent with your outcomes, and to consider transitioning to another phase of organizational evolution, if necessary.

Leadership behavior is the last, but not the least, important factor that affects the dynamics of organization life. All the variables we have looked at are powerful forces operating in an organization. However, it is leadership behavior that is the most powerful variable of all. Action will speak louder than all the espoused values and organization mission statements. A leader's behaviors act as living proof of what the organization wants and expects from its staff members. The issue of congruency is critical in leadership behavior. If a leader's behavior is congruent with the stage of organizational evolution, the values, the mission/goals, and the systems of the organization, it is almost certain that the behavioral outcomes will match expectations. If there is incongruence in this chain, the actions of the organization and its leaders will speak louder than all the words used.

Putting This All Together Through the Eyes of the Leader

This chapter has been written to explain the forces at play inside organizations and the relationships the forces have with one another. As a leader, you can control and affect some of these forces to create a working environment that will produce the behavioral outcomes you desire. You can create mini-organizations within the larger context of the health care system. These mini-organizations can mimic the stage of evolution of the larger system, or they can take on their own phase of evolution. This is particularly evident in research arms of larger systems that are structured quite differently than the host system and consequently get a considerable different set of behavioral outcomes. You can also express values and mission statements that your own department or function can represent. You may not always have a hand in the development of psychological and technical systems, but you may have an impact on how those systems are used. The external competition and its impact may or may not be out of your control, but you can have a better understanding of how those variables create stress in the organization and consequently can manage the stress' repercussions more congruently. Ultimately, this chapter can be reduced to two simple organizational theories.

- There are a number of variables that affect organization life and the behaviors of staff. The more congruent they are with one another, the easier it will be to understand.

- As a leader, you are one of the most powerful variables in this dynamic chain. How you behave can and does make a difference.

Robert J. Inguagiato, MBA, is a training and organizational development consultant in Kauai, Hawaii. He can be reached at bobi@aloha.net.

Chapter

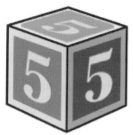

The Roles and Responsibilities of Clinical Department Heads

by Charles E. Hollerman, MD, CPE, FACPE

The roles of the clinical department head include being, first and foremost, a leader and a communicator. Other roles depend on the situation and the circumstances, e.g., arbitrator, negotiator, enforcer, counselor, disciplinarian, innovator, advocate (for both patient and organization), visionary, change agent, influencer, planner, evaluator, ad infinitum. The department head is a manager—in reality, a physician manager who is an interface professional, [1,2] whether employed or voluntary. This requires the attainment of new skills—management skills—so the department head can provide effective leadership within the hospital community.

The role of the clinical department head is, in a word, leadership. The essentials of "leading the way" are well captured in an article with that title.[3] Critical job components for the clinical department head include:

- Energizing the organization.

- Sharing responsibility for outcomes.

- Resolving conflicts.

These three components are effectively articulated in the article mentioned above and also are covered in other chapters of this book. This chapter will concern itself with the more pragmatic aspects of this leadership position.

The day-to-day roles of clinical department heads will vary according to a number of factors, including but not limited to:

The Size of the Hospital[4]

In a survey of hospitals ranging in size from 50 to more than 600 beds, the responsibilities of the clinical department head included quality assurance and supervision of physicians in all reporting institutions. However, responsibilities for budget development, recruitment, and supervision of other employees were added as the size of the hospital increased.

Whether the Hospital Is a Teaching or a Nonteaching Institution

If the hospital is a teaching institution (defined as being involved in medical student or residency training programs), the clinical department head's role will depend on whether it is a community teaching, nonuniversity-affiliated hospital; a community teaching, university-affiliated institution; or a university-based teaching hospital. The institutional designation may also result in different priorities in relation to patient care, education, research, and administration. In all hospitals, high-quality patient care is obviously a prime attribute. However, in teaching hospitals, and especially in university institutions, the attainment of high-quality patient care is derived from an emphasis on education and research that subsequently enhances patient care. In a nonteaching hospital, patient care might be the sole attribute, whereas in a community teaching hospital, patient care is primary, with teaching relegated to a secondary role and research a distant third. In all institutions, the administrative role is integral to accomplishing departmental goals and objectives.

The Method of Selection of the Department Head

In perhaps the majority of hospitals, department heads are elected by members of the departments. The term of office may be two years, and they may be able to succeed themselves. In other hospitals, they may be full-time employees of the hospital, appointed by administration with the approval of the governing board. The length of tenure in office in such instances may be defined by contract, and the roles of department heads may be beyond those usually found in medical staff by-laws.

The Medical Staff Structure

The traditional medical staff model is structured along divisional (departmental) lines—e.g., medicine, surgery, pediatrics, etc.—with subspecialty sections within each major department (or, in some instances, with a subspecialty, e.g., neurology, being a separate department). Other models, however, do exist. One author[5] has delineated three alternative models:

- The independent-corporate model, in which the medical staff is totally independent.

- The divisional model, of which there are three variants. One variant is based on the integration of major functional areas within medical divisions (departments), an arrangement sometimes referred to as the Hopkins Model.[6,7] In this model, hospital functional areas, such as nursing, finance, planning, marketing, housekeeping, etc., are included within each department and report to the head of the department. Alternatively, there could be divisional models structured into such areas as primary care, maternal-child health, chronic diseases, and so on, or along product/services lines, such as oncology, cardiovascular, neurological, etc. In all the divisional models, the functional hospital areas are integral to the division. In the nontraditional divisional models, the role of the department head becomes blurred or nonexistent. Many of the traditional roles of the department head, such as quality assessment and credentialing, are performed by the division itself.

- A medical staff organization is developed that runs parallel to the traditional medical staff structure. This structure is directed by a steering committee composed of both hospital and medical staff members. Examples of such parallel organization include IPAs, joint ventures, and physician-hospital associations.

In some hospitals today, there are examples of all of the above alternative models developing and/or coexisting with the traditional medical staff organization.

In many community hospitals today, the number of departments has been dramatically reduced. Currently some hospitals have only two departments—medicine and surgery. Consequently, the opportunity to achieve leadership positions as clinical department heads has been drastically reduced. Other changes have also occurred, e.g. in required attendance requirements for medical staff members that result in greater challenges for the clinical department leader, as will be noted later. Another limiting aspect of available leadership positions is the merging of hospitals and possibly of their medical staffs. The Joint Commission on Accreditation of Healthcare Organizations recognizes that reality in its Standards for Hospitals in the Medical Staff Standards section.[8] Basically, the hospital organization may have one or multiple medical staffs, the basis for each depending on factors of patient population served and geographic proximity. A recent article notes that there have been many health care consolidations in the past few years; it deals specifically with medical staff issues arising in such consolidations.[9]

Positional Relationships with President/Chief of Medical Staff, Medical Director, and/or Dean of Medical Schools

There is virtually always an elected leader of the medical staff. In increasing numbers, there are also medical directors whose function may be purely liaison between the medical staff, administration, and the board or may include operational duties. The latter usually includes direction of quality management and utilization review staff, as well as administrative direction of the medical staff office. However, operational areas are being added, such as direct reporting and budgetary authority for clinical departments and for medical support areas such as admissions and medical records. In university hospitals, the head of the department is usually the head of the associated medical school department and reports directly to the dean of the school of medicine. Within that framework, the head of the department may also be responsible for directing an associated faculty practice plan. Such plans are also being developed in teaching, nonuniversity affiliated hospitals. In teaching hospitals with full-time faculty, the head of the department takes on an additional duty: managing town-gown interactions. One article expresses concerns regarding the transition from a voluntary hospital to a teaching hospital with full-time compensated faculty.[10] The specter of the leadership and control of the medical staff being assumed by paid department heads, resulting in an evolution to a predicted full-time multispecialty group practice is highlighted in the article.

Despite the organizational diversity and complexity described above, one author has described a key functional role for the department head: "Be a 'Communications expert'— amplify and translate the needs of the department into language that is understandable by those governing the institution; at the same time chairmen must interpret and communicate institutional and strategic goals to their departmental colleagues."[11] The reader is referred to other articles expanding on the diversity of roles in a variety of institutional settings.[12-18] This chapter will attempt to review, within broad categories, the common roles of department heads, primarily within the traditional medical staff model. These categories will not follow the outline of responsibilities typically contained in medical staff by-laws.[19] The chapter will conclude with an overview of the relationships that may exist between the department head and other managers, especially the medical director.

Roles (Duties and Responsibilities)

Quality Improvement and Credentialing

These intertwined responsibilities constitute a significant role for the department head in virtually all institutions. The term quality improvement is used rather than the prior terms of quality assurance or quality assessment. Some would use the term total quality management (TQM), of which continuous quality improvement (CQI) is a component; others would have CQI be premiere. It is not the purpose of this chapter to review the changes occurring in the area of quality management; the reader is referred to selected publications[20-29] on that topic; it is also discussed in this book in Chapter 15.

The following items capture the essence of the department head's role in these areas:

- Be accountable for all professional, educational, and administrative activities within the department, particularly those related to the quality of patient care rendered by members of the department, and for effective implementation of the hospital's continuous quality improvement program and other quality improvement functions delegated to the department.

- Develop and implement short- and long-term departmental plans that include incorporation in the credentialing and privileging process for members of the department an evaluation of individual quality improvement activities, utilization of resources, and continuing medical education, as well as evidence of appropriate professional conduct and competence. Specifically, this means the department head has responsibility for appointment, reappointment, and granting of clinical privileges, including evaluation of the applicant/department member's professional competence, conduct, and cost-effective practice of medicine. In the appointment process, the department head must focus on:

❏   The preapplication process (where one exists).

❏   The application process, particularly in regard to verifying information, gathering references, and interviewing applicants. In most hospitals, verifying information and obtaining references is the responsibility of the medical staff office, often under the direction of a medical director. It is important to recognize that credentialing, e.g.
appointment to the medical staff, and privileging are separate.
Credentialing results in appointment; privileging is the authorization
granted to the physician to provide specific patient care services. The
privileges fall within defined limits as related to 1) the
institution/facility's capability to offer such privileges and 2) the
physician's qualifications and current competencies. As a simplistic
example of the difference, a psychiatrist qualified to do electroshock
therapy requests the privilege; the hospital does not have a mental
health unit offering electroshock therapy; the privilege cannot be
granted, yet the psychiatrist may be appointed to the medical staff
(and with appropriate privileges). The department head must analyze
the data and the applicant and provide a recommendation. This role
cannot and should not be delegated to a committee or to the department as a whole. Such delegation may raise questions related to
antitrust or economic competition. Assistance from subspecialty division chiefs is appropriate when the clinical area is outside the department head's expertise; nevertheless, the department head is accountable for validating the applicants' competence.

The department head is responsible for developing criteria for clinical privileges. Today, interdepartmental negotiation to establish criteria for privileges that cross-traditional departmental lines is common. Aid in establishing such criteria is available.[30]

❏   Monitoring the applicants' performance. The initial appointment is
often termed provisional or probationary for a period. While the
applicant is in that status, the department head should arrange for
monitoring of the appointee's performance in terms of competence as
well as professional conduct.

A new issue of credentialing that may face clinical department heads is the
granting of permission to provide services to providers of complementary or
alternative medicine modalities. A recent article describes these modalities in
general and the approaches that may be considered.[31] The medical staff generally needs to be involved in credentialing only practitioners who are employed
or contracted by medical staff members. Practitioners employed or contracted
by the hospital may be the responsibility of the department of human resources.
Each hospital will need to develop, with the collaboration of the medical staff, a
privileges policy for practitioners who are not members of the medical staff.
These practitioners include such familiar ones as certified registered nurse
anesthetists and some relatively unfamiliar ones, such as reflexologists. A directory classifying and describing more than 250 complimentary and alternative
modalities and therapists is available as an aid in the credentialing process.[32]

In the reappointment process, examination of the quality aspects of the practitioner's care is mandated. The Joint Commission on Accreditation of Healthcare Organizations (JCAHO) requires documentation that reappointment decisions are based on measurement of quality and on a review of the care provided by the appointee since the prior appointment/reappointment period.[33] The hospital, through its quality management staff and/or medical staff office, should provide staff support for this role of the department head; however, the data requirements and the analysis are the responsibility of the department head.

The ultimate responsibility for quality of care, for appointments to the medical staff, and for credentialing for clinical privileges resides with the governing board. However, the board delegates the process to the medical staff, which in turn holds the department head accountable.

As noted previously, one role of the department head is to evaluate appointees in terms of cost-efficient practice of medicine. This provision raises the specter of economic credentialing.[34,35] What is intended is that the practitioner deliver high-quality patient care without under- or overutilization of resources. Examples of poor quality of care include such factors as unnecessary surgery, unnecessary laboratory tests or x-rays, incorrect treatment, or improper prescriptions. These and other aspects of quality-cost relationships are discussed in an article outlining a generic model of these relationships in health care.[36] The point is that a practitioner should not be credentialed on the basis of economic factors alone. Quality of care must be paramount, but efficient use of resources should be considered. Finite resources must be shared among many patients.

General Medical Staff Affairs

The following items delineate the role of the department head in general medical staff affairs:

- Be responsible for all clinical activities of the department. In the past, such responsibility was discharged through monthly department meetings. Although such meetings now generally occur quarterly, some departments continue with monthly meetings, alternating business meetings with quality/performance review sessions. This review is required by JCAHO. It directly relates to the areas of quality improvement and credentialing discussed above. The business meeting involves the communication expert role. Further, it is at this meeting that long-range plans for proper growth, expansion, and diversification of the department can be discussed and prepared for implementation. A major role for the department head in these meetings is to manage change: change in department direction, change in quality measurement, change in hospital-medical staff relations. However, a complicating factor today is that, in many hospitals, attendance by members of a department is no longer mandatory. This creates a significant challenge for the communication and change agent roles of the clinical department head.

- Enforce the hospital and the medical staff by-laws, rules, regulations, and policies within the department, including initiating corrective action and investigation of practitioners' clinical performance and determination of whether consultations were ordered when necessary. The major roles played in this arena are those of enforcer, disciplinarian, and investigator. This area includes identifying impaired physicians, counseling disruptive physicians, and dealing with complaints, such as sexual harassment. Policies for dealing with all these issues should be contained in the medical staff by-laws or rules and regulations.

- Be a member of the medical executive committee, give guidance for the overall medical policies of the hospital, and make specific recommendations and suggestions regarding his or her department and divisions. This role is usually delineated in medical staff by-laws. It includes quality measurement, credentialing, and corrective actions previously outlined. This role has been deemed legislative by some.[15]

- Establish and periodically review and revise plans for effective emergency operation of the department in the event of an institutional or communitywide disaster. The accomplishment of this role requires interdepartmental and intra-institutional collaboration. No single department is capable of providing all the activities in a disaster. This role mandates that the department head be a team player, not an autonomous entity.

General/Administrative/Hospital Affairs

Staff development may consist of two components:

- Medical staff development, in the organizational sense of recruitment and retention of appropriate physicians to further the breadth and the depth of patient care.

- Development of individual medical staff members, e.g., for leadership roles.

Recruitment should be consistent with the hospital's and the department's goals and in accordance with the medical staff by-laws and medical staff development plan. This role may be shared with the medical director or with another administration/board designee responsible for the medical staff development plan. The department head should be aware of physicians who are being recruited by members of his or her department. Additionally, through departmental meetings, the department head should be working with department members to identify new programs/services that, in concert with the hospital's plan, would entail the recruitment of physicians with disciplines and/or skills similar to or different from those of physicians currently on the medical staff. The department chair has the responsibility to communicate department recommendations and to express its views to administration.

The department head also has an obligation to the department, the hospital, and individual medical staff members to assist in the development of department members' abilities. This role may simply call for identifying potential leaders. It may involve being a mentor, or it may involve counseling an appointee on available avenues for personal/professional growth.

If the department head has budget responsibility, the administrative role that is required in such circumstances includes:

- Preparation and implementation of business and marketing plans based on approved strategic plans.

- Formulation, justification, and administration of the department budget in accordance with institutional policies and department goals.

- Management of human and fiscal resources of the department to maximize achievements in service, as well as in teaching and research if within a teaching hospital.

- Cooperation and collaboration with other hospital departments and with hospital administration in matters affecting patient care, including personnel, supplies, standing orders, and techniques.

Paperwork accompanies the role of the department head. Generally, reports need to be provided to designated hospital administrative staff, usually the medical director if there is one, regarding departmental activities and strategy. Annual departmental reports may be required by the president/chief of the medical staff and, although not usually in the same format, by the medical director, hospital president, or the board. Being a "communication expert" requires skills in both oral and written presentation.

Education and Research

If the institution is involved in teaching and/or research, the department head role includes the following duties and responsibilities:

- Serve as, or select, program director of associated residency program.

- Create opportunities for residents to participate in performance improvement and other interdisciplinary problem solving teams.[37]

- Lead and guide members of the department in developing, maintaining, and enhancing intra- and interdepartmental educational programs that support high academic standards, are current, and are responsive to learners' needs.

- Lead and guide members of the department in establishing high, but realistic, goals for intra- and interdepartmental research programs in relation to such factors as staff expertise, availability of funding, needs for equipment, availability of space, and number of support personnel needed.

- Submit and have articles accepted in peer-reviewed publications.

- Aid in identifying public and private funding sources for instruction and research; encourage grant applications and cultivation of private donors.

- Be responsible for ensuring that department members are aware of and in compliance with institutional policies and procedures in the conduct of research.

Institutional and Community Relations

The department head is expected to be a role model within the department, the medical staff, the hospital, and the community. This role carries with it the obligation to carry out the duties and responsibilities of the position in a manner consistent with the vision, mission, goals, and values of the institution. Further, there is a responsibility to the community to promote service by members of the department. Additionally, the department head must show leadership in his or her chosen field; this could include service on relevant task forces or committees at the institutional, local, state, regional, or national levels.

Relation to Other Hospital Managers

The relation of the department head to other hospital managers, including the medical director, will depend on the organizational structure of the hospital. In some institutions, for example in the divisional models mentioned earlier, the department head will be the leader of the management team. The much more likely relationship, however, will be that of being a team member. The latter position is not a familiar or a comfortable one for many physicians, because they are accustomed to being the captain of the ship. No one person, no one department, can provide the answers to the cross-disciplinary issues that exist in today's health care institutions; indeed, it is unlikely that such was ever the case. The department head must work in a collaborative fashion with other hospital managers to accomplish the goals of the hospital as well as those of the department. Suppose, for example, the head of an emergency department wishes to have patients admitted in a more timely manner. That admission process will depend, at least, on registrars, medical records personnel, ancillary departments such as radiology and laboratory medicine providing expeditious turnaround times on x-rays and tests, escort personnel, housekeeping providing ready beds, and floor nurses able and willing to accept patients. The accomplishment of the department head's desire demands input and involvement of a variety of services. The department head cannot just order it to be accomplished.

In general terms, the department head's relationship with the medical director encompasses information sharing, i.e., communication. The department head should keep the medical director apprised of department/medical staff needs and concerns, as well as recommend changes. Conversely, the medical director should not only keep the department head aware of plans and decisions of administration that will affect the department, but also serve as a link between department heads. Further, the medical director is most likely the person held accountable for overall medical quality improvement and credentialing. In the area of quality, the medical director provides oversight and direction. In the area of credentialing, the medical director must often serve as staff to the department head. The medical director, through the medical staff office, assembles all the information required for appointment/reappointment, which is then provided to the department head for analysis and recommendation. In situations in which the department head manages the budget and reports to a medical director, the latter is responsible for overseeing budget formulation, implementation, and monitoring.

Finally, the department head's relationship to the president/chief of the medical staff is usually through the medical executive committee and other committees of the medical staff. The president/chief of staff is responsible for ensuring adherence to the medical staff by-laws. The department heads are, therefore, accountable to the president/chief of staff in carrying out by-laws requirements.

Projections

It is likely that the future will see more full-time medical directors and department heads. At a minimum, there will be an increase in part-time positions, with compensation for administrative duties. The clinical linkage with the administrative activities of the hospital will be the major factor in the success of hospitals. The department head can no longer be selected on the basis of being a nice person, willing to do the job, or a superb clinician. The selection, whether by election or appointment, must be based on administrative skills that are in balance with clinical and political skills. Obviously, in teaching institutions, educational and/or research skills would be added qualifications. Increasingly, institutions will compensate clinical department heads, with or without concomitant financial contributions from the medical staff. Moreover, it is likely that institutions will also provide reimbursement to clinical departments heads for continuing medical education offerings in medical administrative skills/education.

References

1. Kaiser, L. "Key Management Skills for the Physician Executive." In *New Leadership in Health Care Management: The Physician Executive,* Curry, W., Editor. Tampa, Fla.: American College of Physician Executives, 1994, pp. 95-119.

2. Cordes, D., and others. "Management Roles for Physicians: Training Residents for the Reality." *Journal of Occupational Medicine* 30(1):863-7, Nov. 1988.

3. O'Connor, E., and Fiol, C. "Leading the Way." *Physician Executive* 23(8):6-13, Nov.-Dec. 1997.

4. Curry, W. "Hospital Size Determines Department Director Policy." *Physician Executive* 16(6):24-5, Nov.-Dec. 1990.

5. Shortell, S. "The Medical Staff of the Future: Replanting the Garden." *Frontiers of Health Services Management* 1(3):3-48, Feb. 1985.

6. Heyssel, R., and others. "Decentralized Management in a Teaching Hospital." *New England Journal of Medicine* 310(22):1477-80, May 31, 1984.

7. Brady, T., and Carpenter, C. "Defining the Management Role of the Departmental Medical Director." *Hospital and Health Services Administration* 31(5):69-85, Sept.-Oct. 1986.

8. *Comprehensive Accreditation Manual for Hospitals. The Official Handbook.* Oakbrook Terrance, Ill.: Joint Commission on Accreditation of Healthcare Organizations, Medical Standards.

9. Maynard, G., and others. "Medical Staff Consolidation Issues and Concerns." *Hospital and Health Services Administration* 40(3) 348-61, Fall 1995.

10. Davis, W. "One Community Hospital 2000 A.D." *Physician Executive* 16(2):31-2, Mar.-Apr. 1990.

11. Popp, A. "The Neurosurgeon as a Chairman of Surgery." *Surgery Neurology* 31(2):92-5, Feb. 1989.

12. McKhann, G. "Clinical Department Manager: Manager or Scholar." *Annals of Neurology* 26(61):779-81, Dec. 1989.

13. Betson, C., and Pedroja, A. "Physician Managers: A Description of Their Job in Hospitals." *Hospital and Health Services Administration* 34(3):353-69, Fall 1989.

14. Johnson, E. "Managing Physician-Directed Departments." *Hospital and Health Services Administration* 24(3):96-101, Summer 1979.

15. Angermeier, I., and Booth, R. "Establishing an Appropriate Role for Physician Involvement in Hospital Department Operations." *Hospital and Health Services Administration* 28(6):59-76, Nov.-Dec. 1983.

16. Dallman, J. "Hospital Department Chief Administrator or Brother's Keeper?" *Hospital Physician* 24(15):13,17, May 1988.

17. Walt, A. "The Surgical Chairmanship in a Corporate World." *Archives of Surgery* 123(7):805-9, July 1988.

18. Mayer, T. "The Emergency Department Medical Director." *Emergency Clinics of North America* 5(1):1-29, Feb. 1987.

19. *By-Laws Guide for Hospital Medical Staffs.* Chicago, Ill.: American Medical Association, 1984, pp. 37-38.

20. Berwick, D. "Continuous Improvement as an Ideal in Health Care." *New England Journal of Medicine* 320(1):53-6, Jan. 5, 1989.

21. McLaughlan, C., and Kaluzny, A. "Total Quality Management in Health: Making It Work." *Health Care Management Review* 15(3):7-14, Summer, 1990.

22. Merry, M. "Total Quality Management for Physicians: Translating the New Paradigm." *QRB* 16(3):101-5, March 1990.

23. O'Leary, D. "Accreditation in the Quality Improvement Mold-A-Vision for Tomorrow." *QRB* 17(3):72-7, March 1991.

24. Laffel, G., and Blumenthal, D. "The Case for Using Industrial Quality Management Science in Health Care Organizations." *JAMA* 262(20):2869-73, Nov. 24, 1989.

25. Marszalek-Gaucher, E., and Coffey, R. *Transforming Healthcare Organizations: How to Achieve and Sustain Organizational Excellence.* San Francisco, Calif.: Jossey-Bass, Publishers, 1990.

26. Blumenthal, D. "Quality of Healthcare. Part 1: Quality of care—What Is It?" *New England Journal of Medicine* 35(2):891-4, Sept. 19, 1996.

27. Brook, R., and others. "Quality of Healthcare. Part 2: Measuring Quality of Care." *New England Journal of Medicine* 335(13):966-70, Sept. 26, 1996.

28. Chassin, M. "Quality of Healthcare. Part 3: Improving the Quality of Care." *New England Journal of Medicine* 335(14):1060-3, Oct. 3, 1996.

29. Blumenthal, D. "Quality of Healthcare, Part 4: The Origins of the Quality of Care Debate." *New England Journal of Medicine* 335(15):1146-9, Oct. 10, 1996.

30. "Current Challenges in Delineating Clinical Privileges." *Quality Letter for Healthcare Leaders* 2(10):1-16, Dec. 1990-Jan. 1991.

31. Vincler, L., and Nicol, M. "When Ignorance Isn't Bliss: What Healthcare Practitioners and Facilities Should Know about Complementary and Alternative Medicine." *Journal of Health and Hospital Law* 30(3):160-78, Fall 1997.

32. Greeley, H., and Banas, D. *Directory of Complementary and Alternative Medicine.* Marblehead, Mass.: Opus Communications, 1999.

33. *Comprehensive Accreditation Manual for Hospitals.* Oakbrook Terrace, Ill.: Joint Commission on Accreditation of Healthcare Organizations, Medical Staff Standards.

34. Lang, H. "Economic Credentialing: Why It Must Be Stopped." *Medical Staff Counselor* 5(2):19-25, Spring 1991.

35. Greene, J. "System Pioneers Credentialing." *Modern Heathcare* 21(17):32-4,36, April 29, 1991.

36. Klint, R., and Long, H. "Cost/Quality Relationship: A Generic Model for Health Care." In *New Leadership in Health Care Management: The Physician Executive,* Curry, W., Editor. Tampa, Fla.: American College of Physician Executives, 1994, pp. 183-99.

37. Weingart, S. "House Officer Education and Organizational Obstacles to Quality Improvement." *Journal of Quality Improvement* 22(9):640-6, Sept. 1996.

Charles E. Hollerman, MD, CPE, FACPE, is Regional Vice President, Physician and Clinical Integration, Mercy Health Partners of Southwest Ohio, a component of Catholic Healthcare Partners, Cincinnati, Ohio.

Chapter

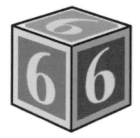

Effective Communication

by Barbara J. Linney, MA

Communication is a two-way street; if another person is determined not to communicate, no attempts can be successful. However, for most situations, the physician executive with well-developed communication skills can ensure that his or her messages are both received and understood. The key is in acquiring the requisite skills. None are automatic; all must be learned and reinforced on a regular basis.

The role of the chief of service and department chair varies from organization to organization, but it is always a physician who has been thrust into a leadership role. Whatever the specifics of their roles, chiefs of services and department chairs have to be able to communicate effectively with a wide array of individuals and groups—administrators, doctors, other department leaders, nurses, and the public, to name a few.

The chief of neurology may want to convince administration that his or her department is the best one to run the sleep laboratory. The chairman of obstetrics and gynecology may need to convince physicians in the department to cooperate and adhere to surgical standards—if someone is doing hysterectomies that do not meet prescribed criteria, the department and the hospital will be in trouble with regulators. The chief of orthopedics may need to talk to the head of physical therapy about procedures in that department. The chief is not that person's boss, an assistant administrator is, so he or she would need to tactfully make suggestions, not give orders, to get things done. The chair of obstetrics needs to cooperate with the chair of pediatrics because the departments often share the same patients.

Good communication is needed in all these situations. The main skills needed for good communication are talking so that people will want to listen to you, listening so that people will want to talk to you, and writing so that people will want to read what you have written.

There are ways to improve these skills and enable communication to take place. If someone absolutely does not want to communicate with you, nothing will work. It takes two people putting forth energy for a good interaction to happen, but if you will work on your techniques, you will find more people will respond to you in a positive way.

Talking

What will make people listen to you when you talk?

- Pronounce your words clearly. Enunciate. Don't mumble. You need to use energy to project your voice to the other person. He or she should not have to strain to hear you. It is very annoying to try to have a conversation with someone you cannot hear or understand. But neither should you yell at them.

- Don't talk too quickly or too slowly. Southerners sometimes have to speed up. Northerners sometimes have to slow down. Midwesterners usually have it about right.

- Look at the other person. Look as if you are enjoying the conversation. You don't have to stare the person down, but if your eyes wander all over the room or you always look over their shoulders, listeners have a hard time paying attention to what you are saying. They secretly speculate about what you are looking at rather than listening to what you are saying.

- Use average size words. If you sling around a lot of jargon or large words that most people do not know, you alienate them. Patients do not always know what MRI or myocardial infarction means.

- Don't talk longer than a couple of minutes without letting the other person talk. Taking turns was a valuable thing to learn in preschool, and we never outgrow the need to do it. "Most people fade fast and lose interest if they don't feel like an equal partner in a conversation. Talking too much is like weighing down a seesaw so that you cannot bob up and down with your playmate. It takes all the fun out of the activity."[1]

  According to Jung's concept of extrovert and introvert, extroverts talk and then figure out what they think; introverts figure out what they think and then talk. The introverts have valuable information if you give them time to say it. It's the job of any physician executive to be sure he or she gets ideas from both kinds, or unneeded resentment builds in the organization. It requires restraining the quick talkers some and encouraging those who do not speak up quickly.

- Be willing to tell what you feel about a subject as well as what you think. Give a personal example. "I think we would have better meetings with the doctors if we met at 6 p.m. instead of 9 p.m. Frankly, I'm just too tired to concentrate at 9 p.m. after I've worked a 12-hour shift."

- Avoid teasing. People fear others will humiliate them for the way they look, for what they say, or for what they have done. They cope with this fear in several ways. Some try to talk a lot and thus control the words. If they are doing the talking, they may not be hurt by someone else's words. Others do not speak up for fear of saying something wrong. The very witty and those able to come back with a quick retort are usually the only ones who enjoy teasing.

Teasing can be fun between equals, but often it is a secret form of aggression, and it strips its victim of power unless both parties are equally good at the quick barb. Teasing usually allows the one doing the teasing to feel one up. This occasionally feels good, but it eliminates closeness and builds resentment. A doctor's teasing nurses is not good unless the nurses feel equally free to tease the doctor. The latter is rare. If you tease your children a lot, you may want to rethink that. You are not equals. The child usually feels very bad, even though he or she may be laughing.

- Don't overuse big emotions, such as anger or tears. There are times when we are angry and the other person must know it, but those times are rare. It's similar to the little boy who hollered "wolf." If you are angry in most of your exchanges, people will learn to tune you out or will automatically scream back at you. If you cry often at work, people will not listen to you or take you seriously.

Big emotions usually interfere with communication. The listener is often threatened, frightened, or repulsed by a show of uncontrolled emotion, and he or she cannot hear the words being spoken. The person raging or crying also cannot hear when the listener responds.

What can you do when emotions are raging?

When you are the speaker, "Writing in a journal about people or situations that have evoked in us anger, anxiety, or a sense of defeat helps to stabilize our psychological situation and strengthen our ego. It helps us to 'get a handle' on our emotions without repressing them, and to get a look at the giant that threatens to swallow us. If we do this before we get into a discussion that might become highly emotional, the chances are good that we can express our feelings to the other person and not be consumed by them."[2]

When you are the listener, if you are feeling strong and collected, it is helpful if you can let the emotional person vent for a few moments. You might then respond, "I can see that you are angry, and I'm not surprised. What can I do to help?" If you are not up to being in the presence of so much negative energy, you might say, "I'll be glad to talk about this when you are calmer."

- Know what you want. It is a good idea to prepare for important conversations. By writing ahead of time, you can clearly focus on what you want and on what price you are willing to pay to get it. The following questions can help you think through an important interaction ahead of time. It is not cheating to prepare; it is wise.

What do you think about the situation?

What do you feel about the situation?
What do you want?
What will be the good or bad consequences if you get it?
What are you willing to do to get what you want?
What do you think the other person wants?
Can you give any of what he or she wants?

The following is an example of using these questions. I was in the middle of a business interaction between two friends of mine. They did not know each other. Bill wanted Joe to put on a program for a group he was in. Bill was outraged at the price Joe asked and wanted me to pass a nasty message back to Joe.

What do you think about the situation? I think Bill got angry when I would not do something he asked me to do. I would not call Joe and tell him that instead of Bill's paying him to speak, Joe would have to pay Bill's group thousands of dollars for it to even let him speak to it.

What do you feel about the situation? At first I felt angry. Now I feel hurt by the rejection. Bill has not talked to me for three months.

What do you want? To have lunch together occasionally, to talk, and to share ideas but not to have him start trying to tell me outlandish things to do again.

What will be the good or bad consequences if you get what you want? Good—I'd have his stimulating mind spurring thoughts in me again. Bad—He'd get into the bossiness again, or I'd get tired of laughing at his jokes, if we had too much contact.

What are you willing to do to get what you want? Call him and say, "Could we have lunch and talk about why we don't talk anymore?"

What do you think the other person wants? To be one up. Maybe an apology. I'm not sure what he wants—that's what I could find out if we talked.

Can you give him any of what he wants? I can apologize and say I didn't handle the situation well, but I can't be in a friendship where he slips into giving me orders.

- Use good body language. How you say something and how you look when you say it are as important as what you say. What causes someone to understand you and respond well to you? Psychologist Albert Mehrabian suggests that 7 percent of understanding depends on the words you use, 38 percent depends on your tone of voice, and 55 percent depends on your nonverbal body language.[3]

Facial expression and voice communicate much more than you realize. A listener understands and interprets your message more through the tone of your voice and the look of your body than through your words. "No, I'm not angry!" said harshly conveys the message that you are angry. "I really love that!" said sarcastically implies that you don't like it at all. People complain about getting mixed signals when words, tone of voice, and body language send different messages. They will believe the tone of your voice and the look on your face much more than the words you say.

Alexander claims people have a hard time accepting these facts. "The reality is that few people accept responsibility for anything more than their words. They have never learned that a harsh tone can deny the gentlest of words...."[4] Most people refuse to believe it if they are the ones doing the talking, but they quickly believe it if someone else is doing the talking.

A positive voice is cheerful, satisfied, concerned, warm. A negative voice is sarcastic, scared, depressed, clipped, tense, too loud or soft. A positive face has a smile, an occasional head nod, and eye contact. A negative face has a frown, smirk, or boring glare. A positive body is relaxed, leaning forward some, with open arms. Negative body language is pointing, wandering eyes, picking at body.[5]

Be even more careful about your tone of voice when you talk on the telephone. We are often thrown into someone's voice mail unexpectedly if his or her line is busy. Do not leave a stumbling, mumbling message. If you are not prepared, hang up, write out what you want to say and call back. Recruiters and others will make judgments about whether or not you can do a management job by the quality of your voice and the coherence of your message on the phone.

Listening

"...in both business and personal relationships, the consequence of inadequate listening are extraordinarily costly. Simple listening mistakes cost the business world millions of dollars annually."[6]

Most people have heard of Parent Effectiveness Training and the active listening that it recommends. Active listening has gotten some bad press, because people have overused the term, "I hear what you are saying." Also, if someone is rampaging, and I say, "You seem to be angry," a natural response might be, "You're damned right I'm angry." Active listening is a good technique, but how and when you use it needs to vary if you do not want to further alienate the person you are talking to.

"Active listening involves a restatement of either the message or the feeling of the speaker without giving advice, analyzing, or probing.7 It is the place to begin when listening to someone with a problem. You do not want to quickly interrupt and say, "I know how you feel" or give advice. But you do not want to overdo active listening either, because the listener may feel that you are acting like a parrot or a robot.

Listening is an art that starts with attentive silence. When my daughter was young, if I did not look at her when she talked to me, she would say, "Turn your face, Mama." Shortly after she could talk, she knew I had to be looking at her to really be paying attention. Adults know this, too, whether they tell you or not. It's your job to hold your eyes and body so that others know you are paying attention.

Young children talk a lot, so when I couldn't listen anymore, I said so and told them I would listen more later. We need to deal with adults in the same way. If you cannot pay attention, say, "I'm swamped with this project right now, but I can give you my undivided attention at 3 p.m. Could you come back then?" Then be sure to give them the time at 3 p.m.

Try not to make a habit of pretending to listen when you are not. People will come to distrust you. However, all of us have been in long meetings when listening simply was not in us anymore. At that point, pretending to listen is better than throwing your arms back with a deep sigh or closing your eyes in a bored slouch. Such behavior has a negative effect on those who may still be paying attention.

Listening is hard work. "While an average speech rate for many people is about 200 words per minute, most of us can think about four times that speed. With all that extra think time, the ineffective listener lets his mind wander. His brain takes excursions to review the events of yesterday, or plan tomorrow, or solve a business problem...or sleep."[8] You have to work to control your mind and make it concentrate on what is being said. If you are troubled by an impending malpractice suit, a divorce, or a child who is having problems, your capacity to listen will diminish drastically. You will need to be patient with yourself in those circumstances and perhaps say to the person speaking, "I am a bit distracted. Can you tell me that again."

If you decide you are willing to expend the energy to listen, here are some techniques that will help you listen so people will want to talk to you:

- Be quiet. You cannot be listening if you are talking or you are thinking hard about what you are going to say next. If you get very anxious about not knowing what to say when they finish, try putting all your energy into listening and then tell them, "I need to think about this. Can I get back with you in a while to talk more?"

- Use your body to let the person know you are there. Look at him or her. Don't let your eyes wander all over the room. Sit attentively but not tensely, not slouching or lying down. On the sofa watching television or reading the paper are not good positions for listening. Neither is opening your mail in your office while someone tries to tell you something.

- Give an occasional "uh huh" or nod to let people know you are following their train of thought. If you are not, ask them a question before you let them go on for too long, and you are really lost.

- Ask nonjudgmental questions. "Can you say a little more? I'm not sure I understand. Will you try me again?" Don't ask, "Why on earth did you do that?" There is absolutely no decent answer to that question, and the person doing the asking is implying, "You are an idiot!" You may be right, but if you want communication to continue, you will have to discipline yourself not to say everything you think.

- Restate some of what the person has said. "Let me see if I understand. You think Dr. X is showing up for his emergency department shift with alcohol on his breath."

- Make a guess about a feeling you think the person is having if it seems appropriate. "I can see why that would make you sad." They may reply, "I'm not sad, I'm angry." It doesn't matter that you are wrong. They will correct you, and you have gotten to a deeper level of communication when you find out how someone feels about a subject. The person will feel a sense of relief and sometimes release when he or she identifies the feeling.

It is not easy to listen. We would all rather be the center of attention, doing all the talking. This is not a bad fact, just a fact. But if we do not learn to take turns, if we do not learn to listen, we will not have a chance of being heard. Also, "listening lets you shower someone with the exhilarating splash of affirmation. It makes a speaker feel wanted, acknowledged, heard. By appearing intent and interested in what's said, indicating that you understand, and asking follow-up questions, you let people know that you actually want them to speak. There is no better way to establish rapport and lay the groundwork for persuasion."[9]

Conflict

Many people would claim they do behave in ways that make interpersonal communication go more smoothly, but they also might admit that, when situations get hostile, they forget everything and often react in ways that they don't like. Confrontation is difficult. People usually deal with it in one of two ways. They verbally attack, using the energy of anger to spur them on, or they withdraw, say nothing, and often plot revenge.

Confronting someone in a calm, firm voice takes courage. I'd like to suggest a how-to process that may help you control yourself if you tend to explode and may help you get the nerve to confront if you tend to withdraw. I mentioned earlier that it is helpful to prepare for important conversations. That is especially true if you are in a heated situation. Try filling in the blanks in this short formula:

When you (do so and so),
I feel (or react in this way),
Because (I think something).
I'd like you to (do so and so).

Examples:

When you verbally attack me and defend your position when I ask you to do something, I get angry and I avoid telling you what you need to hear, because I think nothing will be accomplished and I dread your reaction. Next time, I'd like you to listen until I finish and think about it, and then we can discuss it.

When you come to me with every emergency department problem you have, I feel angry, because I can only deal with one dying person at a time.

I'd like you to make some of the decisions yourself. I trust your judgment.

Sometimes you take the process a step further and tell what the consequences will be if behavior is not changed.

When you leave your charts unreviewed for two weeks, the rest of the staff and I are frustrated (angry), because we can't properly take care of patients and get our work done. I want you to complete them in three days. If not, I'll alert the medical records committee.

Using the formula, continue to write to find out exactly what you want to say. When you actually speak to the person, the formula will take a slightly different form. The following is what I might actually tell the person concerning the first example:

Sometimes I need to ask you to change a behavior. When I do, you quickly defend your position and verbally attack me. As a result, I dread telling you something. I put it off, and yet I know you are going to suffer in your performance evaluation if you do not change. In the future, when I have something difficult to tell you, I'm going to say, "I have something difficult to tell you." I'd like you to listen until I finish and think about it, and then we can get together to discuss it.

When you get ready to talk to the person, you may not tell them exactly what you have written, but the formula can help you get clear about what aggravates you, what part you play in creating the problem, and what it is you want to happen. If you get angry, you can cuss and vent and scream on paper and then throw it away. When you spill those feelings on people, they are usually either so angry themselves or so frightened that they cannot hear what it is you want them to do. If you are the one who often withdraws from conflict, you can sometimes get the courage to speak up, because you have written out exactly what you plan to say. You don't have to have the notes with you. Your brain has thought them and seen them on paper so it will usually remember them. You can also practice saying the words out loud so that your brain will have also heard them.

Some things you discover when you are writing, you will not want to tell. For example, that you are frightened about something. To say that may make you seem too vulnerable. Someone might say, "She's not tough enough to do this job. Let's get rid of her." So you don't always tell what you feel, but it is very important for you to know what you feel. When you don't know, you can continue to act in unproductive ways (e.g., as an angry or frightened little boy or girl) and wonder why life and your job are not good. When you are aware of what you feel, you can move through it and feel something that is often better than the first impression. When you know, you can remind yourself that you are grown, that you have options, that this person does not have your very life in his or her hands.

If writing seems too disagreeable a task, try telling all of this to a friend before you talk to the one who has annoyed you, but don't leave it there. If the information never gets back to the person who caused you the trouble, there is no chance for the situation to improve.

When someone irritates us, we want to complain to a friend because it feels good to do so. We want to vent. I do not think this human behavior will stop, but if the listener could let the talker vent for awhile and then encourage him or her to prepare to talk to the offending person, office gossip would sometimes have a productive end rather than just fueling the "poor-me" fire.

Writing

In the area of communication, there will probably come a time when you have to write. What will make people want to read what you have written?

- Make it short. We may or may not be getting lazier, with shorter attention spans as some sources claim, but we are all definitely busy. Even the brightest executives want documents to be short, because they need to get through them in a hurry.

- Have enough areas on a page where there are no words. Do you remember when, in the seventh grade, you started to read that larger geography book with more words on a page? You struggled through two columns of heavy words and then turned the page to find a picture that took up half the page. Weren't you happy, relieved? When we grow up, we pretend that we get over that thrill, but we don't. None of us want to look at a page that is heavy and mostly black with words. If there are good top, bottom, and side margins, with spaces between paragraphs and perhaps a list in the middle with more white space around it, we are invited to read what is on the page rather than repelled by it.

- Avoid needless repetition. Do not repeat the same word many times. The reader begins to hear the singsong repetition of the word rather than your message. It is fine to repeat the same word when you are first generating your thoughts, but you need to cut them later.

  Writing needs to be a two-part process. First, you come up with ideas without criticizing them at all. If you judge every word as you go, the creative part of you will get tired and will stop sending messages. Just write down or dictate the words as they come to you. Become very critical when you edit. Circle all the repeated words and try to eliminate most of them, unless you are repeating the word to emphasize its importance or changing the word would confuse the reader.

- Don't be verbose. Don't write the same idea a second time using different words: end result, final conclusion, personal opinion, unexpected surprise. Always use fewer words rather than more. "In the event that" can simply be "if." "In view of the fact that" can be "Because." Elbow says, "Every word omitted keeps another reader with you."[10] It is especially important for physicians to use simple words and phrases whenever they can because so often they must use the long technical words of their profession. Too many words of three syllables or more make for heavy reading. Resist using complicated medical terminology unless you are communicating with your medical colleagues.

- Use nonsexist language. Avoid words that imply only a man or a woman could do the job. Instead of businessman, write business executive, manager, or business person. Instead of chairman say chair or chairperson. When writing to a woman, use the title "Ms." unless you know she would prefer "Mrs." or "Miss." "Mr." indicates the person you are addressing is a man but explains nothing about his marital status. "Ms." does the same for a woman. Instead of using the masculine pronoun (he, his, him) when referring to a group that includes both men and women, make the subject of the sentence plural and thus neutral. Ex. Employees must submit their travel expenses by Monday. Sometimes you will have to use the singular pronoun. When you do, write "he or she" or "he/she." Too many of these expressions will sound awkward, but it is no longer acceptable to use just "he."

- Always choose precise words over vague words. Instead of "nice house" say "brick house." Instead of "circumstance" put "Hurricane Floyd." Use strong verbs rather than ones hidden in many words. "Decide" is stronger than "make a decision." "Buy" is better than "make a purchase." "Help" is clearer than "give assistance."

- Don't use jargon unless you are absolutely sure the listener understands it. Jargon, in its broadest definition, is any language that is hard to understand. Sometimes it acts as a shield for those who don't have much to say. It can be specialized vocabulary that a particular group of people understand. Teenagers find a different set of words every two or three years that, they hope, will confuse their parents. Accountants, chemists, bankers, doctors, and others have special terms that must be defined when they are working with the general public. Abbreviations that the listener does not understand are jargon. It's the writer's job to find out what the reader knows and doesn't know. When it comes to abbreviations, if you are in doubt, write it out.

    Often jargon is phony, inflated, and uselessly complex language. A client told me once, "If I speak and write so others understand me, they will steal my job." The opposite is more often true—jargon interferes with communication and could cause you to lose your job. People get angry if you use difficult words without explaining their meaning. They put your memos in the trash and do not do what you have asked them to do.

- Avoid trite phrases. Overworked expressions make a reader switch from paying attention to your message to being irritated that you are saying the same old thing. "The bottom line," "the whole nine yards," and "I need your input" are phrases that need a few year's rest. If you can finish the following statements, they have probably been overused.

    Enclosed
    We're sorry for any
    It has come to our
    Please call at your earliest
    If you have additional questions, feel

Try substituting new words. Examples for the first and second phrases might be, "Here is the information you asked for in your letter of June 5," and "Thanks for your patience with this delay.[11]

- Tone or manner of expression is as evident in the written word as it is in the spoken word. Business correspondence used to have a stuffy, legalistic tone. Now companies like a conversational, friendly tone that sounds as if a person, not a machine, wrote the letter. Pretend the reader is standing beside you. If you wouldn't say "per your request" to his or her face, don't write it in the letter.

Use a positive tone whenever possible. "Saying that someone is 'interested in details' conveys a more positive tone than saying the individual is a 'nitpicker.' The word economical is more positive than stingy or cheap."[12]

Electronic Mail and Voice Mail

E-mail is a quick and efficient way to communicate with people, and, in many offices, thankfully, it has completely replaced the inner-office memo. You can be more informal than we used to advise on hard-copy memos, but don't get so routinely lax that people make judgments about your ability to spell and use proper grammar. A few mistakes here and there are acceptable but if all your messages are riddled with them, people will draw negative conclusions about your intelligence and competence. Do not use all capital letters just because it is easier than dealing with the shift key. All caps are equivalent to yelling at someone, and they are very tiring to read. Do not criticize or correct people on e-mail—do it in a one-on-one conversation. Never type in e-mail or even in your office word processing program anything that you would not want everyone to read. You could accidentally hit the wrong button and send the message to everyone on the mail system, and people who have even a minimal knowledge of computers can go in your files and read what you have there. Some have told me that computer experts can get to files you have deleted if they choose to.

I've given you several do's and don't's, but what if you hate the whole writing process. Is there anything that would make you dread it less? The answer is writing more, but in a different way. Write 10 minutes a day, five days a week, on any subject that pops into your head. Use a kind of paper and pen that you like or type it on a word processor if that's easier for you. (Whatever paper or instrument you decide to write on I'll now refer to as your journal). Don't worry about spelling, punctuation, grammar, or anything that some English teacher told you to worry about. There is just one catch—you must start writing and not stop until the time is up. If you can't think of anything to write, just write, "I can't think of anything. I can't think of anything. This is one of the dumbest things I've ever done," but keep writing. Ideas will pop into your head if you keep writing that simply will not occur to you if you just sit and think.

If you were going to run in a 10-kilometer race on the weekend, you would need to do some daily running to get ready. The same is true for writing. You need to grease the machinery of your hand and brain to make them readily give you words when you need to write something.

This writing exercise will not only make the writing process easier but also can enhance your verbal communication skills and benefit you in other ways. It can help you organize your day. You probably already make a "to do" list. Expand it. Gripe—"month end report for Mr. Jones. I hate the way he makes red marks and gives it back to me to do again just to show he has the power to do that. Performance appraisal for Dr. Thomas. QA meeting—they go on and on without making a decision." You will think of the items to do much quicker if you write comments about them as you go. When you finish the journal entry, circle the tasks that came up that need to be done that day and assign them numbers in order of importance.

Writing in a journal can help you get rid of frustration. Anger is a physical phenomenon. You feel it somewhere in your body—knotted stomach, clinched fist, stiff neck. You cannot always avoid getting angry, but you need to get it out of your system for good health, and you don't want to dump it on the wrong person. You can dump it in your journal. Peter Elbow says, "Garbage in your head will poison you. Garbage on paper can safely be put in the waste paper basket."[13]

Writing quickly without stopping taps your right brain creativity. Most of us judge our ideas quickly. As soon as they pop into our heads, we think, "That will never work. Someone will think that is stupid." If you continue to write, the censor who seems to sit on your shoulder is thwarted and cannot continue to judge every thought. Thus, the right brain will keep sending you fresh thoughts because you are receiving them and showing respect by writing them down. Some of the ideas will be useful, but not all. You have to get a fair number of ideas out to have a few that are good.

While writing, you can find creative solutions to relationship problems. If you and your boss or spouse or child disagree over the same topic repeatedly, write out the scene in your journal. Often you wish you had said something differently or had not cried or had not lost your temper. Write the scene the way you wish it had happened. Next time you'll be amazed at how the interaction is similar to what you wrote, because you stayed calm in your half of the conversation.

If you decide to write in a journal, keep it hidden or tear up any incriminating evidence. Writing will take you places you didn't know you were going to go. If you momentarily hate your boss, it is helpful to write about it but harmful if anyone sees it. You do not have to keep what you write in order to benefit from having written it.

If you've recognized a communication skill you would like to improve, what activities will help you change?

- Practice on a friend.

- Practice in front of a video camera.

- Write about it in your journal.

- Put little reminder notes to yourself where no one else can see them—in your desk drawer or the medicine cabinet. Examples: I will let others have a chance to talk. I am a good listener. I am a strong energetic speaker.

- Relax and talk to yourself. The brain is much like a computer. It can be programmed and reprogrammed. If you don't like what you are doing, start to talk to yourself about a positive change. Learn some kind of relaxation or meditation technique. Do the exercise every day for three weeks. Each time you finish doing the exercise, say a positive statement to yourself about some desired change. Examples: I can control my temper. I can speak up when I choose to. The subconscious is more receptive when your body is relaxed. After several weeks, you'll be aware that you are interacting with people differently. Changing the way you communicate is not easy. It requires practicing new behavior that will feel awkward for a while, but the effort's worth it. "Nothing is more essential to success in any area of your life than the ability to communicate well. Nothing can compare to the joy of communicating love, of being heard and understood completely, of discovering some profound insight from another's mind, or of transmitting your own thoughts to a rapt audience."[14]

References

1. Stettner, M. *The Art of Winning Conversation.* Englewood Cliffs, N.J.: Prentice Hall, 1995, p. 82.

2. Sanford, J. *Between People, Communicating One-to-One.* New York, N.Y.: Paulist Press, 1982, p. 37.

3. Malandro, L., and Barker, L. *Nonverbal Communication.* Reading, Mass.: Addison-Wesley Publishing Co., 1983, p. 278.

4. Alexander, J. *Dare to Change.* New York, N.Y.: New American Library, 1984, p. 138.

5. Swets, P. *The Art of Talking So That People Will Listen.* Englewood Cliffs, N.J.: Prentice-Hall, Inc., 1983, p. 59.

6. *Ibid.,* p. 40.

7. Carr, J. *Communicating and Relating.* Menlo Park, Calif.: Benjamin/Cummings Publishing Co., Inc., 1979, p. 152.

8. Swets, P., *op. cit.,* p. 42.

9. Elbow, P. *Writing Without Teachers.* London: Oxford University Press, 1973, p. 41.

10. Laura Brill and Associates. *How to Sharpen Your Business Writing Skills.* New York, N.Y.: American Management Association, 1985.

11. Kolin, P. *Successful Writing at Work.* Lexington, Mass.: D.C. Heath and Co., 1980, p.13.

12. Elbow, P., *op. cit.,* p. 8.

13. Swets, P., *op. cit.,* p. 4.

Works Consulted but not Cited

Goldberg, N. *Writing Down the Bones*. Boston, Mass.: Shambala, 1986.

Gordon, T. *P.E.T.* New York, N.Y.: Peter H. Wyden, Inc., 1973.

Horton, S. *Thinking Through Writing*. Baltimore, Md.: Johns Hopkins University Press, 1982.

Klauser, H. *Writing on Both Sides of the Brain: Breakthrough Techniques for People Who Write*. San Francisco, Calif.: Harper and Row, Publishers, 1986.

Maltz, M. *Psycho-Cybernetics*. Hollywood, Calif.: Wilshire Book Co., 1960.

Milo, F. *How to Get Your Point Across in 30 Seconds—or Less*. New York, N.Y.: Simon and Schuster, 1986.

James, M., and Jongeward, D. *Born to Win*. Philippines: Addison-Wesley Publishing Co., Inc., 1971.

Barbara J. Linney, MA, is Vice President of Career Development for the American College of Physician Executives, Tampa, Florida.

Chapter 7

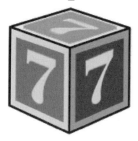

Negotiating Skills

by Howard E. Rotner, MD, FACPE

No individual in an organization is better suited to engage in negotiations involving physicians than the physician leader, whether new or of long standing And in the rapidly changing health care world, negotiations of one kind or another are certain to be an ongoing need. While relationships are vital to your success, one should discard the notion that being a good negotiator places relationships at risk. The concept of principled negotiation advanced in this chapter can enhance the power of the physician leader; create new, unimagined opportunities; and minimize the risk of disturbing relationships.

Negotiation skills rank among the highest priorities for the successful physician leader. It is safe to predict that not a day will go by when, as a physician leader, you won't encounter some negotiation, large or small. Regrettably, however, many new physician leaders are extremely wary of negotiations, perceiving that participation results in exposure to unnecessary and unwanted risk. You may perceive that relationships that you have worked hard to build and value highly might be threatened by the fear of rancor associated with negotiation.

Moreover, lacking significant experience in formal negotiations, you may imagine that you have no business "playing with the big boys." Perhaps, you think, physician negotiations should be conducted by other members of the management team, such as the CEO, the vice president for operations, or the vice president for medical affairs. The purpose of this chapter is to dispel these ideas and allow you to become comfortable in a skill that you cannot and should not avoid. It is a skill that has the potential to considerably elevate your stature and add immeasurably to your power. The alternative is to not engage in negotiations and proportionately diminish your power. If you see negotiations as opportunities to attain commitments never before imagined or proposed, you will enhance the fortunes of your organization many times over.

Opportunities for negotiation for the physician leader are legion. Requests for office space cannot all be accommodated. The part A contract for pathologists is being negotiated, and you know that they are being grossly overpaid, according to the standards of surrounding hospitals in the area. The paid director's position of the ambulatory surgicenter has just become available, and four surgeons approach you for the position. You are attempting to recruit a large internal medicine group to use your hospital's facilities, but they are resistant thus far. Your medical records delinquencies do not fulfill JCAHO standards, and your survey is coming up this year. Much of the physician leader's work is consumed by persuading other people to act in a way that meets the needs of the institution. Each of these efforts becomes, in one way or another, a negotiation. Your success is very much connected to how effective you are in the art of persuasion and in using negotiation skills.

Can Someone Else Do It Better?

All of us have been exposed to the necessity of negotiating on many levels throughout our lives. If you have been selected to be a physician leader in your organization, it is safe to assume that you have already achieved a record of success. Intuitively, you have negotiated on many levels, such as the purchase of your house, the salary and benefits of your job, numerous expectations and needs within your family, and agreements with your colleagues, to name just a few. On balance, it is safe to say that you have applied your knowledge, values, and convictions to arrive at fundamentally sound solutions. In your organization, there probably is no person who is more qualified to comprehend the interests of both parties, or who is more interested in a principled agreement, than you. The real question is not, "Can someone else do it better?" It is, "Who can possibly negotiate better than you?"

Am I Placing Myself at Undue Risk by Participating in Negotiations: The Concept of "Principled Negotiations"

Generally, the physician leader highly values relationships because they are the cornerstone of performance effectiveness. It has been pointed out by many observers that relationships play a major role in the conduct of negotiations. There is no question that one ordinarily negotiates much more forcefully when there is no current or future relationship between the two parties (for example, negotiating the purchase a car). However, the physician leader is very concerned about ongoing and future relationships in practically every negotiation. Nevertheless, that should not compromise your negotiating stance significantly if you utilize the concept of principled negotiation, as described by Ury and Fisher.[1] Principled negotiations include requirements that:

- A fair agreement be reached that meets the interests of both parties.

- The issues involved in the negotiations not be confused with the people who are negotiating.

- The outcomes meet standards that are generally established and accepted by most people.

There is a very useful criterion for evaluating any negotiated agreement: Will the outcome, should it be revealed to others, bear the scrutiny of your peers? Sisela Bok, in her book Lying: Moral Choice in Public and Private Life, strongly promotes the notion of scrutiny by peers when evaluating the quality of your agreement.[2] Physician executives should make an absolute commitment to telling the truth when engaging in negotiations, although you need not disclose information that might place you at a disadvantage. One must assess carefully the difference between withholding information, at the risk of being deceptive, and disclosing information that would weaken your negotiating posture. Because most negotiations conducted by physician leaders are part of a series, it is essential that you establish yourself as an individual who tells the truth and who does not withhold information that should legitimately be disclosed.

If these rules are closely followed, there is little likelihood that relationships will suffer. In fact, relationships will likely prosper, because you will be perceived as a principled, fair individual who is able to find resolutions that have eluded others.

Know Thyself

Just as a psychiatrist must intimately understand his own biases when conducting analysis, so must physician leaders intimately understand themselves. What is your most comfortable behavior? Are you hard-driving and competitive, or are you accommodating and primarily concerned with achieving good will? Are you bold and imaginative, or are you more comfortable with facts and figures, prone to careful analysis and favoring outcomes for which there is previous precedent? Do you try to persuade by using logic and rationale, or do you tend to be more assertive, to dominate and have a need "to win?" Perhaps you are idealistic and persuade by "inspiring" people to your point of view. Do you actively try to understand the other person's perspective, as reflected by engaging in questions such as "Do I understand you to say?" or "Could I restate your argument as follows?" In other words, are you a good listener? If not, you had better learn!

What does your body language say? Does it portray doubt and resistance, or does it encourage open-mindedness? Is it overbearing or intimidating? Do you convey arrogance or condescension? Does it reflect sincere interest and concern? Your body language can be just as communicative as your verbal language in determining the outcome of a negotiation.

If you understand your biases, your behavior, and your body language, you are more likely to make the necessary adjustments in order to reach the desired outcome. Differences in language and style, as insightfully described by Tannen, are based on gender, ethnic background, and social and economic class.[3] These differences frequently cause misunderstanding and a failure to communicate effectively.

Finally, choose your words carefully. Try to avoid words that have a pejorative or judgmental connotation. My involvement recently in an ethical consultation concerning the withdrawal of life support dramatically illustrated to me how individuals focus on a particular word. The son of the patient repeatedly focused on the use of the word "cruel." This word was used by the attending physician when discussing the futility of continuing to provide care to the mother, who was hopelessly and terminally ill. The son reacted defensively and resisted strongly any intimation that continuing to provide life support for his mother was "cruel." While I fully agreed with the attending physician's objective assessment, the choice of words in this case was detrimental to persuading the son to agree to withdraw life support for his terminally ill mother.

Another example is a mistake I made recently. In attempting to persuade radiologists at our hospital not to designate their contribution to the physicians' fund-raising campaign for radiology projects, I described the action as "self-serving" when viewed by others. The radiologists reacted negatively to this "accusation," focusing especially on the word "self-serving." I was not successful in my effort.

Know Thy Opponent

You should make every attempt to understand the individual with whom you are negotiating. Consider your opponent's biases, behavior, body language, and background in the same manner that you have tried to understand your own. What are that person's values? Are they economic, or do they reflect values of social justice? Is the person most interested in power, or do ethical issues have a higher priority? Are intellectual attainments, such as research or publications, driving the individual with whom you are negotiating? Values are primarily what motivate people to do the things they do, and your conceptual understanding of values is essential to understanding the art and science of negotiation. We tend to think of negotiations as being dominated by economic values, but other values often have a higher priority from the viewpoint of the person with whom you are negotiating. Not only should you understand your opposite's values, but you also need to get them on the table. What better way to find out than to ask openly, "What is really important to you?"

Information is critical. Every time you have information on what your opponent might want, you have more "currency" with which to negotiate. That is, you have discovered other "interests" that might be brought to the table and be offered as part of a negotiated agreement. A tug of war over financial positions, for example, can be resolved by providing other opportunities that are not financial but are, nevertheless, highly valued by your opposite. Such opportunities might include additional access, recognition by title, control of resources, etc. The admonition of Charles Dwyer is helpful to remember.[4] "Never expect anyone to engage in behavior that meets your needs unless you give them adequate reason to do so," i.e., behavior that they perceive as being in their best interests. Adequate reason can only be offered by thorough understanding of the issues, interests, values, and needs of the individual with whom you are negotiating.

The Plan

It is most helpful to have a plan when you enter a negotiation. Such a plan is really no different than the system or the outline that most physicians follow when obtaining a history. Many effective negotiators follow the concepts described by Ury and Fisher.[1]

Understand the issues as thoroughly as possible, and separate the issues from the people involved in the negotiation. The quickest way for a negotiation "to go South" is for the negotiators to attack the people involved rather than to concentrate on the issues attendant to the negotiation. Past history has to be discreetly put aside. Accusations attributed to motive, character, or past behavior will create friction and make a negotiation very difficult or, most likely, impossible. A thorough understanding and discussion of the issues will frequently reveal information that can be used later in the negotiation to achieve agreement. Moreover, the proper atmosphere for the negotiation is established as points of view are expressed and a good deal of listening is established. It is in this part of the negotiation that listening skills reflecting attention, questioning, understanding, and empathy are critical.

Discuss interests and not positions. How many times have you been involved in a disagreement and your adversary says, "My position is...." Consider that opening gambit. Does it not promote a certain obstinacy and rigidity? Frequently, the opening is followed by a long-winded rationalization and justification of the position. It is very difficult to have an effective meeting of the minds when this strategy is used. It places on the listener the obligation to state his or her "position" in equally strong terms and with equal justification. When a negotiation follows this path, the lines of battle are drawn, and the negotiators are usually far apart. Inordinate time is expended to bring the negotiating parties together.

Ury and Fisher suggest that negotiators concentrate on interests rather than on positions. Consider the following example of a recent negotiation conducted with our internists and cardiologists concerning the interpretation of ECGs on Medicare patients in the hospital. Recently, HCFA determined that it would not compensate physicians for professional interpretation of these ECGs. The interests of the cardiologists and internists were that they be reimbursed for the performance of a legitimate service at a reasonable amount. They also had an interest in not having the ECG interpretation put out to bid, either to a service outside the hospital or to a small group from within. The hospital's interests were that the ECGs continue to be interpreted by qualified individuals (a quality and safety interest), that it spend as little as possible (an economic interest of high priority because this represents incremental nonreimbursed expense for the hospital), and that it preserve its relationship with the internists and cardiologists (critically important for a hospital tightly engaged in competition). The expression of these interests by both parties to the negotiation resulted in a favorable agreement.

Imagine how different the results would have been if the internists and cardiologists had opened the negotiation with a statement of their "position": that the hospital should pay them x dollars to interpret ECGs on Medicare patients. Most likely, the hospital would have responded with a lower amount and a tug of war and bilateral threats would have begun. When there was clarification and understanding of mutual interests, agreement was much easier to achieve and both parties felt more fulfilled by the outcome.

The example above demonstrates that statement of positions frequently pre-empts discussion of interests. It places the outcome of the negotiation ahead of the discussion that should lead to the outcome. The importance of this discussion is not only to expose the interests of the negotiating parties, but also to provide the essential ingredient of participation in the process. Experienced negotiators will often tell you that the outcome of their negotiations was not very different from what they wanted prior to entering negotiations. Imagine how a participant would receive a resolution if appropriate discussion and participation had not occurred. A goal of principled negotiation is to get "buy in" of the agreement, and this can only be achieved through a participative process.

In summary, statement of positions draws lines of battle. Statement of interests opens doors for understanding and a sense of ownership of the agreement.

Consider alternative options. It is this stage of the negotiating process that often opens previously "locked doors." It is here that an imaginative and creative negotiator can be invaluable. Creative solutions are arrived at only when negotiators thoroughly understand the values and the interests of the parties to the negotiation. Ury and Fisher[1] have described a useful list of needs that are common to most people:

- Security.

- Economic well-being.

- A sense of belonging.

- Recognition.

- Control of one's life or domain.

Why is it important to understand needs, and how do they open your imagination to alternative options for agreement? Superficially, many disputes confronting the physician leader appear to be economic in nature. For example, on behalf of the president of the medical staff, the Medical Executive Committee requests from administration an increase in salary from $15,000 to $30,000. The fact that the president is spending precious time on hospital affairs and could otherwise be earning money in his office is given as the ostensible reason. Consider the possible other options, using the concept of needs. Would recognition by the administration or the board of trustees be valuable in lieu of increased salary? Would a vote on the board of trustees give the medical staff a greater sense of participation and control of the decision-making process? Would a longer term in office be valuable to the president? Would more staff support that would enable the president to be more efficient be a substitute for more salary? From administration's point of view, is this an opportunity to extract from the president more scheduled time with which to meet with the CEO or board committees? Would greater salary achieve more commitment from the president's partners to utilize the hospital rather than split patients with its competitor? Do the staff physicians achieve a greater sense of belonging because the president is being treated more respectfully? You may agree or disagree with any of these concepts as having relevance, but if you don't think about them or create others, you will continue to have tunnel vision regarding helpful options and alternatives.

To illustrate needs even more vividly, consider a dispute that the author witnessed between a radiology group and a group practice. The two parties were negotiating the salary for the radiologists who performed x-ray interpretations for films taken at the group practice location. On the surface, it appeared that the dispute was simply over money. However, it became obvious to me that, from the radiologists' perspective, the dispute had at least as much to do with recognition, belonging, and control as it did with financial remuneration. Repeatedly, the radiology negotiator complained that communication to him was conducted through a staff manager rather than a physician. The radiologists did not have input into ordering or purchasing of equipment. They had no control over the transcription of reports and, because they were not allowed to have a key to the building, they frequently could not access the radiology suite to perform readings early in the morning or after the office had closed in the evening. Moreover, the radiologists much preferred to do their own professional billing rather than be salaried employees of the group practice. Had these issues of professional control been addressed, most certainly the outcome of the negotiation would not have been as protracted or nearly so bitter. Moreover, one can easily see that a number of different options and alternatives could have been introduced to the negotiation proceedings that would have considerably ameliorated the dispute over money and met the interests of both parties to the negotiation.

When considering options, it is essential to open your mind and not prejudge what initially appear to be hopeless and useless suggestions. It is a time for brainstorming and not critiquing. In fact, essential to the brainstorming process is that ideas are thrown on the table and not judged until later. Ury and Fisher use a circular chart[1] that emphasizes the description of the problem, the causes and symptoms of the problem, possible solutions that can be applied to fix the problem, and actions that can be taken to address the solution. In medical terms, this is analogous to the chief complaint and history, the physical exam, the diagnosis, and the treatment. Just as there frequently are many options and alternatives to treating a medical problem, there are numerous options and alternatives that can be applied to resolve disputes.

Apply reasonable standards to the negotiated agreement. I have observed that, when a negotiated agreement reflects reasonable standards and objective criteria, it is generally a good one and is not likely to be broken. The agreement by the negotiators to apply such standards at the outset of negotiation immediately establishes the foundation for a principled agreement. If it appears early in negotiation that reasonable standards are not being requested by one of the parties, it becomes an effective strategy for the other party to indicate that he or she is going to insist upon reasonable standards and objective criteria.

Earlier in the chapter, it was mentioned that a principled agreement will bear the scrutiny of your peers. This is an effective litmus test for negotiated agreements and can be an internal standard frequently helpful as a guideline to your own flexibility in negotiations. While one would always attempt to maintain the confidentiality of agreements achieved through negotiation, one should also assume that information could become public. Agreements should never be a source of embarrassment to either party. As you negotiate, ask yourself, "How would this agreement be viewed by others should it become known?"

What kind of standards are appropriate to negotiated agreements in the context of health care? Agreements should be ethical. They should be legal. They should be within the norms of the industry and meet marketplace criteria. They should not establish precedents that you don't wish to repeat with others. They should be sensible in that they reflect legitimate pay for legitimate work. In summary, they should be fair and reflect common sense.

What If You Cannot Reach Agreement?

Sometimes, despite your best efforts, you are not successful in achieving agreement. It is critical not to make a bad deal simply in the interests of resolution. A bad deal will always come home to haunt you sooner or later. If it doesn't haunt you, it is likely to haunt your successor!

Ury and Fisher have popularized the acronym BATNA, "best alternative to a negotiated agreement."[1] The purpose of establishing a BATNA is that it forces you to consider your options ahead of time should you not be able to achieve an agreement. This exercise is critical, because it gives you negotiating confidence and forces you to examine a "worse case" scenario. That examination may well result in consideration of options and alternatives not previously examined. Failure to create a BATNA causes you to negotiate from weakness. You might make agreements that will not serve your best interests, and such agreements usually cause tremendous resentment at a later time. A BATNA differs from a "bottom line," which sets limits but doesn't examine alternatives and options. To illustrate, let us consider the ECG negotiation referred to earlier in the chapter. The hospital could have established its BATNA as follows: If we cannot reach agreement at a reasonable level of reimbursement to the ECG readers, what will we do? Possible alternatives, each with advantages and disadvantages, are to do nothing and allow each physician to interpret his or her own ECGs, have physicians obtain consultation to interpret ECGs, have the ECGs read by a computer and pay a cardiologist to "overread," put out for competitive bid ECG interpretation among groups within the hospital, or have an outside service read at a very low fee. One can see that, simply by considering a BATNA, a whole host of alternative options are raised. Just considering these solutions allows you to internally evaluate the solution that you reach. One should be very suspicious of any agreement that is not as attractive as options created by reviewing your BATNA.

As in poker, you must know "when to hold and when to fold." When you fold in poker, you are out of that hand. However, you are not out of the game, and the next hand offers you new opportunities. Herb Cohen, author of You Can

Negotiate Anything, puts it another way: "I care...but not that much."[5] If you "care too much" in a negotiation, the result will be the same as staying in a poker game with a poor hand.

If you cannot reach agreement in a negotiation, it is often useful to arrange for a third party to mediate. While one can formally request that an outside mediator be engaged, in health care organizations the third-party mediator is frequently an individual who also has an interest in having the negotiation succeed. One can easily imagine that, in a dispute between two physicians, it is in the hospital's best interests to reach satisfactory resolution. In the example of the dispute between the medical group and the radiologists, it was clearly in the hospital's best interests to have the dispute favorably resolved. Indeed, when asked to assist in the resolution, the hospital was able to bring options to the table not previously available to the two negotiating parties. These options served the interests of all three parties.

Finally, consider the time-worn physician's axiom of "tincture of time." Frequently, a negotiation is not successfully concluded because the timing is not right. Generally, it is not advisable to force conclusion of a negotiation because of time pressures. This is especially true when the time pressures are imposed by the other negotiating party. It is critical to evaluate the advantages and the disadvantages of delay against those of quick closure. For example, consider your decision to buy a house. Are you getting the best price now, or will prices go down over the next few months? Will the house still be available if you wait? What alternatives will be available if waiting causes you to lose this house? Will mortgage rates rise or fall in the near future? Is this the house that you really want, or are you willing to consider other locations, styles, sizes, price ranges, distance from work, etc? With the passage of time, change occurs. Evaluate the consequences of change carefully when negotiating.

Summary

While relationships are vital to your success, one should discard the notion that being a good negotiator places relationships at risk. The concept of principled negotiation enhances the power of the physician leader; creates new, unimagined opportunities; and minimizes the risk of disturbing relationships. Moreover, no individual in the organization is better suited to engage in negotiations involving physicians than the physician leader.

It is very important for you to understand yourself in terms of your behavior, your language, and your body language. What messages are you sending, consciously or unconsciously? It is equally important that you understand your counterpart and "read between the lines." What is he or she really saying? Values that motivate people and common needs that require satisfaction have to be addressed in the context of understanding alternative viewpoints and facilitating new options for agreement.

The concepts of principled negotiation are straightforward: separate the people from the issues, discuss interests and not positions, examine many alternatives and options, and reach agreements that reflect acceptable standards and criteria. In addition, any agreement must pass the test of "scrutiny by your peers." Principles of truth-telling and fairness are fundamental to favorable, durable agreements. A systematized approach, using a negotiating plan, is recommended when entering a negotiation.

Finally, if all avenues are exhausted and agreement cannot be achieved, the strategy of the BATNA (best alternative to a negotiated agreement) is recommended. Advantages of bringing in a third party to the negotiation should be evaluated, as well as the options of mediation or arbitration. Resorting to legal action generally reflects a failure of the negotiation process.

References

1. Ury, W., and Fisher, R. *Getting to Yes*. Boston, Mass.: Houghton-Mifflin, 1981.

2. Bok, S. *Lying: Moral Choice in Public and Private Life*. New York, N.Y.: Random House, 1979.

3. Tannen, D. *You Just Don't Understand*. New York, N.Y.: William Morrow & Company, 1990.

4. Dwyer, C. *The Shifting Sources of Power and Influence*. Tampa, Fla.: American College of Physician Executives, 1992.

5. Cohen, H. *You Can Negotiate Anything*. New York, N.Y.: Bantam Books, 1982.

Howard E. Rotner, MD, FACPE, was formerly Vice President for Medical Affairs at AtlantiCare Medical Center, Lynn, Massachusetts. He is now engaged in the private practice of endocrinology.

Chapter

Conflict Management

by James M. Richardson, MD, FACP, FACPE

Communication is the essential ingredient that allows people to relate to one another. It is essential on both personal and business levels. When effective communications fails, one of the things that often occurs is conflict. The conflict may be a simple disagreement in regard to ideas, issues, or interests, or it may be more complex, extreme, and destructive. The latter case of communication failure is called dysfunctional conflict. It is never desirable or necessary. It is always bad, even at its best. Managers cannot afford to have dysfunctional conflict in their organizations, but unless they manage conflict by being effective communicators, recognizing situations that will convert simple conflict into more complex conflict, dysfunctional conflict will be inevitable.

Simple Conflict

Conflict is a naturally occurring phenomenon. It is to be expected in individual or group situations. Conflict resolution is a common and time-consuming process. Being able to effectively deal with conflict episodes depends on how well the manager understands the dynamics and how well he or she can identify the features on which intervention can occur.

Effective conflict management requires skills that have to be learned. The skills required are in oral, written, and nonverbal communications; in preventing, recognizing, and removing barriers to communication; and in active listening and feedback.

Conflict is a subjective phenomenon. Depending on how it is perceived in the minds of the individuals involved, it becomes objective only in the sense that its manifestations are real, through the acting out, the anger, the attacks, etc. Because conflict is subjective, it is emotional. One can, therefore, understand how, during conflict episodes, basic communication is impaired, reasoning and perceptions are distorted, attacks become personal, and the overall situation tends to deteriorate.

It is easy to automatically consider conflict to be negative. When this occurs, the consequences are predictably adverse. If conflict is viewed as being a positive force, a completely different outcome is possible. With this latter view of conflict, a process can be initiated that can result in full identification of problems, understanding of the points of view of others, evaluation of alternatives, stimulation of interest, involvement of people in such a way that they will become committed, and willingness to devote the energy necessary for implementation of a successful project. In other words, the positive consequences of conflict can include the evolution of new or modified goals, closer interpersonal relationships, effective problem solving, and results that are far superior to those originally envisioned.

Dysfunctional Conflict

Dysfunctional conflict is a negative force. It occurs at a high price. Not only do emotions run high, but anger and hostility are exhibited; the primary problem or issue becomes subverted; stress is created; efficiency, effectiveness, and productivity are lowered; there is damage to interpersonal relationships, with respect and trust being lost, at least for the short term; and time, energy, and money are wasted.

In order for conflict to occur and develop, there must be an underlying cause or condition of which both parties are aware. The involved parties respond to the condition with feelings of tension, irritation, actions, and counteractions. Finally, the end defines the type of result that comes from the conflict episode. Was it satisfactorily or unsatisfactorily settled? Were the issues in the conflict resolved? If not resolved, the conflict episode is sure to recur.

Causes of Conflict

There are six major causes of conflict in organizations:

- **Basic failure in communication, including a misconception of information**—Just as effective communication can affect the organization's efficiency and effectiveness and the quality of its products or services, a failure to communicate effectively can cause organizational conflict.

- **The threat of change**—Because everything is in a state of change, change is inevitable, and no change is final. Change involves the future, and the future is unknown. We fear the unknown. When the unknown involves us personally and adversely, we feel insecure. This insecurity provokes in us a negative action that is manifested in an emotional way. This action further provokes a spiraling series of counteractions. Each person responds differently to the stresses caused by change, making for different outcomes, which are unpredictable.

  The results of change have differing impacts, depending on whether external or internal forces affect the organization. External forces often are in the form of constraints. They may include changes in laws, regulations, funding, competition, etc. They can affect the individual, but they are more likely to have a direct impact on the organization and its resources.

Internal forces are more likely to affect the power structure or organizational arrangement. Issues of authority, power, control, position, economics, and security come into play.

In an organization, change can best be dealt with in a systematic fashion. At the time of an anticipated significant change, there needs to be a determination of the scope of the problems that will develop as a result of the change. This cannot or usually should not be done by the manager alone. Neither should the development, analysis, and selection of alternatives or the implementation and evaluation of the change be the responsibilities of the manager alone. With the participative style of management, the goal is to have appropriate staff involvement. With commitment, there is acceptance of decisions made, and, with acceptance, there is the required energy and time necessary to make it possible for decisions to be successfully implemented. These are advantages over the autocratic style of management, which institutes change independently by oral or written communication.

- **Competition for limited resources**—Resources are always limited. In most organizations, critical limitations of resource allocation are a frequent reason for competition among individuals, groups, or departments and are a source of conflict. The resource may be money, space, equipment, etc.

- **Differences regarding organizational goals**—Such differences are a frequent cause of organizational conflict. The differences occur in spite of the fact that it is clear to most employees that top management or the board of directors determines the mission of the organization and sets the organization's policies and goals. It is the responsibility of middle management, through strategic planning and with top management's approval, to establish department goals and objectives by which organizational goals can be achieved. It is lower level management's responsibility to develop procedures to achieve day-to-day goals and objectives that will produce products or services. In spite of the best efforts, differences occur in the perception of the overall goals, priorities, methods, resource utilization, etc. When these ideas are the same, there is no conflict.

- **Ambiguities in organizational structure**—The structure of the organization may be poor, allowing for overlapping responsibilities, gaps in responsibilities, and inconsistent and conflicting policies.

- **Differences regarding performance standards and expectations**—Although performance standards and expectations initially affect individuals and can cause conflicts, they eventually affect the entire organization and the products or services that are to be delivered.

Avoiding Conflict

Before delineating specific ways to avoid conflict in organizations, two characteristics of vital importance must be discussed. They are frequently underemphasized and involve shared values and having trust in the persons or groups with whom you are dealing.

Organizational Values

Just as values and value systems are important to individuals, they are also important to organizations. Values represent the desirability or worth of a thing; they are a moral precept. The organization's value system not only influences its ethical standards, but also is the foundation for its code of ethics. It influences staff behavior. The value system determines how hard and how long a person will fight for something. Values are very hard to change. When our values are threatened, our integrity is threatened. But values are just an abstraction until choices have to be made. Hard decisions are value judgments. The quality of an organization's value system is seen in the types of hard decisions it makes. An organization's budget also is representative of its values.

Because personal and organizational values are so basic, if one party knows the other party's values, the behavior and the decisions of the other party can be, to some degree, predicted. In decision making, the individual or organization should determine the value of a significant point at issue and then make the decision. This is value-based decision making. It can make decision making easier, especially if there is no incongruence between values and the actions taken. And, as expected, core values make up the organization's mission statement. It is differences in values that are often the sources of conflict.

Trust

Good interpersonal relationships are essential to any effective communications process, and fundamental to good interpersonal relationships is the need for trust between individuals and groups. Trust is a feeling of being safe, confident, accepted, respected, reliant, consistent, and devoid of fear, even in the presence of disagreement. Trust is a subjective feeling. Being trustworthy is based on a summation of things—what we say, how we say it, what we do, how we do it, honesty, integrity, our behavior, actions, responses, sensitivity, empathy, etc. We cannot set as an objective the creation of a sense of trustworthiness. Being trustworthy comes from an inner quality and strength, namely, good ethical and moral character, the absence of which cannot be covered up for long.

Personal Issues

Also of great importance in avoiding conflict is to keep issues nonpersonalized, which means to avoid focusing on principles, morals, religious beliefs, or ethical issues. Once any one of these four issues is raised, it usually becomes a win/lose situation. We naturally tend to defend our self-image and issues of principle, morals, religion, and ethics uncompromisingly. "Losing face" or sacrificing integrity is at stake. An impasse in conflict resolution usually results. Sometimes the only way to get beyond this impasse is for both parties to agree to disagree.

Other Ways to Avoid Conflict

Other ways to avoid conflict in management are:

* Remain calm.

- Disarm the other party by not responding as he or she does.

- Disclose something that will be interpreted as a positive move.

- Avoid statements that begin with "you."

- Avoid accusations such as "you always" or "you never."

- Avoid the "no" word.

- Avoid judgmental statements such as "Why did you do that?"

- Avoid insults to the other party's ego.

- Avoid words or actions that will escalate the conflict episode.

Beginning Conflict Resolution

The purpose of the process of conflict resolution is to:

- Present thoughtful alternatives so that conflict will be converted into collaboration.

- Validate the values of the other party.

- Appear fair.

- Accept some responsibility.

- Promote a spirit of understanding and cooperation.

- Look for opportunities to improve interpersonal relationships.

Perceived Differences

If there is a significant perceived difference in strength, authority, or technical advantage in either party's favor, the resolution process is likely to be more difficult. This situation can exist between manager and subordinate, manager and colleague, or management and union representatives. The difficulty may be that the stronger party may be more likely to want to impose a solution or that the weaker party, because of his or her situation, may have to accept a solution that is far from satisfactory.

Managers, by their very positions, have authority and power. How much authority and power depends on many factors. One's authority will depend on the job description, but, just as important, it depends on how the person in the position executes authority. The person may gain or give up authority that is inherent in the job.

Power can be considered the perception of others about how well someone can influence or effect change, about the person's ability to exercise control. Because authority and power are necessary for managers in their decision making, it is only a matter of time before managers generate conflict. This is because managerial decisions will eventually restrict the autonomy of some colleagues and subordinates. It is therefore essential for managers to use their abilities, authority, and power to the utmost in managing conflict in order to minimize the possibility that dysfunctional conflict will develop.

Unreadiness

The two parties involved in a conflict episode must perceive that a conflict exists, but, before they are ready to resolve the conflict, there is an escalation phase when resolution is impossible. This is the period when accusations, insults, hostility, and anger are prevalent. It is not until at least one of the parties wants to seek a resolution to the conflict that there can be attempts at successful conflict resolution.

Confrontation

In addition, there has to be confrontation during a conflict episode if there is to be conflict resolution. Otherwise compromise, postponement, or avoidance will usually occur. The word "confrontation," from one aspect, is similar to the word "conflict." It can and should be looked at in terms of possible positive consequences. Confrontation in regard to issues in conflict can and should result in an improved outcome. If the conflict worsens and dysfunctional conflict occurs, the process has failed.

Confrontation in conflict resolution usually involves six major steps, according to Newstrom and Davis.[1]

- **Awareness**—There is recognition by at least one person or group involved that a conflict exists, and they are willing to initiate the confrontation.

- **Confrontation is decided**—Both persons or groups decide that the issue is important enough not to be avoided and that confrontation will resolve the differences.

- **Confrontation occurs**—The response of the opposing persons or groups will determine if there is acceptance of the confrontation, denial, a reduction in the seriousness of the conflict, escalation, or resolution of the conflict.

- **Determination of the cause of the conflict**—At this step, if the issue is focused and the opposing parties share information and describe their opinions and feelings, the cause of the conflict can be determined.

- **Development of solutions**—Here, the opposing parties work toward eliminating or reducing the causes of the conflict.

- **Follow-up**—For long-term success of the solution, both parties must make regular checks to verify that agreements are being kept.

When this process has been successful, the positive aspects of conflict episodes are exemplified, because the two parties have worked together to solve problems.

Strategies in Conflict Resolution

If conflict is to be resolved satisfactorily, it must be approached and dealt with correctly. An unsatisfactory strategy will most likely result in an unsatisfactory outcome. The strategy can be goal-directed (what benefits both parties) or outcome-directed (who gets what). Filley's studies describe three forms of conflict strategies—win/lose, lose/lose, and win/win.[2] These are the same strategies recommended for formal and informal negotiations.

Possible Outcomes

The strategy selected will determine if the conflict episode will be:

- Positive or negative.

- Personalized or objective.

- Goals- or outcome-directed.

- Satisfactory or unsatisfactory.

- Resolved or unresolved.

- Finished or recurring.

Win/Lose

Individuals as well as departments within organizations often oppose one another in order to gain prestige, power, or resources or to show dominance. If the win/lose strategy is selected, one party will be the winner, the other the loser. The loser will likely be angry and hostile and will not be a fully committed and involved participant in the implementation of solutions. The winner is, therefore, not a true winner, because friendship and future cooperation by the other party may be lost. It is noteworthy that the practice of voting in these circumstances formalizes the win/lose strategy and should be avoided.

Lose/Lose

Just as the lose/lose strategy suggests, neither party wins, the conflict is not resolved, and a solution is not reached, even though each party may have gained something.

Win/Win

The win/win strategy to resolve conflict is most desirable. The solution is agreed upon and is satisfactory to both parties, even though neither party may have received all of what it initially sought. The parties commit to implementation of the solution and involve themselves with the energy necessary to achieve success.

The win/win strategy usually results in solutions by consensus or by integration. When this happens, alternatives have been thoroughly examined. True consensus is ideal, but it usually takes a long time, requires a lot of energy, and is difficult to achieve. The larger the opposing parties, the greater the difficulty. When consensus occurs, the focus is on problem solving, not the solution itself.

The Integrative Approach

When the integrative approach is used, goals and values, not solutions, are stressed. Filley describes several characteristics necessary for the integrative approach[2]:

- Clearly defined issues.

- A focus on goals and objectives.

- A genuine search for alternatives.

- A lack of time constraints.

- A truly interactive process.

- Sharing of information.

- Open-mindedness.

- Flexible leadership.

- Trust.

- Acceptance of solutions.

Third-Party Intervention

When a conflict episode has resulted in a win/lose confrontation, a third party may have to intercede through mediation or arbitration. Facts alone and attempts at persuasion are usually ineffective. In this situation, a change in attitude or position is necessary if there is to be movement toward resolution of the issues.

The mediator should be neutral, prestigious, trusted, and respected by both parties. He or she can provide the forum for new information to be shared; for the feelings of the opposite person or group to be known; for reasonable and constructive stances to be taken; and, ultimately, for there to be a change of attitude or position.

Mediation is preferable to arbitration, because arbitration is usually judgmental and often results in a win/lose or a lose/lose conclusion. Mediation provides the opportunity for true conflict resolution and a win/win conclusion.

Conflict Resolution in Large Groups

The process for conflict resolution in large groups can be quite different from dealing with a small number of individuals. The mediator usually meets independently and dually with representatives of each group and, according to Newstrom and Davis,[1] often functions in the following manner:

- **Prepares**—Before the opposing groups meet, the mediator prepares them for meeting one another, in part by encouraging an approach that is positive, open-minded, frank, and constructive.

- **Controls discussion**—The mediator controls the content and the pace of meetings and maintains the peace.

- **Permits role reversal**—Each side learns to understand the position of the opposition.

- **Defuses tension**—The mediator facilitates the expression of feelings, including anger and frustration, in a constructive manner.

- **Transmits information**—Information is given to each side to facilitate the communication process.

- **Formulates proposals**—At the appropriate time, the mediator suggests possible solutions.

Methods for Implementing Strategy

After a satisfactory conflict-reducing strategy is developed, implementation of the strategy is necessary. According to Blake et al., this step can involve five methods[3]:

- **Compromising**—This is a process of problem solving using mutual concession.

- **Confronting or Problem Solving**—Facing the problem head on, rather than avoiding it. The cause for conflict is identified and eliminated during this process.

- **Forcing**—This method uses physical, intellectual, ethical, and moral pressures.

- **Smoothing**—Decreasing the harshness, crudeness, unpleasantness, and distasteful component of the conflict episode is attempted.

- **Withdrawing**—This involves withdrawing, retreating, or disengaging from the conflict.

Confronting and smoothing result in constructive handling of the situation. Withdrawing and forcing result in adverse outcomes. The impact of compromising is relatively neutral in regard to reducing conflict.

Other Components of Strategy

There are other components of strategy that are necessary for successful conflict resolution:

- **Preparation**—This is achieved through learning a wide variety of interpersonal communication skills, understanding the dynamics of organizational conflict, managing change and the resistance to it, overcoming dysfunctional individual and group behavior, and keeping dialogue open and frank.

- **Early intervention.**

- **Keeping issues focused.**

- **Depersonalization of the problem**—When a problem becomes personalized, all the dynamics of defensiveness come into play, resulting in intensification of the seriousness of the problem. When the focus is on persons or personalities, the conflict is sure to continue.

Know the Other Party

It is essential to know the parties with whom you are dealing. Learn their values, personalities, emotional makeup, likes, and dislikes. If the parties involved in a conflict have worked together successfully in the past and will have to work together in the future, they are more likely to approach the situation from a win/win perspective. On the contrary, if this is a first encounter and they are not likely to be involved in future relationships, a win-lose perspective will more likely be followed. The conflict will be more difficult to resolve, and, at the conclusion, one party will be dissatisfied.

Cooling Off

Early on in the conflict episode, there may be a need for a cooling-off period in order for there to be calm, reasoned, and rational discussion. The length of the cooling-off period (minutes, hours, or days) will depend on a number of factors:

- The seriousness and duration of the conflict.

- How hardened opposing views are.

- The level of the emotional state or tension.

- Past experience the opposing parties have had in dealing with one another.

- How they feel about one another at the time of the current conflict episode.

Summary

Conflict in organizations is inevitable, but every effort should be made to prevent dysfunctional conflict and its costly consequences. Prevention is possible only if the manager develops good interpersonal relationships, learns effective communication skills, and recognizes and manages conflict episodes when they first begin.

References

1. Newstrom, J., and Davis, K. *Organizational Behavior.* New York, N.Y.: McGraw-Hill Book Co., 1989.

2. Filley, A. "Conflict Resolution: The Ethic of the Good Loser." In Huseman, R., *et al.,* Editors, *Readings in Interpersonal and Organizational Communication,* Third Edition. Boston, Mass.: Holbrook Press, 1977.

3. Blake, R., and others. *Managing Intergroup Conflict in Industry.* Houston, Tex.: Gulf Publishing, 1964.

Further Reading

Dubrin, A. *Fundamentals of Organizational Behavior—An Applied Perspective*. Elmsford, N.Y.: Pergamon, 1974, p. 312.

Huseman, R., and others. "Interpersonal Conflict in the Modern Organization." In *Readings in Interpersonal and Organizational Communication*, Third Edition. Boston, Mass.: Holbrook Press, 1977.

Keating, C. *Dealing with Difficult People—How You Can Come out on Top in Personality Conflicts*. New York, N.Y.: Paulist Press, 1984.

Montana, P., and Charnov, B. *Barron's Business Review Series*. New York, N.Y.: Barron's, 1987, p. 300-29.

Pondy, L. "Organizational Conflict: Concepts and Models." *Administrative Science Quarterly* 12(9):299-306, Sept. 1967.

Rasberry, R., and Lemoine, L. *Effective Managerial Communication*. Boston, Mass.: Kent Publishing Co., 1986, p. 377-94.

Richardson, J. "Communicator, Know Thyself." *Physician Executive* 14(3):19-21, May-June 1988.

Richardson, J. "Defensive Barriers to Communications." *Physician Executive* 16(5):37-8, Sept.-Oct. 1990.

Richardson, J. "Management of Conflict in Organizations." *Physician Executive* 17(1):39-42, Jan.-Feb. 1991.

Richardson, J. "Listening and Feedback: Two Essentials for Interpersonal Communication." *Physician Executive* 17(2)35-8, March-April 1991.

Selye, H. *Stress without Distress*. New York, N.Y.: New American Library, 1975.

James M. Richardson, MD, FACP, FACPE, is retired as Medical Director of Fairmont Hospital, San Leandro, California and Assistant Clinical Professor of Medicine, University of California, San Francisco. He is a Distinguished Fellow of the American College of Physician Executives and a Fellow of the American College of Physicians.

Chapter

Making the Most of Conflict: Its Value, Sources, and Opportunities

by C. Marlena Fiol, PhD, and
Edward J. O'Connor, PhD

After many months of continuous debate, administration has decided to move forward in implementing a new computerized OR scheduling system. You believe that it promises to streamline patient flow and lead to more efficient use of resources. However, resistance and conflict in your department regarding the new system appear to be growing.

Dr. Adams, one of the most vocal opponents of the new system, is also one of the most powerful physicians in the department. He has been holding private meetings with others, engaging their support in blocking this effort. His negativism is contagious. Even those initially in favor of the new scheduling system are now beginning to question its value.

Other leading surgeons appear to be withdrawing. Dr. Wright, for example, publicly says little about the new system, but he has failed to come to the meetings you have scheduled to discuss the system's value and how it will work. In addition, surgeons in his group appear to be scheduling more of their cases with your major competitor, and their relationships with you and department nurses are becoming strained.

The situation is becoming increasingly uncomfortable. You know you must deal with the differences among your people, but the strong feelings that have been aroused are threatening personal relationships and making it difficult to look at the situation objectively. While you want people to express their individuality and opinions so that you can engage them in developing new options, it also seems important to reconcile these conflicts so that harmonious pursuit of objectives can be restored. As you ponder the situation, you wonder whether there is any value in the current conflict, what its sources are, and what actions to take to make the most of the current opportunities.

Value of Conflict: Friend to Be Embraced or Curse to Be Avoided?

Picture yourself as part of a management team being judged in terms of the quantity and the quality of solutions you generate. Your group has a member who regularly challenges conclusions and forces others to critically examine both their assumptions and the logic of their arguments. Would this ongoing source of conflict be embraced as a contributing friend or expelled as a troublesome foe?

Research conducted by Boulding[1] demonstrated that groups containing confederates who played this "devil's advocate" role generated more and superior alternative solutions than groups without such an individual. However, when given permission to eliminate one member, high-performance groups consistently expelled their unique competitive advantage because the person made others feel uncomfortable. These results demonstrate a widely shared reaction to conflict: a recognition of its positive impact on outcomes and an acknowledgment that, for many, it is not personally comfortable. While improved decisions can emerge when conflict leads to identification and consideration of alternative solutions, it also breeds dissatisfaction, discomfort, and reduced cooperation. Leaders often recognize the "need to simultaneously embrace conflict to improve decision quality and shun it to improve the chances for consensus and efficiency."[2] As a leader, how can you assess whether the benefits will outweigh the consequences resulting from the conflict you are facing?

Too Little or Too Much

Some level of conflict appears to be both inevitable and valuable. Certainly it can enhance the creative identification of alternative solutions, increase understanding among those willing to listen, force assumptions to be clarified, and provide a mechanism for the cathartic airing of emotions.

The efforts of neither Dr. Adams nor Dr. Wright seem to be having these desired effects, however. While each is taking a very different strategy, both seem to be contributing to stress, a decrease in productivity, impaired decision making, poor working relationships, and possible misallocation of resources to a scheduling system that may be doomed to failure without their support. In addition, while Dr. Adams' meetings may be consuming excess time, Dr. Wright's efforts are also contributing to an unpleasant emotional experience as well as ensuring that relevant information is not shared. While the form of resistance each has chosen is different, both are producing a high level of conflict that will have a negative impact on organizational performance and on the way people feel about being in the department.

Obviously, a lack of conflict would not solve the problem. When people follow their leader over the cliff, no matter what, new ideas are seldom generated and old ideas are not effectively reviewed and tested against current demands. It has long been recognized that too much agreement among top management is one of the leading causes of business failures.[3] It may matter little whether the absence of conflict results from blind allegiance to a leader, intimidating consequences for nonconformance, excessive homogeneity among department members, or the absence of incentives encouraging effective organizational performance. In all cases, new ideas will be lost, and performance is likely to suffer during rapidly changing times.

As a leader, therefore, it is critical to seek an optimal level of conflict within your organization. Too little conflict and lethargic adherence to the past will destroy your organization. Too much conflict and the crippling impact of dissension will destroy relationships, reduce productivity, destroy attitudes, and lead to the loss of critical personnel. The optimal level varies across organizations and depends on both the nature of the conflict and the manner in which it is expressed.

Overt or Covert: Which Way Would You Like It?

Dr. Adams opposes the new scheduling system, and it isn't hard to find out why. He'll tell anybody what's wrong with it and how it would need to be fixed to gain his support. Dr. Wright has taken a very different approach. While he and his friends say little publicly about their concerns, they regularly discuss them among themselves and are taking the actions necessary to demonstrate their quiet opposition.

Which way would you like to have your conflict—overt or covert? Zero conflict is not an option in our rapidly changing environment. A lack of evident conflict generally means that either you do not yet have their attention or that they see no value in discussing the situation openly. With Dr. Adams' open opposition, you at least know where you stand. While it might be more desirable to receive his open opposition privately in your office, he is providing the information necessary to identify the problems that must be addressed if the scheduling system is to succeed. Just as it is preferable not to ski or drive a car blindfolded, it is also preferable to obtain critical information from those who are upset during conflict.

Cognitive or Affective: Not All Conflicts Are Created Equal

Conflict can affect the quality of decisions made in an organization as well as the degree to which those decisions are accepted and effectively put in place. Both Dr. Adams and Dr. Wright appear to be challenging the quality of the scheduling system decision and thus are making its successful implementation unlikely. While conflict between your desire to implement this system and their support for other alternatives appears inevitable, the form this conflict takes will affect your chances of success. Conflict can either be cognitively focused on issue-related differences in perspectives or affectively directed in an emotionally charged manner at individuals who oppose your views. While both are forms of conflict, they lead to radically different outcomes.

Cognitive conflict generally enhances people's understanding of issues, allows identification of problems/solutions, and improves the chance of acceptance of decisions. When it is openly shared, relatively high levels of cognitive, issue-based conflict lead to desirable results (performance level Z in figure 1, page 101). Affective conflict generally leads to poor decisions, lower levels of decision acceptance, and disruption of group cohesion.[4] When conflict is covert and not openly shared, its negative effects are exacerbated, and relatively low levels of conflict can lead to poor organizational outcomes (performance level X in figure 1). It is your job as leader to steer the focus back to clarifying the issues involved, generating alternative solutions, and building acceptance for these decisions.

Who and What Are the Sources of Conflict?

Both Dr. Adams and Dr. Wright appear to be sources of significant problems for implementing the new scheduling/patient tracking system. Because they are the visible sources of conflict, it would seem that one would either need to understand their motives or write them off as defects that should be isolated from the system. While the nature of each of these individuals may well contribute to current tensions, broader ways of thinking about both the sources of and the solutions to conflict are valuable to the effective leader.

Who: Individual Contributions to Conflict

Both personal values and resulting differences in individual goals contribute to conflict within organizations. Sometimes diverse histories and education result in disagreements over ethics, moral considerations, or assumptions about fairness and justice. Such differences may be particularly evident between individuals or groups who have chosen different careers and have been shaped by diverse training. For example, a chief financial officer may be drawn to efficiency and cost containment, while a physician may be more concerned with clinical outcomes and patient satisfaction.

Differences in values and beliefs may lie dormant—unspoken or even unrecognized—until they are confronted by opposing beliefs. My belief that I am underpaid may be only a mild irritation until I go to my class reunion and find peers earning twice my current salary. It is often the presence of organizational conditions (e.g., task relationships, scarce resources, competition) that stir beliefs and move people forward into conflict. The independent, autonomous physician's short-term time perspective, for example, may lie dormant and unnoticed until confronted by the collaborative, participative long-term time perspectives of an administrator during their mutual development of an integrated delivery system.

What: Situational Contributions to Conflict

A common misperception about conflict is that it is primarily personality driven and the result of defective individuals. Two problems exist with this view:

- Our increasingly specialized and diverse work force means that we can't just get rid of people who see the world differently.

Figure 1. Effects of Conflict on Performance

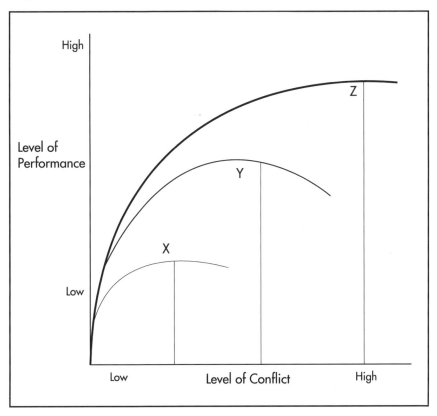

Note: "X" and "Z" denote optimal level of conflict under three different conditions:

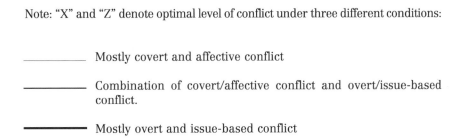

_____ Mostly covert and affective conflict

_____ Combination of covert/affective conflict and overt/issue-based conflict.

_____ Mostly overt and issue-based conflict

- Personality differences are not typically the immediate source of conflict at work. Such differences usually lie dormant until they are triggered by an organizational catalyst.

Organizational catalysts likely to trigger conflict include differential information, incompatible task relationships/incentives, and competition for scarce resources.

Differential Information. Orientation or status differences may result in differential information. To the degree that people have different definitions of the problem, either because they are aware of different pieces of relevant information or because they bring divergent interpretations to the facts that are present, conflict is a likely outcome. The situation is exacerbated by inadequate communication systems creating levels of uncertainty and tension during rapidly changing times. The resulting anxiety leaves people prone to conflict. While administrators may be expected to view the new scheduling/tracking system as a great way to trim costs by identifying and rectifying process problems, both Dr. Adams and Dr. Wright may see the system as a mechanism for interfering with their ability to make decisions based on patient well-being.

Incompatible Task Relationships/Incentives. To the extent that people in work settings depend on each other to get the job done, separation is not possible. When different authority structures overlap (e.g., surgeons, anesthesiologists, administrators, nurses), tensions naturally rise. To the degree that incentive systems push these groups to pull in inconsistent directions, conflict is a likely outcome. Differences in personal values frequently lie dormant until structural forces come into play and heighten these inconsistencies.

Competition for Scarce Resources. Conflict is more likely to result as the supply of resources becomes noticeably smaller. The threat of loss generates stress and brings old assumptions into conflict with one another.

While the debate between administration and both Dr. Adams and Dr. Wright may seem to be about the new scheduling/tracking system, circumstances surrounding that system (e.g., fear of losing resources when the health care resource pool is shrinking) may have much to do with both the level of conflict and the alternative methods these physicians have chosen to deal with their concerns. The normal tendency is to attack individuals who appear to be sources of conflict. It is more effective to understand organizational catalysts and make adjustments. Structural conditions can be more readily manipulated than the values or beliefs individuals hold.

Conflict Management Strategies: Taking Advantage of the Opportunities

While many leaders seek to avoid the discomfort associated with conflict, this strategy may deny them the potential creative innovation and enhanced performance that can result from opposing viewpoints. There is no one right way to deal with the naturally occurring differences in views that exist within organizations. However, a conscious understanding of alternative approaches to conflict and their consequences is critical to successful leadership. Choices exist for both general strategies and specific action steps fundamental to effectively utilizing the most potentially rewarding of these approaches.

General Strategies

People's responses to conflict can be classified into five general strategies: competing, avoiding, accommodating, compromising, and collaborating.[5,6] These responses can be organized on the basis of the degree to which they are focused on the conflictive issue as opposed to the relationship among conflicting parties, as shown in figure 2, page 104. Accommodating strategies, in the lower right corner of the triangle, focus on the importance of the relationship among involved parties and are intended to satisfy the other parties' concerns. Competing strategies, in the lower left corner of the triangle, focus on the importance of the issue and are intended to ensure that one's own concerns are satisfied. Avoidance and compromise represent differing levels of non-attention to both the relationship and the issue. Collaborating strategies, at the top of the triangle, encompass full attention on both the relationship and the issue.

Competing is a command and control approach designed to overpower other groups, ignore their concerns, and promote one's own position at the expense of others. It can be carried out using one's formal position or manipulative ploys. While the possibility of behaving as if you are right and getting your way is sometimes appealing, the approach is inappropriate when long-term relationships are important, one's power base is not sufficient to force one's will upon others, or one needs innovative ideas from the other people involved. If immediate action is required (e.g., business turnaround with limited cash flow, avoidance of an impending clinical crisis) and you have the power to ensure compliance, this strategy may be highly effective. Competing may also be necessary when needed solutions (e.g., downsizing) are likely to be unpopular to some of the people involved or when it is necessary to demonstrate your conviction to those who would take advantage of non-competitive behavior.

These conditions are often not present in professional organizations. For example, in dealing with either Dr. Adams or Dr. Wright, it is unlikely that formal authority exists to impose one's wishes on them. In addition, ignoring their concerns is likely to lead to a worsening of current conditions. The resulting hostility, resentment, and backlash, even if the new scheduling/tracking system could be imposed, would be detrimental to your future success as a leader.

Accommodating, at the opposite extreme, is an appealing approach for many. By satisfying the other parties' concerns, one appears to be caring for the relationship, building rapport, and creating the right to claim favors at a future time. This strategy may also be appropriate when you recognize that you are wrong, wish to appear reasonable, or lack the power necessary to achieve your desired outcomes. While the strategy can be highly effective in reconciling differences with minimal time investment, its reoccurring use in

Figure 2. Conflict Resolution Strategies

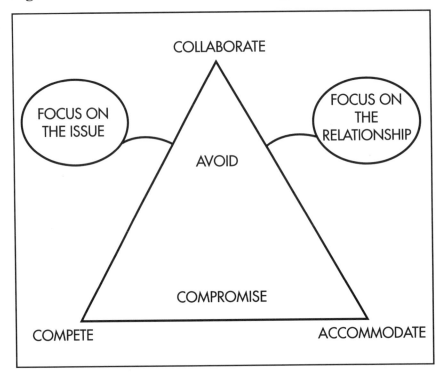

the name of maintaining harmony can result in others' learning to take advantage of you. In addition, all involved may actually lose as a result of not critically appraising issues and selecting optimal solutions if the sources of the conflict are of significant importance to the organization. In the case of the scheduling/tracking system, accommodating the needs of Drs. Adams and Wright would ignore the need for efficiency, cost containment, and enhanced access to medical technology. Accommodating, under such conditions, not only would result in loss of esteem but also would make it more difficult to deal with future issues.

A strategy of **avoiding** conflict has the advantage of saving time and removing oneself from unpleasant circumstances in the short run. This strategy may also be appropriate when conditions suggest that you have no chance of achieving your objectives and that the potential disruption of conflict outweighs any benefits likely to occur. This approach is most useful when the issues are not relevant to organizational performance (e.g., religion, politics, or loyalty to sports teams), no need exists to reach agreement, and the parties involved are not dependent on each other to produce effective performance.

Unfortunately, this approach neglects both one's own needs and those of the other parties involved. Such an approach may be appropriate if the issue and the relationships are unimportant to you and/or circumstances suggest that others who are currently engaged can better handle the conflict. However, assuming that disagreements are inherently bad because of their negative impact on harmony or that this is someone else's problem can have detrimental consequences. Problems don't get solved, and frustration often mounts. As a result, the organization in the long run is in a weaker position to handle ongoing challenges that arise. Further ongoing avoidance of conflicts regarding the scheduling/tracking system seems impossible. Battle lines have been drawn in different ways by both Dr. Adams and Dr. Wright in response to this administrative imperative. Differences of views must be resolved if confusion, negative feelings, and reduced performance are to be avoided.

Compromising often appears to be an appealing solution that partially avoids both the demands of the issue and the relationships. It allows one to reach an agreement relatively quickly by providing partial satisfaction for all involved by splitting the difference and spreading the pain. Compromising may be most effective when other approaches have been unsuccessful and it is essential to minimize further disruption in your organization. The approach may also be appropriate when you must reach a solution rapidly, the parties involved are of roughly equivalent power, and all must agree to support the new decision. The regular use of this approach can be counterproductive, however. Conflicts may be postponed and prolonged as each side continues to bemoan its losses and seek further satisfaction of its needs. All involved may simply learn to ask for more in the future so that compromises are closer to their initial desires. Some form of compromise regarding the scheduling/tracking system may work in the short run (e.g., postpone implementation until further fact finding can occur) if this approach is used to allow time for more effective data gathering and problem solution. Given the importance of the issue to all involved, it is not likely that it will provide a long-term solution to the problem, heal relationships, build trust, or meet the needs of the parties involved on a long-term basis.

Collaboration, the conflict-handling strategy at the top of the triangle in figure 2, focuses on addressing both the issue and the relationship. It is most appropriate when it is important to satisfy the needs of all parties by working through differences and seeking win-win solutions. When both relationships and issues are critical, investing time and energy in this approach will improve future performance. When it is important to combine ideas, gain commitment, and improve the capacity to work together on future challenges, this approach is most likely to channel differences into increasing the range of alternatives, encouraging trust, focusing on issues rather than personalities, and enhancing long-term performance. Given the need to repair relationships, encourage trust, and reach solutions with Drs. Adams and Wright, collaboration appears to be the strategy of choice. In addition to bringing the issues to the surface, it is likely to enhance open as opposed to covert communication and to build a base for resolving both the scheduling/tracking system and future problems.

Collaborative Action Steps

Presuming you wish to resolve an important issue while maintaining or enhancing the relationships among the parties to the conflict and have the time necessary to focus on future success, a collaborative approach seems most appropriate. A number of collaborative action steps are important to the effective implementation of this strategy:

1. Create a context for success.

2. Embrace the conflict.

3. Encourage communication and trust.

4. Clarify critical issues.

5. Work within other people's perspectives.

6. Clarify processes to be followed.

7. Protect and enhance relationships.

8. Ensure support, follow-up, and commitment.

Create a Context for Success (versus focusing on the problem). "Most dissenters won't stand up and shout at you that they hate what you're doing to them and to their comfortable old ways. Instead, they will nod and smile and agree with everything you say—and then behave as they always have."[7] A leader's job is to create circumstances in which people will choose to come forward, contribute their ideas, and work to achieve mutually agreed-to solutions to conflict situations. Such conditions demand a mutual understanding of where the organization and its members can go as a result of reconciling this conflict and why they should wish to participate in these outcomes. The presence of goals that cannot be achieved without working together provides a framework of common objectives that inspires searching for potential solutions.

Beyond knowing where you might go, it is also essential that people understand why you are going there if they are to be energized to resolve conflict and work together to produce these future outcomes. Describing the future in terms of the individual benefits to be achieved or of the consequences of failure is important in focusing people's attention on the need for reconciling differences. Making these descriptions personal (e.g., impact on their career, earnings, power, prestige) energizes people toward action.

Embrace the Conflict (versus punishing those who verbalize differences). As noted above, most people intellectually assent to the value of conflict while behaviorally avoiding it to the best of their ability. Not only is conflict unpleasant for most of us, but also it violates our basic desire to be nice and not create pain and discomfort for others. Without leadership intervention, people will typically avoid open expression of conflictive concerns to those who they know will disagree. In order to embrace conflict and encourage others to engage in the pursuit of mutually acceptable solutions, it is important that a leader openly acknowledge that the conflict exists. If steps are not taken to encourage acknowledgment of concerns, the conflict strategies pursued by Dr. Wright will most likely continue. Under these conditions, people are not involved in a process designed to find mutually agreeable solutions. As a result, productivity will suffer and relationships will become increasingly strained.

Encourage Communication and Trust (versus repeatedly being logical, telling people they don't understand, and pushing harder). Abraham Lincoln said, "When I am getting ready to reason with a man, I spend one-third of my time thinking about myself and what I am going to say, and two-thirds thinking about him and what he is going to say."[8] While it is not necessary to ignore your own position, it is critical to put yourself in others' shoes/heads if you are going to get to mutually acceptable solutions. The ability to see the situation as others do, while difficult, is essential to conflict resolution. Others will believe their views are right just as strongly as you believe yours are right. These views are usually based on prior learning and assumptions, not on the facts involved in the situation.

Trust cannot be demanded or required. The building of trust and a shared understanding of reality involves listening in order to understand rather than telling over and over again how you see things. The building of trust requires an investment in demonstrating understanding and respect for the views of others involved in the conflict. It involves active listening, using open-ended inquiries to elicit further information, and accepting what others have to say while probing for additional clarification.

Active listening and inquiry into the concerns of Dr. Adams and Dr. Wright are essential to beginning to build a bridge that involves them in the process of identifying acceptable solutions to the current scheduling/tracking conflict.

While Dr. Adams is more than willing to express his ideas, it will be important to demonstrate your commitment to understanding and then clarifying potential solutions to meet the full range of challenges faced. Having demonstrated your understanding of Dr. Adams' views and your willingness to build them into revisions of the planned systems, you will have increased the likelihood of his being willing to examine outcomes you must produce and engage with you in the development of creative means of reaching these ends. Dr. Wright has demonstrated the desire for a less open approach, and it may therefore be necessary to create anonymous processes for gathering information about his concerns regarding the scheduling/tracking system. Through the use of anonymous surveys, third-party interviewers, or electronic question and answer systems, one may gather initial information from Dr. Wright and others who have concerns.

Clarify Critical Issues (versus pointing out why they are wrong and you are right). Frustration arises when participants are focused on different aspects of a conflict. For example, administration may be primarily concerned about the goals to be achieved by the new scheduling/tracking system; Drs. Adams and Wright may be much more interested in discussing the methods to be used in achieving those goals. It is important to clarify the issues as the two parties see them. By managing the discussion effectively, a leader can move the focus toward the issues and away from personality clashes. Maintaining attention on issues rather than on personalities shifts the conversation to descriptive rather than judgmental issues. For example, attention focused on reducing the duration of emergency department visits will be more productive than complaints regarding the slowness of those performing laboratory tests. The former approach allows you to identify process problems while the latter will create defensiveness and an inability to communicate in a manner that generates innovative solutions.

Work within Other People's Perspectives (versus focusing on specific demands). Focusing on specific positions or demands minimizes the likelihood of successfully resolving conflicts. In contrast, coming to understand each party's interest or the reasons behind his or her demands—what is really at stake for the person—opens up the possibility of finding creative solutions. Once you better understand the interests of the parties involved, and they feel understood, brainstorming ways to satisfy all of the needs involved becomes a possible strategy. When a demand is placed before you, it may be appropriate to ask what that demand would get the person that he or she really wants. While it is clear that Dr. Adams and Dr. Wright are upset regarding the new scheduling/tracking system and opposed to its implementation, little has been done to date to clarify the critical issues involved. Until that step is taken, the likelihood of reconciling the conflicts remains low.

Clarify the Process to Be Followed (versus doing the same thing over and over and hoping for a different result). One of the best predictors of future behavior is past behavior. When one is unhappy with the outcomes produced by past behavior, it is usually wise to try something new. While you may hope that others will change their behaviors, taking the lead in reconciling conflict necessitates that you alter your own behavior patterns first. For example, to the degree that the situation continues to be emotionally entangled and based on positions, it may be valuable to suggest the use of objective criteria. Progress may be made through a discussion of what standards could be used or what data could be collected to clarify which of the opposing proposals is most likely to be successful. The conversation may then shift from a focus on getting "what I want" to a focus on deciding what makes the most sense given the agreed-to criteria.

If it has become clear that a disagreement is over facts, progress may be made through validating existing data or developing additional information regarding which of the alternatives best meets the agreed-to criteria. Alternatively, in a situation in which righteous indignation about the moral correctness of values is at stake, it may be useful to move from abstractions to a description of what the values mean in operational terms. Because the same words and concepts mean different things to different people, the process of clarification can lead to a deepened understanding and the possibility of mutually acceptable solutions.

Protect and Enhance Relationships (versus focusing on getting what you want at any cost). Crisis offers you the opportunity to redefine, through your behavior, how you will do things from this point forward. While words about involvement, listening, and participative decision making are interesting, a leader's behavior during crises speaks far more loudly regarding commitment to these issues. If conflict is to be transformed into problem solving, people's feelings, interests, and general well-being must be protected in the process. By looking for ways to meet their needs and suggesting areas in which parties can make concessions of value to others with little impact on themselves, steps can be taken toward further establishing conditions of caring and trust. For maximum impact, a leader may have to go beyond keeping parties informed about progress and challenges and take the lead in being vulnerable if others are to do the same. This may involve recognizing publicly your contribution to current problems and taking steps to demonstrate your commitment to correcting past inadequacies.

It may be, for example, that Dr. Adams and Dr. Wright, having witnessed your prior refusal to consider their views regarding other issues, have come to conclude that it is useless to engage in a dialogue with you regarding the new scheduling/tracking system. If so, it may be necessary for you to recognize with each of them that you now see the consequences of your prior behavior. In addition, genuine interest in repairing the situation can best be demonstrated by your taking actions to implement some of the suggestions that they have previously provided.

Ensure Support, Follow Up, and Commitment (versus hoping for the best). The appearance of agreement can leave a leader so relieved that final steps in reconciling the conflict are overlooked. It is essential to verify that all parties have a common understanding of their commitments to specific actions. Beyond simply settling for their verbal assent to your summary, it is important to establish mechanisms for follow up. Benchmarks and specific time lines for measuring progress will make the plan tangible and will ensure accountability. While it may be important to encourage flexibility and to adjust the plan to meet emerging circumstances, original agreements regarding measures of success help people recognize that they are agreeing to the same thing.

If benchmarks are not achieved (e.g., if Dr. Adams or Dr. Wright continue with their current course of action with respect to agreed-to adjustments), it is necessary to demonstrate your commitment to the agreed-to decisions. If you fail to do this, others will recognize that the scheduling/ tracking agreements, as well as other organizational arrangements, have low credibility and are subject to arbitrary change. The lack of consequences for violating agreed-to plans will lead to a lower state of harmony and productivity than existed prior to the conflict. Clarity regarding consequences of not supporting the agreed-to objectives is an essential part of this last step in successfully resolving conflict. Such consequences, if they occur, will not be seen as arbitrary impositions. They will be recognized as a choice made by those who did not keep their agreements.

Clearly, the processes followed by Dr. Adams (e.g., holding private meetings to engage others in blocking the effort) or Dr. Wright (e.g., withdrawal from the situation) are not ideal vehicles for reaching mutually acceptable solutions. Progressing with them through the steps outlined above may create a context and understanding in which new processes can be put into place.

References

1. Boulding, K. "Further Reflections on Conflict Management." In Kahn, R., and Boulding, E., Editors, *Power and Conflict in Organizations*. New York, N.Y.: Basic Books, 1964.

2. Brockmann, E. "Removing the Paradox of Conflict from Group Decisions." *Academy of Management Executive* 10(2):61-2, May 1996.

3. Argenti, J. *Corporate Collapse: The Causes and Symptoms*. New York, N.Y.: Wiley, 1976.

4. Amason, A. "Distinguishing the Effects of Functional and Dysfunctional Conflict on Strategic Decision Making: Resolving a Paradox for Top Management Teams." *Academy of Management Journal* 39(1):123-48, Feb. 1996.

5. Rubble, T., and Thomas, K. "Support for a Two-Dimensional Model of Conflict Behavior." *Organizational Behavior and Human Performance* 16(1):143-55, June 1976.

6. Whetten, D., and Cameron, K. *Developing Managerial Skills*. Glenview, Ill.: Scott, Foresman, and Company, 1995.

7. Fisher, A. "Making Change Stick." *Fortune* 131(7):121-8, April 17, 1995.

8, Charlton, J., Editor. *The Executive's Quotation Book*. New York: St. Martin's Press, 1983.

C. Marlena Fiol, PhD, is Associate Professor and Edward J. O'Connor, PhD, is Professor, University of Colorado at Denver. Both are Principals of the Implementation Institute, Denver.

Chapter

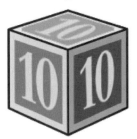

Time Management

by Douglas P. Longnecker, MD

Time management for the administrator presents a list of problems that are unimagined by the clinician. The time demands are no more or less rigorous than those for the clinician, but they are very different. The physician wishing to succeed in management will have to exercise a great deal of personal control over the use of his or her time.

There are as many experts in the field of time management as there are people who have written on the subject. In thinking of the management of time, it is perhaps more appropriate to consider personal management rather than time management. It is critical to balance personal versus professional time in any endeavor, whether medical practice, administrative medicine, or other professions.

Table 1, below, compares and contrasts practice time and administrative time for physicians. In the clinical arena, the physician's time is practice-driven. Time is consumed by the requirements of patients, procedures, paperwork, phone calls, mail, and third-party payers. Administratively, the physician's time is organizationally driven through meetings, interventions,

Table 1. Contrasts and Similarities for Practice vs. Administrative Time

Clinical Practice (Patient-Driven Needs)	Administrative (Organization-Driven Needs)
1. Patients	1. Meetings
2. Procedures	2. Interventions
3. Paperwork	3. Plenary Sessions
4. Phone Calls	4. Phone Calls
5. Mail	5. Mail
6. Third-Party Payers	6. Administrative Structure

plenary sessions, phone calls, mail, and administrative structure. Many other areas could be included in this list, but these are the most significant factors.

As can be determined by asking any patient waiting in a physician's office, physicians are perceived as poor time managers. Clinical practice dictates that time management be patient- and practice-driven. Consequently, a significant amount of activity falls in what may be described as the crisis arena. Even though many activities can, and must, be scheduled, because of the press on the physician's time from surgery, procedures, etc., a great deal of the practicing physician's time is driven by patients' needs and not by the physician. Physicians who do not pay close attention to tight time allocations have gained the reputation not only of being late, but also of being poor time managers.

There are specific differences between clinical and administrative time. In the clinical arena, as briefly listed above, time segments are largely patient- and schedule-driven, either by office visits or procedures. In the physician's administrative time, the system is management-driven. The administrative physician must be able to organize his or her time through self-discipline, have the time to interact with peer groups, and provide specific time for productive thinking and planning.

To explore more closely the contrasts between clinical and administrative activity and time, let's look at an example of scheduling of clinical time.

Medical practice scheduling is well known to all physicians who have moved from a clinical to an administrative arena. Appropriate scheduling in a medical office or a medical practice is dictated by the medical specialty. However, it is well known that the schedule may be constructed either in specific time blocks or on a wave method. Additionally, practice time is affected by specific procedures, be they surgical or other, related to outside scheduling availability. Appropriate staffing within the physician's office or practice arena is extremely important. Sufficient secretarial, nursing, and general office personnel are critical to an efficient medical practice. The layout of the office facility and of procedural rooms and the way in which the facility is equipped will greatly facilitate or hamper the physician's efficiency.

In administration, the physician must appropriate sufficient time for management. If the physician is both a practicing and an administrative physician, time must be rigorously scheduled for management activities. The support staff from an administrative aspect is equally important as the support staff from the physician's practice aspect. Because physicians in clinical practice commonly use their support staffs for scheduling not only their offices but also their procedural time, it is imperative for the administrative physician to effectively use his or her secretarial and administrative staff in an efficient manner.

Delegation of duties in both the clinical and the administrative arenas is of utmost importance. This is accomplished through many mechanisms. However, the ability to specifically observe and supervise the delegation once it has happened is crucial. Administratively, this presents many problems for some physicians, as delegation to this depth is not frequently done in clinical practice.

In analyzing administrative and clinical physician's time, it is quite apparent that "something has to give." Management time cannot be squeezed between clinical activities. Management time must be specifically scheduled. It must be time that is used during a productive period of a physician's day. For most practicing physicians, the use of management time appears grossly inefficient when compared to clinical activities. As mentioned earlier, practicing physicians are familiar with scheduling of patients and procedures for their clinical specialties. Most physicians going from clinical practice to management positions are much less prepared for scheduling of their time and for allocation of priorities.

A brief overview of the phases of time management are in order at this time (see table 2, below). The first phase may be described as developing notes and checklists to which frequent reference is made during the course of the day. The second phase would be the establishment of calendars and appointment books. The third phase is prioritization of time. This is apparent to all practicing physicians. A clinical example would be, given a busy office schedule, the time prioritization that would be required because of the appearance in the emergency department of a patient requiring immediate attention. Administrative time prioritization is somewhat different, but the basic elements are the same.

Table 2. Phases of Time Management

1. Notes/Checklists
2. Calendars/Appointment Books
3. Prioritization of Time
4. Personal Management

One must also recognize the fact that there are "crisis" interventions that are necessary throughout the course of an administrative day. This is frequently referred to as "putting out fires."

The fourth phase listed in table 2 is that of personal management. The concept of personal management changes one's philosophy from management of time to management of people. I can think of no better example of a paradigm shift than for a practicing physician to enter the administrative arena. Stephen Covey, in his book *The 7 Habits of Highly Effective People,** goes into great detail discussing paradigm shifts.

---

*Covey, S. *The 7 Habits of Successful People.* New York, N.Y.: Simon and Schuster, 1989.

He divides daily activities into four specific categories: urgent, nonurgent, important, and not important. He also describes, as shown in table 3, below, the interactions within the four quadrants. Quadrant I activities are crisis problems, pressing problems, and deadline-driven projects. Quadrant II activities are prevention, production capability activities, relationship building, recognizing new opportunities, planning, and recreation. Quadrant III activities are interruptions, some phone calls, mail, meetings, proximate pressing matters, and popular activities. Quadrant IV activities are trivia, busy work, some mail, some phone calls, time wasters, and pleasant activities. Quadrant IV activities are perceived by many managers to be wasted time.

To repeat, I can think of no better example of a paradigm shift than a practicing physicians assuming an administrative position. This is further exemplified by looking at table 3 in regard to clinical practice activities. Practicing physicians, on a daily basis, must deal with crises, pressing problems, and deadline-driven projects in their clinical activities. From an administrative aspect, Covey, and many others, feel it is extremely important to shift as many activities as possible into Quadrant II. This transition is a difficult task for the practicing physician. It requires the new administrative physician to change attitudes and philosophies, either totally or partially, from a clinical to an administrative posture (a paradigm shift). It has been shown that Quadrant I activities, to the exclusion of other activities, result in a high rate of stress, burnout, and crisis management. This is more graphically depicted in table 4, page 117.

Table 3.

Urgent	Not Urgent
Important	
I **Activities** Crises Pressing problems Deadline-driven projects	II **Activities** Prevention, PC activities Relationship building Recognizing new opportunities Planning, recreation
Not Important	
III **Activities** Interruptions, some calls Some mail, some reports Some meetings Proximate, pressing matters Popular activities	IV **Activities** Trivia, busy work Some mail Some phone calls Time wasters Pleasant actvities

Table 4.

I **Results**	II
• Stress • Burnout • Crisis Management • Always putting out fires	IV
III	

In table 5, below, one can see that, with physicians' predominant activity centered in Quadrant III activities, the results are short-term focus, crisis management activities, reputation of a chameleon character, and planning and goals of little value. The physician functioning in Quadrant III feels victimized, out of control, and shallow in relationships. Many clinical activities lie in Quadrant III, although they do not relate specifically to "out of control activities."

Table 5.

I	II
III **Results:** • Short-term focus • Crisis Management • Reputation-chameleon character • See goals and plans as worthless • Feel victimized, out of control • Shallow or broken relationships	IV

Table 6, below, relates to Quadrant IV activities, which can lead to total irresponsibility, termination from employment, total dependency on others, or dependency on institutions for basics. This behavior is contradictory to what a practicing physician must exhibit in his or her daily activities, as well as what he or she must produce in regard to administrative duties.

Table 6.

I	II
III	IV **Results:** • Total irresponsibility • Fired from job • Dependent on others • Dependent on others or institutions for basics

Activities located in Quadrant II—prevention, production capabilities, relationship building, recognizing new opportunities, planning, and even recreation—are the areas in which the administrative physician must focus his or her physical and intellectual energy. The results of these endeavors would be increased vision and perspective, the balance of idealization, self-discipline, control, and diminution of administrative crises. These concepts are depicted in table 7, below.

Table 7.

II	II
	Results: ● Vision, perspective ● Balance ● Discipline ● Control ● Few Crises
III	IV

Where the paradox occurs for the physician administrator relative to the clinical physician is the transferring of activities from Quadrant I to Quadrant II. It is a total impossibility for practicing physicians to transfer all of their activities to Quadrant II. In fact, it may be quite difficult for a predominance of clinical activities to be transferred to Quadrant II because of the nature of clinical practice. Consequently, the physician who is engaged in both the clinical and the administrative fields of medicine must develop and maintain the ability to "shift gears" or "paradigms" between the administrative Quadrant II and the clinical Quadrant I activities.

This concept may be expressed by contrasting proactivity versus reactivity. The clinical physician, by the nature of the profession of medicine, must be a reactive individual. The clinical physician must be able to deal with crisis/pressing problems, to shift his or her thinking immediately to the problems at hand, and to plan for the long-term aspects of clinical care.

For the administrative physician, conversely, it is much more appropriate and effective if the proactive mode is employed to produce decisions.

To use a more specific example of the reactive versus the proactive mode, the practicing physician needs to see patients either at his or her office or at the hospital. The physician must immediately form the most appropriate plan of action and envision medical needs to arrive at a correct judgment. In contrast, the administrative physician faced with a decision should become proactive rather than reactive, because there may be more than one decision that would be appropriate. Furthermore, in an administrative situation, the physician must look at alternatives to a much greater extent, especially in regard to the people who surround and work with him or her in the administrative environment.

In summary, in time management or, more specifically, in personal management, it is apparent that clinical thought processes and administrative decisions may diverge in concept. In addition to the divergence of clinical and administrative physician activity, one must look at differences in the demands on support staff of the practicing physician and the administrative physician. Practicing physicians are accustomed to delegating less critical responsibilities in both the office and the hospital setting. Practicing physicians ask their office nursing personnel, their front office employees, and hospital-based technicians and nurses to assist them in their activities by the delegation of appropriate responsibilities. There is a deeper level of responsibility to be delegated from an administrative position. The administrator must have well-trained and capable individuals who are in a position not only to carry out decisions by the administrator, but also to formulate ideas, concepts, and decision-making processes on their own.

For some physicians, it is difficult to accept delegation of this level of responsibility, but this is a mandated conceptual change or "paradigm shift" for the administrative physician. Practicing physicians have no choice but to reserve significant clinical decisions for themselves, to the exclusion of delegation. In contrast, it is the ineffective physician manager who feels that he or she is the only individual who can make decisions or perform the procedures necessary for appropriate administrative functioning.

These concepts are important for the full-time physician administrator, but perhaps more significant for the part-time physician administrator. The changes in thought processes and conceptual insights from a clinical "action" mode to an administrative "delegating" mode are difficult transitions to make.

It is important for the physician administrator, particularly physicians just leaving clinical practice to join administration, to understand and accept that:

- Time interactions and time utilization present difficulties.

- Administrative physicians cannot expect the immediate gratification seen in clinical practice and must expect and accept long-term gratification.

- Individual decisions are not final, as they are in clinical practice.

- Organizational structure and actions are the basis for administrative medicine.

Douglas P. Longenecker, MD, is Senior Vice President, Medical Affairs, Good Samaritan Hospital and Health Center, Dayton, Ohio.

Chapter

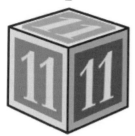

Managing Diversity

by Doreen Moreira, MD, CPE, FACPE

The health care work force is no longer just becoming more diverse—it is more diverse, and profoundly so at that. As long as you manage people at your workplace, effective diversity management will bring a host of benefits. Recent studies show that organizations with highly diverse work forces that manage the diversity well outperform their less diverse peer organizations. In addition, one of the key functions of the physician executive is to increase the effectiveness and productivity of the physician workforce. In order to accomplish this task, it becomes imperative for a physician executive to manage diversity problems well, as the outcome of not doing so can be to encourage, or even create, disruptions among staff members that decrease physician effectiveness and productivity.

Diversity. A small word but one that routinely provokes many different physical and emotional reactions from physicians and physician executives. A roll of the eyes toward the ceiling, A glazed look. Shrugged shoulders and a puzzled face. "What do they want me to do about it?" "Does this mean I have to hire someone who isn't qualified?" "If only white males (or physicians just out of residency, foreign medical graduates, etc.) apply for these jobs, how can they expect me to make the department more diverse?" "Why is human resources wasting our time with this diversity training when we need to be seeing our patients?" "We don't have diversity problems in my department." "I already have the most diverse department in this organization." "Everyone who works for me is a woman." "I've been told that the work force is becoming more diverse but how does that affect what I do?" I have yet to have a person come up to me at the end of a talk on diversity and say "Isn't it great that the work force is more diverse? It sure makes my life easier."

Diversity is neither good nor bad in and of itself. Diversity has a positive influence when people are respected for their differences and when multiple points of view can be used to create innovative and highly competitive programs for the organization. Diversity has a negative influence when multiple conflicting ideas and poor diversity management keep people from working productively.

It's a good bet that, if you let a group of physician executives prioritize their interest in tasks they do, managing diversity would make the top of very few, if any, lists. We should ask ourselves why this is the case, given the evidence that maintaining and managing a diverse workforce can positively affect the organizational bottom line.

The reasons are multifactorial, but one problem we face is that diversity training programs tend to be poorly designed for physician executive audiences. Teaching methods in medical schools develop physicians who can manage large amounts of data successfully but don't usually provide students with exposure to the softer or touchy-feely approaches that diversity trainers and human resources professionals find successful with other groups. While diversity training is useful, it is important that presenters know and understand the physician executive audience and its preferred learning styles. Also, keep this in mind when arranging diversity training for your physician staff.

Perhaps an even more important reason why physician executives shy away from managing diversity is that many immediately associate the word diversity with conflict and the word conflict with something bad. No one likes the negative side of conflict, and, as a result, many people try to avoid any conflict at all. Unfortunately, avoidance of conflict rarely, if ever, improves a situation. While discomfort with conflict can contribute to diversity's being a relatively unpopular subject, it is important to remember that the presence of well-managed conflict can bring many positive results, such as improved morale, communication, and trust among staff members. Therefore, using conflict resolution tools as part of good diversity management can help achieve positive growth or change in an organization. (See chapters 8 and 9 for more on conflict management.)

An Approach to Managing Diversity

Our first step should be to decide what "diversity" means. My dictionary defines diversity as *the condition of being different from all others*. Given this simple definition, it should become clear that all of us in the work force meet this condition. Therefore, we can begin to view diversity not from the point of view of interactions between older people versus younger, Afro-Americans versus whites, or males versus females, but from a more global point of view of interactions between people who are inherently different from one another, *even if they are the same age, race, or sex.*

Also, if we are going to understand diversity, we must know what we mean by the commonly used term "diversity issues." I believe what we really mean by diversity issues is diversity problems. My dictionary defines "problems" as questions raised for inquiry, consideration, or solution and as situations, matters, or people that present perplexity or difficulty.

Therefore, I propose defining "diversity problems" as questions raised for inquiry, consideration, or solution arising from perplexing, disruptive, or destructive situations that result from the condition of each person being different from all others. Ideally, this definition serves to reduce the diversity mystique and points us in the right direction for solutions to our diversity-related problems.

The broadness of this definition gives us the freedom to see that diversity problems are more than matters of race, culture, age, or gender. They also can encompass a number of other concerns, such as sexual harassment, misunderstood or misinterpreted communication, interpersonal conflict, etc.—items not generally viewed as being under the standard diversity umbrella.

Of course, having a clear understanding of what diversity is, and determining what diversity-related problems are, allows us to intervene effectively. Also keep in mind that the appropriate interventions should serve to enhance mutual respect, understanding, and collaboration.

What are three steps a physician executive can take to effectively manage diversity-related problems?

1. *Understand* what "diversity" means.

2. *Notice* problems that arise because of "diversity."

3. *Do something* immediately to resolve the problem.

Understand

Understand that diversity brings both positive and negative consequences. Just as a diverse staff can open an organization to new ideas and allow it access into new markets, having a diverse staff can bring a variety of conflict-filled events that the physician executive will be expected to manage deftly. If diversity means the condition of being different from all others, a staff is diverse even if it is composed of people who are similar ethnically, racially, and by age and gender. Granted, some organizations are less diverse or have fewer diversity-related problems than others, but the only truly nondiverse work setting is the sole proprietorship. Therefore, there will always be some diversity-related problems to manage.

Understand that diversity goes much deeper than having the right demographic mix or being politically correct. With regard to diversity, actions will always speak louder than words. It would be wise to set some private time aside in which to examine contributions to diversity problems that you might inadvertently make. Are all staff requests for holidays given equal consideration? Do two people on the staff make widely divergent salaries even though they have the same education and experience? How are staff members who annoy you the most and the least treated? How do you feel about the employee who takes off time to care for a sick child and about childless staff members putting in more hours to cover for that employee? Do women, disabled individuals, "difficult" physicians, etc. belong in the workplace? Would you honestly prefer to have a staff made up of clones of yourself?

A commitment to successful diversity management is an all or nothing proposition. Remember that workplace diversity deals with interpersonal interactions and, as the saying goes, "While you might fool some of the people some of the time, you can't fool all of the people all of the time." Ignored or unresolved diversity problems ultimately result in decreased staff effectiveness and productivity. If you are not committed to supporting staff members in their endeavors by providing appropriate role modeling and by ensuring that they have the skills to manage their differences, you will be spending much of your working day handling problems that you probably could have avoided.

Notice

If a tree falls in the forest but no one is there to hear it, does it make a sound? If you believe the answer to this question is yes, you have to believe that diversity-related problems exist in your staff *even if you don't hear about them*. It's your job to take a regular walk through the forest known as your workplace to catch the sound of as many trees falling as possible.

Notice what beliefs your employees and patients bring to the workplace because of their culture, gender, age, education, etc. and what their impact is on patients, the rest of your staff, and other employees. For example, in the sexual harassment arena, many problems are caused by someone acting in a manner acceptable to their culture but not in one that would be considered appropriate in the professional American work force. Think about whether or not your providers are aware of the context in which their patients, their peers, and ancillary staff regard them.

Notice how interpersonal conflict manifests itself among staff members. Overt signs of interpersonal conflict include constant arguing with or badmouthing about other staff members. Rarely, there will be an out-and-out refusal to work with another employee. More covert signs of conflict include repeated backstabbing behaviors, withholding of vital information, "forgetting" to follow routine protocols, calling in sick when assigned to work with someone who makes them feel uncomfortable, not meeting deadlines, and general poor work quality. Also, if the staff is of small enough size, try to think about what motivates each one of them and what drives each of them crazy. Use your answers to this question to help you predict potential conflicts among staff members.

Do Something

Immediately. Diversity-related problems not only cause dissatisfaction among those directly affected, but, in the long run, can cause alienation of co-workers around them as well. This will eventually produce general morale problems throughout the staff. The risks of delaying intervention on diversity-related problems are a perceived loss of credibility as a leader and decreased impact of your eventual intervention on the staff. In addition, the likelihood of fostering passive or passive-aggressive reactions to the incident within your staff is greatly increased.

Listen to both sides. This sounds easy, but, in fact, active listening is a difficult skill to cultivate. Not only do you need to listen to what the speakers are saying, but you must convey to them that you understand the content of their story, both factual and emotional. Asking open-ended questions may help a reluctant speaker broaden his or her message. Restate the factual content of the message to ensure that you understand the facts accurately.

Make sure you reflect upon the emotional content of the speaker's message, using phrases such as "You seem...," "What I'm hearing is that...," and "I believe you feel..." Diversity problems can be highly emotionally charged. Acknowledgment of awareness of the speaker's emotions can help tremendously in relieving the speaker's anxiety and in building his or her trust in your ability to handle your job. At the end of the discussion, summarize, factually and emotionally, all that has been discussed. Make the speaker aware that he or she has an opportunity to clarify any misunderstandings.

Be sure to give both sides an opportunity to speak to you about the problem in a private setting. For various reasons, such as fear, embarrassment, etc., a person may be unable to adequately convey his or her side of the story with the other party in the room. Once you feel you understand the story and its implications for those involved, it becomes appropriate to conduct a discussion with both parties present.

At that point, review what you know about the problem with the parties involved. Be clear on the current position or relevant policy of the organization and explain that position or policy to all involved. There are times when the organization may not have a clear position on a particular issue. Don't panic. Remember, you're in charge of your staff, and, within that context, you can set your own rules. If you are concerned about doing that, speak to human resources, risk management, or legal counsel to make sure what you propose is within appropriate legal bounds.

It is also very important to define the future expectations of the involved parties. This may include describing acceptable behaviors and/or desired outcomes. Additional diversity training may be warranted for some staff members. If the problem is such that remediation is possible, that should be requested of the appropriate party or parties. Often, the best remediation is no more than an apology or an admittance of wrongdoing and an agreement that the behaviors leading to the problem won't happen again. Unfortunately, in some circumstances this can be exceedingly difficult to obtain from the people involved. Remediation can also be provided in the form of money or services, depending on the nature of the problem in question.

Occasionally, no matter what you do, the problem cannot be resolved. If the particular issue warrants such action, notify human resources, risk management, or your legal department about the situation and what you have done to rectify the problem. At some institutions, you may be able to request mediation or arbitration to resolve the problem. Find out in advance if such services are available.

Document everything as it occurs. When dealing with human beings in what can be emotion-laden settings, stories can change. Documenting also helps you keep everything clear when you are trying to define and resolve a problem. Also, good documentation is crucial should your problem ever end up in court.

Last of all, don't forget to follow up. The hard work you have had to do to remedy the situation isn't over yet. Just because you've gotten someone to agree to something doesn't make it so. It is your responsibility to check with the parties involved to make sure that what was agreed upon is being followed to everyone's satisfaction, including your own.

Follow up can be as simple as informally asking staff members involved if things are working out the way they intended. Depending on the nature of the incident, you may need to monitor work volume or quality. Also, you may need feedback from those on the periphery—patients, co-workers, ancillary workers, etc. If you do, be sure that any one who speaks with you has no fear of reprisal or compromise of status, position, or confidentiality. Depending on the severity of the problem, follow up may entail weekly meetings with those involved until the problem is resolved to your satisfaction.

Bibliography

Dreachslin, J., and Hunt, P. *Diversity Leadership*. Chicago, Ill.: Health Administration Press, 1996

Focusing solely on diversity within the health care industry and intended for health care executives, consultants and health care management students, this is the most academic of the books listed here. The book presents a framework for diversity leadership, outlining a process of finding common ground and shared purpose in today's diverse health care organizations.

Gardenschwartz, L., and Rowe, A. *Managing Diversity: A Complete Desk Reference and Planning Guide*. Burr Ridge, Ill.: Irwin Professional Publishing, 1993.

A general text on diversity, this book contains numerous quizzes and worksheets to help assess and promote diversity awareness within an organization.

Gardenschwartz, L., and Rowe, A. *Managing Diversity in Health Care*. San Francisco, Calif.: Jossey-Bass Publishers, 1998.

This book takes the authors' general concepts and approaches to diversity and applies them to health care organizations.

Nicarthy, G., and others. *You Don't Have To Take It! A Woman's Guide to Confronting Emotional Abuse at Work*. Seattle, Wash.: Seal Press, 1993.

Although not billed specifically as a book on diversity, this book manages to touch upon every diversity-related problem one can think of. More important, it presents excellent ideas on how to handle yourself when personally confronted with a difficult diversity problem. While addressing a female audience, this book could nevertheless provide some useful insights for male executives regarding problems that women face in the workforce.

Wagner, E. *Sexual Harassment in the Workplace: How to Prevent, Investigate, and Resolve Problems in Your Organization.* New York, N.Y.: AMACOM, 1992.

Everything you need to know about sexual harassment in one short volume. If you're interested in this topic, this book is a superb place to start.

Doreen Moreira, MD, CPE, FACPE, is a Principal and Managing Partner, Conflict Free Workplaces, Cabin John, Maryland.

Chapter

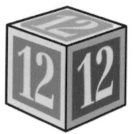

The Economics and Fiscal Management of Provider Organizations

by Hugh W. Long, MBA, PhD, JD, and Mark A. Covaleski, PhD, CPA

Fiscal or financial management covers a broad spectrum of activities associated with the economics of an organization. Fiscal management encompasses tasks such as writing down in monetary terms a record of the organization's actual historical activity; analyzing that past performance; determining a variety of "costs" for a product or unit of service; raising money for short-term or long-term purposes; designing future performance goals (budgeting); forecasting changes in local or national economic environments and assessing how such changes will affect the organization and how the organization should respond to such changes; and, finally, making resource allocation decisions, both small (how much cash should we have in the bank) and large (should we undertake a $50 million expansion).

The purposes of this chapter are to:

- Introduce you to some very basic aspects of fiscal management and what various fiscal specialists do.

- Provide you some familiarity with internal fiscal information, financial statements, and the uses of each.

- Give you some understanding of the economics that underlie organizational financing and resource allocation decisions.

The two major organizational fiscal management domains are accounting and finance, each of which covers a wide and diverse range of activities. While literally "to account" means "to keep a record of," accounting encompasses a great deal more than simply keeping records. Similarly, the literal meaning of "to finance" is to gather money for some particular use (e.g., meet a payroll, buy a piece of equipment), but finance involves much more than simply amassing stacks of money.

Much of what accounting and finance address is quite distinct. For example, the information gathering and processing used to generate traditional financial statements (e.g., income statements and balance sheets) has virtually no overlap at all with the information gathering and processing used for asset acquisition analyses. These two distinct fiscal activities, the first a part of accounting, the second a part of finance, are built on quite separate and different sets of concepts and assumptions. As discussed below, using finance cash-flow concepts to define "income" would be as misleading as using financial accounting mechanisms for asset acquisition decisions. Serious errors, indeed irrational outcomes, would result. Hence, identifying the distinct characteristics and uses of each set of tools is a major priority for managers. At the same time, some areas of accounting and finance are closely related, indeed are highly complementary. Much of what managerial accounting addresses requires the same kind of forecasting, modeling, and "what if" analysis that is also central to corporate finance.

Accounting and Accounting Systems

As suggested above, the field of accounting involves many subspecialties. Internal to health care and other business organizations, one finds financial accounting and managerial and/or cost accounting. Financial accounting has the primary role of keeping records and preparing financial statements; managerial accounting addresses budgeting and control issues (budgeting is really a form of making very short-term resource allocation decisions); and cost accounting identifies costs throughout the organization, allocating those costs to various services or programs (units of output). Other accounting subspecialties include actuaries, who make statistical predictions about the frequency with which certain events (e.g., number of births during a one-year period for a specified population group) may take place; tax accountants, who specialize in working with the income tax code and regulations; and, in the health care industry, accountants, who specialize in the technical aspects of health insurance and payment systems. Accounting firms use certified public accountants (CPAs) to audit the financial statements of client organizations to certify the validity of those statements in accordance with certain rules. CPAs, and often certified management accountants (CMAs), also provide consulting services related to the fiscal management of the organization.

Financial Accounting

The Users of Financial Accounting Information

Financial accounting information is the result of a process of identifying, measuring, recording, and communicating the economic events of an organization (business or nonbusiness) to interested users of the information. This information is summarized and presented in three important financial statements: the balance sheet, the income statement, and the statement of cash flows. Because these statements communicate financial information about an enterprise, accounting is often called "the language of business." An understanding of financial statements provides the users of this information with important insights as to the economic status of the health care organization.

The predominant users of financial accounting information—investors and creditors—have a direct financial interest in evaluating the economic status of the health care organization. Other parties, such as taxing authorities, regulatory agencies, labor unions, customers, and economic planners, may have an indirect financial interest in the economic status of the health care organization and would also be users of financial accounting information. However, our major concern is to understand financial accounting from the eyes of investors and lenders.

Investors typically represent the predominant financial interest in a health care organization. One of the unique features of the health care industry relative to many other industries is that the term "investor" reflects a variety of different forms, depending on the mission of the health care organization. Investors might literally purchase stock in the case of a for-profit health care organization where the shares of stock are sold publicly. However, the term "investors" in the health care industry might also cover situations in which there is no stock as in classic not-for-profit organizations such as religious-based health care systems, community hospitals, or large not-for-profit private systems. These traditional not-for-profit health care organizations have no explicit investor groups (as reflected by shares of stock), but they can represent their communities at large (whether defined in terms of religious, geographical, or common interests) that have donated and generated wealth for the organizations over the years, thus implicitly representing investor groups. While these implicit investor groups do not receive financial remuneration, such as dividend payments, for their investments, the investing community expects not-for-profit organizations to reciprocate through such paybacks as charity care, support of research, community education, etc.

The critical commonality across these different types of investor groups in the health care industry is that they all have boards of directors. And whether the health care organization is for-profit or not-for-profit, or issues stock or does not issue stock, the board of directors has a critical fiscal stewardship responsibility—ensuring the economic viability of the health care organization for the broader investors who own the organization. The relationship of investor to organization through financial accounting information becomes crystallized or operationalized in the relationship between the board of directors and the management of the health care organization. Exploiting charitable assets for personal gain can take place in health care organizations if fiscal stewardship by board members is not upheld. Someone has to be watching the store.

Lenders constitute the second broadly defined group that has a direct financial interest in the economic status of the health care organization in the form of the resources that the lending group has provided to the organization. As one of the two dominant sources of financial capital for the health care organization, lenders expect remuneration. Such remuneration is not in the form of a cash dividend, enhancement of economic value of stock (capital appreciation), or a metaphorical dividend such as charity care to the community that the investor group might receive. It is in the form of interest payments received by the lenders from the health care organization. Lenders represent their direct financial interests through the contract of the debt instrument (debt covenants), which often specifies financial results that must be achieved by management and clear consequences for failure to achieve them.

Although these two groups—investors and creditors—are critical users of financial accounting information as a result of their direct financial interests, they do not simply read the financial statements. They can also actively pressure management and the health care organization to achieve desired financial results within these financial statements. This pressure eventually becomes translated into the internal management structure of the health care organization in the form of budgets, pricing strategies, cost cutting strategies, and the like.

Regulation and Standards in Financial Accounting

As a consequence of the Great Depression of the 1930s and the resultant widespread collapse of businesses and the securities market, the federal government intervened and began regulating financial statements and accounting standards. A direct result of this collapse in the financial markets was the creation of the Securities and Exchange Commission (SEC) as an independent regulatory agency. The SEC has the legal power to enforce the form and content of financial statements for companies that wish to sell securities to the public. To do this, the SEC has developed a common set of standards, called generally accepted accounting principles (GAAP), to govern preparation and presentation of financial statements. These principles apply to the area of financial accounting as distinct from other areas of accounting, such as managerial accounting and tax accounting. If a company does not follow GAAP, it will not be allowed to issue securities. The SEC believes that financial statements that follow GAAP provide investors, creditors, and other interested parties with useful information to make informed decisions.

For the most part, the SEC has delegated responsibility for establishing GAAP to a rule-making body called the Financial Accounting Standards Board (FASB). FASB is a private organization whose mission is to establish and improve standards of financial accounting and reporting. Just because FASB has the authority from the SEC and the private resources to study and rule upon different financial reporting issues does not guarantee that those in the accounting profession will carry out their work in the manner prescribed by FASB. The American Institute of Certified Public Accountants (AICPA) derives the actual rules and documents (for example, there is an Audit Guide for the Health Care Industry) that public accounting firms and individual CPAs follow when auditing an organization's financial statements. The auditor's report is a letter from the outside auditor giving an opinion on whether or not the firm's financial statements are a fair presentation of the firm's results of operations, cash flows, and financial position in accordance with GAAP. Essentially, these AICPA rulings and audit guides govern the accounting profession and align the work of professional accountants with GAAP. Public accounting firms or individual CPAs who choose not to follow AICPA rulings and documents are subject to strong sanctions by AICPA. In turn, if AICPA rulings and documents stray too far from GAAP, the profession runs the risk of facing the wrath of the SEC.

The Accrual Concept

A critical issue in the financial accounting model pertains to the measurement of the economic event. For example, let us say that an organization provides $700 worth of services in November and does not receive payment until February of the next year. Because the delay crosses over the December 31 fiscal year end, there will be two different accounting results, depending on whether one is using the cash or the accrual basis of accounting.

Under the cash basis of accounting, the organization does not recognize the revenue until the cash is received in February. The argument here is that the critical event is the receipt of cash. The accrual concept states that earned revenue does not necessarily correspond to the receipt of cash. Earned revenue is recognized when a service has been provided and there is a corresponding economic obligation by the purchaser. The asset received in exchange for the services performed may be cash (or some other thing of value), but more often it is accounts receivable. The accrual basis of accounting calls the critical event the provision of service in November. The concern under the accrual accounting method ties back to our discussion of the objectives of financial statements. The argument is that the cash basis of accounting has failed to portray the economic status of the organization. In this case, it can be argued that the cash basis of accounting has understated revenue by $700 in November and overstated it by $700 in February.

So how does the accrual basis propose to remedy this problem. First, the accrual basis will recognize $700 in revenue in November, even though the cash has not yet been received. The asset that will be booked in lieu of cash will be accounts receivable, which, in theory, is almost as good as cash. This recognizes revenue when the service has been provided and matches revenue with the proper period. The slight tradeoff the accrual basis has made is in terms of objectivity; that is, the $700 in accounts receivable may not all eventually translate into cash because of bad debts. Nonetheless, the accounting profession is comfortable enough with the benefits of the tradeoff to recommend accrual basis accounting over cash basis accounting in GAAP. In short, we book (make an entry, in this case debit) $700 to the balance sheet as an asset in the form of accounts receivable and book (credit) $700 to the income statement as revenue in the form of patient services revenue.

Taking this illustration further, when the cash does arrive in February, the accrual basis of accounting can handle this fairly easily in its bookkeeping. Most important is not to double count the revenue. The bookkeeping entries go like this: we book (debit) $700 to the balance sheet as an asset in the form of cash and book (credit) $700 to the balance sheet in the form of a deduction from accounts receivable, thus bringing our accounts receivable balance down to $0. Accounts receivable serves as a bridge (setting it up in November, taking it down in February) that divorces revenue recognition in November from receipt of cash in February. When we receive the cash in February, we do not book revenue again but simply exchange assets—bring in (increase) cash and take down (reduce) accounts receivable.

Let's follow the accrual versus cash basis debate through on the expense side. Let's assume that the organization had payroll obligations of $400 for the last two weeks of December that did not get paid until January. Since this delay crosses over the December 31 fiscal year end, there will again be two different results. The cash basis of accounting does not recognize the expense until the cash is paid—January. The argument here is that the critical event is the payment of cash. The accrual basis of accounting argues that the critical event is the economic obligation related to services provided to the organization by its employees in December. In this case, it can be argued that the cash basis of accounting has understated expenses by $400 in December and overstated these expenses by $400 in January. So how does the accrual basis propose to remedy this problem? First, in December, the accrual basis will recognize a $400 expense even though the cash has not yet been paid. The item that will be booked in lieu of the take down of cash will be a liability—accrued expenses—which, in theory, is a short-term obligation that will need to be paid from cash. This recognizes the expense when the service has been provided and matches expenses to the proper period. We book (debit) $400 to the income statement in the form of salary expense and book (credit) $400 to the balance sheet in the form of accrued expenses.

When the cash does get paid out in January 2000, the accrual basis of accounting can handle the transaction fairly easily. Most important is to not double count the expense. The bookkeeping entries go like this: We book (credit) $400 to the balance sheet as a deduction from an asset (a deduction of cash) and book (debit) $400 to the balance sheet in the form of a removal from the accrued payroll expense liability, thus bringing our accrued expenses balance down to $0. The accrued expenses account serves as a bridge (setting it up in December, taking it down in January) that divorces the expense recognition in December from the receipt of cash in January. When we pay out the cash in January, we do not book payroll expense again but simply make exchanges in the balance sheet—pay out cash (decrease assets) and take down accrued expenses (decrease liabilities).

Managerial and Cost Accounting

As important as the statements produced by financial accounting systems are, other analyses of the information amassed by the accounting system are even more important for internal managerial purposes. In addition, organizations typically engage in various extensions of financial accounting activity in the form of cost accounting and budgeting. Although cost accounting is sometimes viewed as a subset of managerial accounting, managerial and cost accounting together deal with formulating budgets, analyzing actual fiscal performance in comparison to what was budgeted, projecting the effects of management decisions on future financial accounting statements, identifying actual costs of producing services, calculating "full" costs of services using cost allocation formulas, and dealing with other related issues of cost and payment (e.g., internal transfer pricing, income distribution mechanisms, and maximizing third-party payments). The sections that follow offer a survey of managerial and cost accounting activities.

Cost Concepts

Cost Behavior

Preparation of a budget requires a basic understanding of cost behavior in relation to volume and, as will be discussed later, in terms of responsibility centers. Costs can be expressed as they relate to changes in activities, such as occupancy rates, patient visits, patient mix, services provided, etc. Costs described in terms of activity levels (volume) are usually separated in terms of fixed and variable components. A fixed cost is a cost that does not change within the relevant range of alternative levels of activity.[1] For example, the manager's salary will not typically change with the number of patients. This does not mean it cannot be changed, but it changes as a function of management decisions rather than of activity level. Variable costs, on the other hand, are costs that vary directly with volume. For example, raw food costs will vary with the number of meals served, the costs of pharmacy items can vary with the number of procedures performed, etc. These types of costs are illustrated graphically in figure 1, below.

The manager must work with per unit comparisons in addition to the total costs approach displayed in figure 1. Costs are typically expressed on a per unit basis for reimbursement, rate setting, and billing activities. Total costs are a combination of variable and fixed costs; total costs per unit are a combination of variable costs per unit and fixed costs per unit. On a per unit basis, variable costs are the same for each individual unit of service. For example, if the reagents required for one test are $2.00, they are $4.00 for two tests, $6.00 for three tests, etc. Of course, the average or per unit cost remains at $2.00 regardless of volume. This cost relationship can be expressed graphically, as shown in figure 2, page 136.

Figure 1. Total Cost Curves

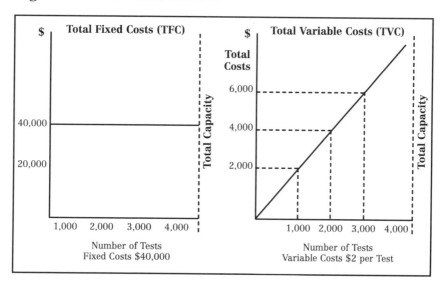

Figure 2. Per Test Variable Cost Curve

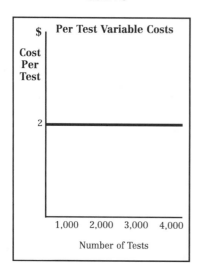

Number of Tests

Figure 3. Per Test Fixed Cost

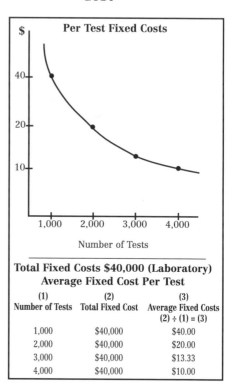

Total Fixed Costs $40,000 (Laboratory)
Average Fixed Cost Per Test

(1) Number of Tests	(2) Total Fixed Cost	(3) Average Fixed Costs (2) ÷ (1) = (3)
1,000	$40,000	$40.00
2,000	$40,000	$20.00
3,000	$40,000	$13.33
4,000	$40,000	$10.00

In determining the total costs per unit, the determination of the fixed costs component presents a more difficult challenge, complicated by the large proportion that fixed costs represent of total costs in the health care industry. Because fixed costs per unit are obtained by dividing total fixed costs by the level of activity, the more units provided, the lower the fixed costs per unit. Continuing our test example, suppose the laboratory supervisor is paid $40,000. At a volume of 1,000 tests, this calculates to $40 per test. But fixed costs per unit for 2,000 tests would be $40,000 divided by 2,000, or $20 per test. As most experienced managers have observed, volume is of vital concern for financial well-being because of the heavy fixed cost nature of most health care services. The relationship of per unit fixed costs to volume is illustrated in figure 3, sbove.

Average (Full) Cost Determination

Determination of what a test costs is typically based on the average cost of providing the test (total costs divided by volume = average cost, where total costs = total variable costs + total fixed costs). As discussed above, fixed costs per unit will vary as the level of output or volume changes. Therefore, it is impossible to determine per unit costs without first estimating the level of

Figure 4. Average (Full) Cost Determination

(1) Estimated Number of Tests	(2) Average Variable Cost	(3) Average Fixed Cost $40,000 : Col. (1)	(4) Full Cost Per Test Col. (2) + Col. (3)
1,000	$2	$40.00	$42.00
2,000	2	$20.00	$22.00
3,000	2	$13.33	$15.33
4,000	2	$10.00	$12.00
5,000	2	$ 8.00	$10.00
6,000	2	$ 6.67	$ 8.67
7,000	2	$ 5.71	$ 7.71
8,000	2	$ 5.00	$ 7.00

output. Figure 4, above, presents an analysis of the laboratory example discussed above in which capacity is now assumed to be 8,000 tests for the period covered by the analysis.

Computation of full costs per unit is an important element in establishing prices or rates. The computation depends on the planned fixed costs and estimated volume, because the variable costs component is usually not sensitive to changes in the level of output within the relevant range of output. Hence, if one wants to establish a price or rate that covers the costs (total or per test), the price or rate necessarily relies on the underlying fixed costs and volume assumptions.

Related Cost Definitions

Management must be aware of cost classifications in addition to the fixed and variable cost behavior dichotomy. One of the more useful categorizations is direct and indirect costs. Direct costs can be traced directly to the cost objective being measured. For example, the costs of the laboratory test, whether fixed or variable, are direct costs. Conversely, costs that are necessary but are not directly involved with the test are indirect costs. Examples of indirect costs include senior management salaries and the cost of running the business office. These are part of the total costs of providing the test, but they cannot be traced directly to the test (and, in fact, support other outputs in addition to this test). Still, they must be allocated to this test through some mechanism. The distinction between direct and indirect costs is crucial in responsibility accounting and reporting. By separating costs into direct and indirect categories, managers and supervisors can be held accountable for costs they can control. An example of this type of report is illustrated in figure 5, page 138. In figure 5, even though an overall loss is reported, a $270 positive controllable operating margin has been achieved in terms of direct costs over which departmental personnel have control.

Figure 5. Responsibility Center Reporting

Department Activities for the Month of May 199x		
	Dollars	**Percentage**
Net Revenues	$3,000	100
Controllable Operating Expenses		
Variable Costs	<u>450</u>	<u>15</u>
Contribution Margin	$2,550	85
Controllable Fixed Costs	<u>$2,280</u>	<u>76</u>
Controllable Operating Margin	$270	9
Allocated Costs	<u>1,500</u>	<u>50</u>
Net Operating Margin (Loss)	**($1,230)**	**(41)**

Cost Estimating Techniques

Considerable progress has been made in the recent past in using statistical modeling techniques to estimate costs and cost behavior in health care settings. Most of these techniques involve a form of regression analysis in which independent variables such as patient days are used to predict dependent variables such as nursing hours and supply costs on the basis of historical relationships. For example, a relationship between volume of laboratory tests and supervisory hours could be presented on a scatter diagram as shown in figure 6, below. The relatively flat nature of the curve indicates that supervisory hours are fixed for the range of tests covered. The slope of the regression line in figure 7, below, indicates that technician hours increase with volume of tests, as common sense would suggest. Supervisors are involved with administration and supervision of the technicians, while the technicians perform most of the direct work. Statistical techniques can be used to estimate the fixed and the variable portions of the technician hours.

Those who wish to explore these techniques in greater detail are encouraged to review the references for this section at the end of this chapter.

Figure 6.

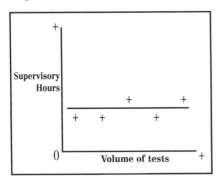

Figure 7.

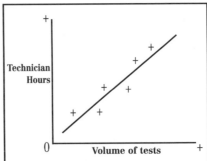

Overhead Costs

Overhead or indirect costs can represent a significant part of the total costs of the health care provider. Costs that cannot be traced directly to the provision of individual patient services typically fall into the overhead area. The salaries of senior management, clerical staff, and accounting staff and general maintenance/housekeeping costs are examples of overhead costs. These costs are difficult to control, because, while they are necessary, they are typically not directly related to the provision of patient services and thus to revenues.

In addition, because there is no direct relationship between revenues and costs, it is difficult to determine the "correct" amount of these costs, i.e., should they be expanded or should they be cut? What should be the size of a business office? How many accountants, clerks, and administrators are needed? What type of equipment do they require? How much space should be allotted to them?

These decisions—and their resultant costs—are not directly related to the number of patient visits, the number of discharges, or the number of procedures performed, but they are an essential part of providing high-quality service to patients. In order to determine the full cost of providing services, it is necessary to devise some method of allocating a "fair" share of overhead costs to each activity being performed.

Allocation Methods

Allocation of overhead costs to the various activities of the organization requires development of an overhead charge per unit of service. Overhead charges are basically "average" shares of total overhead costs that can be applied to the service performed. Total overhead costs can be determined from the budget before the period of operations begins and from the accounting system after the period of operations ends. These total overhead costs are divided by the activity base selected to obtain the overhead charge (total overhead costs divided by volume). Each unit of service receives an estimated share of the overhead cost through this average rate. For example, business office costs could be allocated on the basis of the number of employees in each section. Nursing administration costs could be allocated according to the number of FTE nurses or the level of patient activity. Social service costs could be allocated according to the number of users or the total hours of service received by patients.

Allocation of overhead requires that the health care provider be divided into patient care centers and patient support centers. Patient care centers are departments that provide direct care and for which revenue can be recognized. Support centers are all other activities or cost centers, such as the business office, housekeeping, or marketing.

Summary

In order to determine what a service or an activity costs, it is necessary to define exactly the purpose for which the cost information is being collected.

Because of the effect of fixed costs on per unit costs, such cost figures are appropriate only for the volume selected. Statistical techniques are available to assist managers in estimating costs and cost behavior. Overhead costs present special challenges, and choices surrounding overhead allocations can significantly affect calculated per unit total costs.

Pricing Strategies and the Role of Managerial Accounting

An important part of managerial decision making pertains to establishing or accepting a price for health care services. For example, in a fee-for-service environment, health care organizations need to determine whether they should offer discounts for large volume to valued payer groups such as large HMOs or business coalitions. In a capitated environment, the health care organization needs to determine the premium amount within which it is willing to risk responsibility for the provision of health care services. And in the case of payers such as Medicare and Medicaid, for which the health care organization is basically a price taker, the organization still needs to know the impact of this de facto decision to sell services to the government. Understanding how to analyze product costs, such as costs by services, costs by DRG classification, or costs by enrollment population, is important for making such pricing decisions. Even when prices are set by overall market supply and demand forces (or by government power) and the health care organization has little or no influence on prices for services, the organization still has to make decisions about the extent and the mix of services offered. In short, an important function of management accounting is to supply cost information that helps support pricing decisions.

Because the financial resources of most health care providers are derived chiefly from revenue received for providing health care services, it is essential that health care managers establish rates or prices that will generate revenues sufficient to meet the organization's total financial requirements. Total financial requirements include the full cost of doing business (operating expenses). However, it is important that revenue provide for the replenishment of existing assets; the costs of assets to expand into new services; and, in the case of a for-profit organization, dividend rewards to investors.

One of the critical underpinnings of past pricing strategies of health care organizations was cross-subsidization, which essentially meant markups (overcharging) on many routine services, such as radiology and ancillary services, and undercharging on other services to support teaching and care for the poor. Such cross-subsidization (also sometimes called "cost-shifting) helped many hospitals to function as full-service institutions. Major purchasers are no longer interested in having cross-subsidies built into their prices to support the provision of health care services to others who are not the purchaser's moral and economic responsibility. Health care organizations that continue to base pricing strategies on extensive cross-subsidization will contribute to two adverse selections:

- Healthier populations will move to providers whose prices reflect the real value to the purchasers.

- Less healthy populations will move to health care organizations that offer services below value (the difference that has historically been subsidized by other groups or services). This adverse selection will challenge the ability of health care providers to function as full-service institutions.

Today, however, the pricing strategies of health care organizations take place in a much more competitive marketplace. As health care organizations begin to understand the competitive forces driving much of the health care industry, one of their important insights is whether they can influence the price of their health care service/product. If the health care organization is one of many providers in its area and there is little to distinguish its services, economic theory suggests that prices will be set by supply and demand. No health care organization can influence prices significantly by its own decisions. In such a situation, the health care organization may well be a price-taker, because it more or less follows prices set in the marketplace. This is probably the case for most health care organizations.

As a general rule, health care organizations that are price-takers need to take the industry price as a given and concentrate on the other two critical variables (cost structure and volume) to affect the fourth variable (profits). This price-taker health care organization should offer as much as it can of its services whose costs are less than the industry price (even if the industry price has become significantly discounted). This appears to be a straightforward comment, but it does raise two important issues regarding managerial accounting. Management needs to decide what costs are relevant to the decision at hand. That is, direct costs are often easy to identify, but how are overhead costs affected by the decision to accept a certain volume level? This is more difficult to determine. It also must be recognized that, in the short term, managers may not have much flexibility to alter their fixed costs. Therefore, only variable costs may be relevant to the pricing decision (i.e., to accept the offered price for services).

In contrast, health care organizations with relatively few competitors, large market shares, and leadership in the industry must decide what prices to set for their products/services. If the health care organization's products/services can be differentiated from others because of enhanced quality, features, service, or other characteristics, the organization has more ability to set prices for them. Such health care providers are price-setters.

As a general decision rule, health care organizations that are price-setters (or price-setters for certain services/products) are in a position to make longer term pricing decisions when full costs are more relevant to the pricing decision at hand. These full costs include not only direct and variable costs but also proportionate burdens of the fixed cost structure and overhead. While such an approach to pricing strategy is desirable for all health care organizations (and, indeed, was basically facilitated by the regulatory environment), price-takers are not in a position to price on a full-cost basis.

It is important to recognize the fluid nature of the price-taker and the price-setter. These positions in the marketplace change regularly. For example, once two price-taker health care providers merge, they may become a price-setter as a merged entity. Also, organizations can have outstanding reputations for certain services and can command a premium to cover their full costs. For other services, however, they may be price-takers. Or, for the same service, the health care organization might be a price-taker in one geographical market and price more on marginal costs and a price-setter in another geographical market where it would price the service on more of a full-cost, premium basis.

Specific Issues Pertaining to Pricing Strategies for Health Care Services

One of the most significant changes in the health care industry in the past 20 years has been a dramatic shift in power from the seller to the buyer of health care services. Buyers are forming local coalitions to increase their financial leverage in negotiating with providers. Some would say that this shift means that revenues health care institutions receive will more and more be dictated by large purchasers of care—monopsonists and oligopsonists. These predominant purchasers of health care—HMOs, business coalitions, insurance companies, and government—have served notice that the marketplace is to be taken seriously in the dynamics that determine the prices of health care services. Furthermore, the seriousness of the marketplace as a formidable buyer is compounded by excess capacity in the health care industry. Dominant business coalitions can change the dynamics of pricing strategies of the health care organizations.

A final example of the seriousness of purchasers of health care services is reflected in the relationship between the auto industry and health care providers. The Big 3 automakers treat health care providers as they do suppliers of windshield wipers, batteries, and brakes, demanding top quality at the lowest cost and telling them exactly how to do it. These manufacturers are actively dispatching their productivity experts to their health care providers to improve productivity. This is important to auto manufacturers because the health bill for active and retired employees exceeds what these companies spend on a car's steel. Those outlays compare with minimal cost per car for the factories of some foreign automakers and almost zero cost for producers in countries with socialized medicine.

Among the concerns about the increasing strength of the buyer in the health care marketplace is the belief that these buyers, despite the rhetoric of cost and quality, will purchase exclusively on a low-cost basis. For example, one health care provider has outstanding mortality data for bypass surgery (1.4 percent). This excellent quality has been reflected in higher charges, with few discounts given to HMOs. The result has been that regional HMOs have chosen an alternative health care provider with a higher mortality data that was among the earliest hospitals to agree to discount prices for HMOs. Similarly, another provider has attempted to market its reputation to health plans at higher prices, such as that for heart surgery, which is at least $2,000 above competition. This provider has been losing business to an alternative health care provider that has lackluster results (mortality rates) but continues to win discounted contracts from managed care plans. NYU

Medical Center is another standout in heart surgery rankings, but it can't get HMOs to pay extra for its services.

According to many benefit managers, the market will become more consumer-driven because of the availability of increasingly useful outcome measurements. Certainly this demand for, and use of, quality information is at the heart of the logical purchasing coalitions. These groups achieves the goals of cost management and improved employee health care by being less prescriptive about health benefits and more proactive in demanding that health plans report better information about patient satisfaction, clinical outcomes, and overall value in delivering health-related services.

The increasing importance of quality in the consumer's decision to purchase health care services has been recognized by Standard & Poor and Moody's, which use quality assessments to determine hospitals' creditworthiness. These credit rating organizations feel that quality assessments are important because they demonstrate the stability of markets and demand forecasts and the ability to control resource use in times of declining reimbursement. For example, a quality measurement and management system helped one major health care provider obtain a double-A rating on a $90 million financing because it showed that the organization was positioning itself as a leader in documenting the quality of services it offered.

Many believe that deregulation and price competition in the health care industry will raise service quality and drive costly excess capacity out of the market, much as they have in the airline, trucking, banking, and railroad industries. Market competition has resulted in the end to managing hospitals as if they were country clubs, void of serious concerns for productivity and effectiveness. Although price elasticity of demand for hospital care is still relatively low, pricing decisions are still important to major purchasers.

Implications of Managed Care and the Assumption of Risk

Managed care covers a range of pricing philosophies: from fee-for-service, where the challenge is in setting discounts, to semi-flat rate such as DRGs and commercial product line pricing, where some risk is assumed by the provider, to fully capitated arrangements that expose the health care provider to significant risk if utilization goes unmanaged. For example, fee-for-service pricing essentially puts the provider at risk for only direct costs of service provision and levels of discounts offered. There is basically a positive incentive for the health care organization to utilize more resources at a micro-level (more tests, more procedures, etc.), keep the patient in the hospital more days, and admit more patients to the hospital. The only way the provider can be hurt in this payment arrangement is if the net revenue after discounting the unit of service fails to exceed the direct costs of that unit of service. DRG payment, or the related commercial product line payment such as fixed-price contract for kidney transplants, now provides negative incentives for the hospital to increase utilization at the micro-level—resource by resource—and/or to increase days in the hospital. However, under this payment philosophy, it is still in the hospital's interest to maximize the number of hospital admissions pertaining to this DRG or commercial product line.

Finally, the capitated payment philosophy provides negative incentives for the health care provider to maximize utilization across all three levels—at the micro-resource use, in terms of intensity, and in terms of encounters.

The whole focus of managed care systems as they move from fee-for-service toward capitation is to change the provider from a revenue center to a cost center. This focus becomes consistent with a target costing approach to pricing strategies in which the provider competes on competitive premium prices established in the marketplace and works backward to get its cost structure in line with market-defined prices. Part of the work on cost structure is dealt with by cascading health care services down to the lowest cost mode of delivery (e.g., moving away from the hospital) while maintaining quality. One CFO from a health system stated "We don't consider ourselves as being in the hospital business....we view our hospital as a cost center, not as a revenue center as in the past." Essentially, the premium dollar has moved outside the hospital toward outpatient, nursing home, and home health care services. As a health care organization moves from fee-for-service to prepaid practice, the primary emphasis moves from revenue production to cost control.

Examples of moving away from a strict fee-for-service pricing strategy to a more risk-assuming strategy can be seen in the development of commercial DRG approaches in which the health care organization commits itself to a price for a defined diagnosis. For example, renowned transplant centers are adapting pricing strategies based on fixed-price contracts that cover nearly all the expenses associated with organ transplants—cost of obtaining the organ, surgery fees, other hospital and physician charges, and a year of follow-up. To gain more HMO patients, these institutions are aggressively marketing their services in terms of these fixed-price strategies.

The switch to DRGs changed many hospital service departments from profit centers to cost centers, but left the entire hospital as a profit center. Further movement toward fixed pricing, such as capitation payment, makes the hospital a service arm of a larger, more encompassing profit-making entity, the managed care enterprise. As a result of this change, the hospital's relationship to the organization changes from a producer to a consumer of revenues. And just as many health care organizations are adapting aggressive fixed-price strategies around product lines to win HMO patients, we also see health care providers adapting even more aggressive pricing strategies in terms of committing themselves to capitated revenues for defined populations. For example, one health care provider, in an unprecedented arrangement, agreed to provide comprehensive cancer care at a fixed price. This is the first contract of its kind in the cancer field. The provider receives a monthly fee per member in exchange for providing the HMO's patients with a full range of hospital, outpatient, and home care services. Similarly, another provider has signed a unique contract to provide oncological treatment under a capitated contract. The provider provides oncological treatment to the membership and is one of only a few contracts nationwide in which oncology has been carved out. Some HMOs believe the method will help shift financial risk and rewards to other specialty medical organizations that try to deliver high-quality care at low cost.

The shift of risks will mandate that health care providers obtain access to better cost and utilization information. While cost and utilization data are important to the management of fee-for-service care, data are critical for a health care organization offering prepaid care. There will be increased scrutiny of what employees are getting for the employer's money, with development of data systems by the purchasers of health care that will match or exceed the information system of the health care organization. Buyers are seeking providers with feedback processes that can provide them with information and data documenting both clinical efficacy and cost efficiency. Health care providers might be well served to develop joint ventures with employers to build databases that can meet the growing demands of accountability. These data (market, financial, utilization, quality, and patient satisfaction) need to be collected and analyzed on a real-time basis. Effective contract negotiation requires that a hospital know its costs and whether the rate structure covers these costs and related margins.

The Roles of Budgeting in Health Care Organizations

Budgeting is an important part of planning a health care organization's economic activity. The budget is probably the most fundamental financial document in a health care organization and is most likely the first encounter that a health care manager has with accounting information. The organizational budget is a basic tool for tying together the planning and the control functions of management. More specifically, budgeting involves detailed plans, expressed in quantitative terms, that specify how resources will be acquired and used during a specified period. The predominant portion of this quantified plan is expressed in economic terms. Because many of these economic terms pertain to costs and revenues, budgeting applies much of our knowledge of cost accounting and pricing.

However, this quantified economic plan is not a detached analysis done by accountants. Derivation and use of the plan should infiltrate the entire organization. Thus, the budgeting process serves to facilitate communication and coordination throughout the organization. Each manager must be aware of plans made by other managers for the organization to be effective as a whole; essentially this process integrates the plans of each manager in an organization. Finally, the budgeting process and the resultant approved budget plan serve to allocate limited organizational resources among competing uses. These three major uses of the organizational budget—quantify economic plan, facilitate communication and coordination, and allocate organizational resources—are the front end of budgeting processes.

The richness and relevance of budgeting, however, is that it goes beyond planning, communicating, and allocating processes. There is also a back end to the budgeting process at which budgets are used in a feedback mode. That is, budgeting serves to help control operations and related profits. Plans are subject to change, and the budget serves as a useful benchmark within this change. Comparing actual results with budgeted results helps to evaluate the performance of individuals, departments, product lines, capitated contracts, etc. Because budgets are used to evaluate performance, they can also be used to provide incentives for people to perform well. Furthermore, information pertaining to what actually happened versus what was planned is incorporated into future plans to improve the accuracy of the planning process. The budget process forms a continuous loop of information—planning, implementing, controlling, and feedback.

It is important, in using the budget as an analytical tool, that analysis of variance between planned results and actual results is approached systematically. The starting point is the static budget, which is simply the original approved budget that has not been adjusted for differences between planned and actual volumes of services provided. The problem with static budgets is that they provide an expected cost, revenue, and profit for a particular volume, hence the name static. At the end of a reporting period, it is highly unlikely that we will have attained exactly the expected output level. If that is the case (as it almost always is), we end up with an apples-to-oranges comparison. For example, we have budgeted costs at one volume level and actual costs at another volume level. Based on the discussion of cost behavior, it should be obvious that, as the volume of patients rises, variable costs must rise. Just as obviously, if volume falls, we would expect that variable costs will fall. However, with the static budget, we do not know if the difference between budgeted and actual costs is due to different volumes of services or some sort of underlying inefficiencies.

To explain what is driving the total variance, we must move from a static budget to a flexible budget. A flexible budget is one in which the approved budget has been adjusted for volume changes. Essentially, flexible budgets are devices to tell what the results (revenues, costs, and profits) would be if a volume level was actually attained. The flexible budget approach places emphasis on the volume of patients actually treated by the organization (or, in the case of capitation, the volume of patients enrolled in the contract). The front-end of the budgeting process is very much like generating pro forma income statements. In preparing these budgets, we could prepare alternate budgets based on a range of possible volume outcomes. Each of these pro forma income statements could be considered to be a flexible budget based on the costs, revenues, and profits that we would expect to incur at a specified volume. The reason for different budgets at different volumes is that fee-for-service revenues should rise or fall with volume of services provided, capitated revenue should rise or fall with volume of enrollees, and variable costs should rise or fall with volume. This last point means that a flexible budget system must be developed on the basis of a knowledge of which costs are fixed and which are variable.

Finance

Finance focuses on matters quite different from those addressed by financial accounting, and of longer horizon than those addressed by managerial accounting. While managerial accounting is clearly focused on the future, the future it addresses is typically short-term. Financial accounting primarily deals with reporting an organization's historical activity in fiscal terms and secondarily makes forecasts of future financial statements and performance.

Managerial accounting, while to a large extent breaking from the structures of financial accounting, still tends to focus on accrual concepts. Further, managerial finance, in contrast to financial accounting, is exclusively future-oriented and, in contrast to managerial accounting, deals with fiscal decision making on sources of financing and resource allocation (uses of financing) over the full range of time horizons. Both accounting and finance make important contributions to managerial processes, but they are very different from each other.

For example, while accrual accounting tries to match dollar figures with physical events, such as "patients served," finance matches dollar figures only with fiscal events, such as the collection of monies for services to patients. As a result, finance is concerned with the accounting accrual concept in only peripheral ways. Finance focuses not on when service delivery occurs but rather on when money associated with that service comes in or goes out the door. Are you going to collect tomorrow, next week, or two months from now? Are you ever going to collect? When does the cash flow occur? Similarly, finance does not associate resource cost with the timing of resource use, but rather with the timing of the payment for the resource. Finance focuses on receipts, not revenue, and on expenditures, not expenses. This is because it is concerned with future cash flows or their equivalents, not past performance, and because, ultimately, only cash matters in capital markets.

Suppose that you order a diagnostic laboratory test today that is performed today and a corresponding charge is generated at the same time. Assume further that medical supplies already on hand were used to obtain and to test the specimen. An accrual system will recognize the revenues from the test today, whether or not any collection occurred today. If there was no collection, the accrual system will recognize a corresponding increase in "accounts receivable" on the balance sheet. Finance will recognize nothing until the actual collection occurs. The accrual system will also recognize the "expense" of the supplies today, reducing an "inventory" (of supplies) account on the balance sheet. Finance will recognize nothing today unless there is a cash outlay today for those supplies.[2] Finance is interested in and will recognize only actual cash inflows and outflows, regardless of when the economic activity that gives rise to those flows takes place.

Finance also treats capital expenditures very differently than they are treated by accounting. If you decide to spend $100,000 for a piece of equipment that is expected to be productive for five years, the $100,000 is gone as soon as you acquire the equipment. Finance "recognizes" the full "outlay" of the equipment when the cash outflow for the equipment takes place. It does not matter if the machine is going to last two years, five years, or 10 years.

The financial accountant will record the expense of the equipment in installments during which the equipment is used. Each installment will be labeled "depreciation expense" and will appear on an income statement covering some part of the time the equipment is being used. The amounts of each installment will reflect various rules and formulas, but will not themselves reflect any cash outflows in those amounts. For this reason, depreciation expense is not, by itself, relevent to finance. Finance pays attention to depreciation expense only if its presence affects some other cash flow, for example, tax payments.

Why does finance place all of its emphasis on cash flows? Because finance focuses on the organization's ability to command resources (goods and services) and capital and its ability to service its capital in the future. At root, these abilities rely directly on the use of cash, of money.

Money is like any other resource, in that an organization must pay for the privilege of using it. Examples include paying interest on a loan or on a bond issue (debt financing), distributing profits (dividends) to partners (stockholders) for profit (equity financing), or providing charity care and supporting teaching and research (not-for-profit equity financing). The organization's ability to make such "rent" payments, plus its ability to repatriate the capital itself directly, affects whether or not it will be able to attract future capital.

Buying resources and servicing capital ultimately requires cash. You cannot meet next Friday's payroll with accounts receivable, revenue, or even income (all accounting measures). You can only meet the payroll with cash or its equivalent, e.g., checks drawn against bank balances. This is why decision making, analysis, and evaluation in finance look at the ability of the organization to meet next Friday's payroll, to buy supplies next month, and to service its capital into the indefinite future—i.e., to generate required levels of cash flow. You can defer some things in the short term by borrowing money, of course, but, ultimately, you must have the cash to repay the borrowing. Thus, while you can shift future cash flows around in time, at some point you finally get to the economic bottom line requiring cash in the bank.

In identifying organizational cash flows, finance focuses on incremental analysis, because it is analyzing the future for the specific purpose of assisting managers in making decisions. That is, finance considers only changes in cash flows that may result from a decision. Should we buy a new computer for the accounting department? Finance analysis will look at the timing and amounts of cash outflows and inflows only to the extent that they differ from what they might be if the new computer is not purchased.

In finance, the time value of money is always explicit.[3] A dollar today is always different from a dollar tomorrow. If you try to add a January dollar to a December dollar, you are doing what your second grade teacher told you never to do: You are adding apples and oranges. From an economic point of view, January and December dollars are not the same thing, partly because the effect of inflation causes their purchasing power to differ. They are also not the same thing for a variety of other reasons having nothing whatsoever to do with purchasing power. Even if a dollar in January bought the same quantity of real goods and services as a dollar would in December, (i.e., there was no inflation or deflation), you would not be indifferent to the choice between these two time-separated dollars. If you receive a choice between a dollar's worth of purchasing power today and a dollar's worth of purchasing power a year from now, you would still choose the dollar today rather than the purchasing-power-adjusted dollar a year from today. If nothing else, you could always take the dollar today and invest it at a risk-free real (after-inflation) investment rate of two or three percent. That two or three percent represents the compensation required to induce people to defer consumption of real resources.

The finance function includes:

- Constructing forecasts of distinct sets of future cash flows, each associated with alternative courses of organizational action.

- Establishing valuation criteria based on estimates of required rates of return.[4]

- Using those criteria to evaluate the relative worth of alternative sets of future cash flows.

- Assisting managers in integrating this economic information into decision-making and planning processes.

Finance forecasts and evaluations are primarily designed for internal, managerial purposes rather than for outside parties. They are not to be relied upon for external applications or as a vehicle for the implementation of public policy as are the outputs of accounting. They are an input to decision-making and planning processes, primarily internal.

There are several broad categories of decisions that are amenable to analysis from a finance perspective:

- Decisions focused on near-term cash flows, so-called "working capital management."

- Capital structure decisions.

- Capital acquisition and disbursement decisions.

- Long-term investment/divestment choices, so-called "capital budgeting" decisions.[5]

The first three of these areas are largely the province of the controller/CFO/treasurer of the organization, while the fourth area is more the province of operational managers supported by the fiscal function. Management of the organization's near-term cash inflows and outflows addresses questions such as: "How much cash should we keep in the bank?" "How big should our inventories be?" "What should our policy be on charging interest on past due accounts?" "What's our collection policy?" "How fast should we pay our bills?" "Should we invest in Treasury bills?" "Should we prepay insurance premiums?" Working capital management decisions are generally based on how variable the organization's cash flows are and on what effect the choices have on an organization's ability to meet its required rate(s) of return.

Capital structure matters are another decision area to which the health care industry has historically paid very little attention. Very few organizations have explicit policy positions on the mix of debt and equity that finances their assets and programs. For each organization, there is some particular capital structure range that offers optimal cost and risk characteristics, and, typically, that structure includes significant quantities of debt and/or lease financing.

Capital acquisition and disbursement decisions address raising and servicing capital. This is different from the capital structure decision, which concerns the proportions of debt and equity capital used by an organization. Capital acquisition, by contrast, deals with how you plan to bring capital into the organization as cash (or, in the case of leasing, as real assets). Capital disbursement involves planning for what goes back out the door as cash or in-kind dividend payments, salary "bonuses" to owners, other distributions of accounting income, and interest and principal payments on debt. For debt capital, should we have level debt service, balloon payments, declining debt service? For equity capital, how much should we retain, how much should we repatriate? Correctly structured, these types of transactions ensure organizational continuity, both in being able to provide health services and in having needed access to capital markets.

The "capital budgeting decision" encompasses all decisions involving the initiation and/or the abandonment of programs and services and the resultant retention and/or the termination of personnel. Should we acquire this equipment, initiate this new service, hire this physician, sell off this part of the business, close this department, not replace persons at retirement? How do we structure a portfolio of assets, people, and programs?

In all four categories of decisions just described, finance provides the economic component, the projection of what will best enable the organization to meet or exceed its capital suppliers' required rates of return, thereby preserving or enhancing organizational value. That is what finance is all about.

The Changing Role of the Chief Financial Officer

In the 1960s, the health care industry had very little competent financial management. Indeed, the state of fiscal management in most health care provider organizations, if it existed at all, was roughly comparable to the level of fiscal sophistication in the rest of American industry in the 1870s. In prior decades, when most health care providers in the private sector were largely supported by philanthropy and public-sector grants and when health care costs were not an item of major national policy concern, fiscal management beyond simple bookkeeping and occasional audits was seen largely as a luxury.

It was only after the advent of the major national entitlement programs, Medicare and Medicaid, that the majority of health care providers instituted double-entry accrual accounting. In the years since 1966, the health care industry developed highly competent financial accounting and, since the advent of Medicare's Prospective Payment System and the rise of prepaid health care in the 1980s and 1990s, has added sophisticated cost accounting. In addition to financial accounting and cost accounting, managerial accounting, especially in the areas of budgeting and control, is also being increasingly used. What is only now emerging, however, is adoption of finance techniques that have been at the forefront of fiscal management for the rest of American industry since shortly after World War II, techniques of such import that they were the basis for two Nobel prizes (in economics) awarded during the 1990s.

Thus, while today's CFO is light years away from the green-eyeshade book-keeper who ran the business office of the 1940s and 1950s, he or she is much more likely to use a cost accounting approach to pricing than one involving net present value (a finance method discussed later in this chapter) and much more likely to rely on balance sheet information on organizational value than to build alternative systems to estimate market values directly. The key to sound fiscal management is to appreciate the strengths and weaknesses of all of these approaches to resource allocation, to appreciate the interrelation-ships between fiscal and nonfiscal elements within an organization, and to communicate broadly within the organization, speaking not in "fiscal" tongues but in common language.

Value: Measurement, Maintenance, Enhancement

This section introduces the following concepts of finance:

- Debt and Equity Capital

- Rate of Return

    ❏ "Pure" interest or "the time value of money"
    ❏ Adjustment for expected inflation
    ❏ Business risk
    ❏ Adjustment for taxation
    ❏ Interest rate risk

- Financial Risk and Capital Structure

- Cost of Capital and Weighted Average Cost of Capital

- Net Present Value

These concepts and the techniques related to them form the foundations for financial evaluation. They are used to evaluate an organization's current financial status and to evaluate what effect, if any, a given proposal or course of action will have on that financial status. The underlying normative princi-ple of finance is that each discrete organizational activity should at least "pay for itself," because, if too many activities are "losers" (without offsetting "win-ners"), the organization will eventually find its survival threatened. Finance is also quite pragmatic. It recognizes that there are times when activities should be supported even though they are not fiscally viable by themselves, if the organization is capable of providing that support. For example, professional personnel might be encouraged to teach at local universities or do research in clinical areas. For these purposes, they receive release time or its equivalent. From a financial perspective, this policy has a direct, measurable cost and no associated measurable income. Yet there is little doubt that their participation in such activities benefits the organization's reputation.

The point is that finance always focuses on the measurable economic consequences of an organization's actions. This analysis is, of course, only one input, although certainly a very important one, into the organization's decision-making and planning processes.

Debt and Equity Capital

The economic foundation of any private-sector organization (in the health care field or in any other industry) is its capital. That capital, whatever its mix of debt and equity, supports the entire structure of assets owned (or resources controlled) and programs engaged in by the organization. The ultimate success, indeed the very survival, of the organization depends on the extent to which its utilization of assets and program activities provides fiscal returns sufficient to preserve and/or enhance the underlying capital base.

Preserving and enhancing capital is a fundamental task of any organization in the private sector. Within the private sector, of course, we have both for-profit and not-for-profit organizations. We may characterize not-for-profit organizations as entities that should, at minimum, preserve (maintain) the economic value of their capital, while for-profit organizations need to go the further step of enhancing the economic value of their capital.

For-profit organizations are created to increase the wealth of their owners. This can happen in two ways. First, economic profits can be returned to the owners in cash. Second, profits can be reinvested in the organization, which increases the market value of owners' equity. In accounting terms, equity is literally the extent to which the value of all organizational assets exceeds the value of all organizational liabilities (debts). In the real (financial) world, owners' equity is the market value of owners' claim on the organization if they wished to sell those claims to a willing buyer.

In the not-for-profit case, "owners" are considered to be parent entities, the community, or the public at large. The return to the community is the services that the organization provides and its ability to continue to provide those services over time. As good stewards, managers of not-for-profit organizations must also attempt to make an accounting profit (i.e., to have revenues exceed expenses).[6] But how large a profit and what the organization does with it are entirely different questions. For example, a not-for-profit provider having a "profit" in a given year might choose to use the portion that a for-profit counterpart might use for dividends or owner wealth enhancing investment to:

- Lower its charges (or, simply hold them constant while competitors' rates go up).

- Offer additional services in non-income-producing areas, such as health education, support of research, or additional charity or deeply discounted care.

- Retain and invest monies in relatively liquid, low-risk assets, helping to carry the organization through lean times.

- Replace or add real assets to improve the quality of or access to services provided.

The key concept here is that all organizations must show an accounting profit (have revenues greater than expenses) if they are to survive in the long run.[7] This is equally true of not-for-profit and for-profit firms. What distinguishes the two is what is done with the profit, if any, that exceeds the amount needed to preserve capital.

Preservation of Capital

The term "preservation of capital" has a very specific economic meaning. What we wish to preserve or maintain is the real value of capital, the claims of the existing suppliers of the fiscal resources supporting the activities of the organization. Because capital comes from an external, competitive marketplace, the ability to satisfy those who have, in the past, supplied capital is the key element to being able to attract new capital from those or other suppliers in the future.

Satisfying capital suppliers means meeting their expectations. All suppliers of capital to the private sector expect some form of return in exchange for their having supplied the capital, and those expectations exist whether the capital was supplied to a for-profit or a not-for-profit organization.

Suppliers of debt capital are readily identified as institutions and individuals having contractual claims against the organization—for example, a commercial bank that has extended credit, an insurance company holding a mortgage, a pension fund holding a private placement of bonds, or individuals holding bonds that were publicly offered. The expectations of suppliers of debt capital as to returns are clear and explicit. They are embodied in the contractual terms agreed to in advance by themselves and the borrowing organization in a loan agreement, mortgage contract, bond indenture, or the like.

Most suppliers of equity capital to a for-profit organization are clearly identifiable. Shareholders of a corporation, the partners in a partnership, or the owner of a sole proprietorship supply equity capital to those organizations. For the not-for-profit health care provider, equity suppliers are somewhat more diverse and, other than when it is the wholly owned subsidiary of a parent not-for-profit entity (e.g., a religious organization), more difficult to identify individually. The list may include private donors of cash, be they major philanthropists, private foundations, or persons contributing a few dollars to an annual fund drive; volunteers who provide wage and salary expense relief to the institution or program; payers of tax monies that flow through a government entity to the provider by grant, appropriation, or designation[8]; and a small number of recipients of health services who, themselves or via third parties, pay more than the economic cost for those services. Because of the breadth and the diversity of these equity capital suppliers, we generally refer to them as "society," "the community," or "the service area."

There is, of course, no written contract concerning specific returns to suppliers of ordinary equity capital. Further financial accounting deliberately excludes all reference to returns on equity capital as an expense (unlike the recognition by financial accounting of interest expense, the return on debt capital). As a result, managers (even of for-profit firms) sometimes fall into the trap of viewing equity capital as free, as having no explicit cost, that is, requiring no returns. Nothing could be further from economic reality.

The shareholders or the partners of a for-profit organization have very clear expectations of dividends or cash distributions and/or appreciation in the market value of their ownership claims. Suppliers of equity capital to not-for-profit organizations also have specific expectations of return. The fact that these returns are not permitted to be in the form of cash distributions or market value appreciation in no way lessens the strength of the expectations or reduces the economic burden on management to meet those expectations. Suppliers of equity capital to not-for-profit health care providers expect those organizations to remain viable into the indefinite future[9]; they expect the social value of the services provided by such organizations to exceed the organizations' charges for providing those services; they expect such organizations to support, as appropriate, relevant educational programs and research; and they expect reasonable levels of free and/or discounted care to be provided to certain segments of the community served. Indeed, the range of equity supplier expectations may be quite large.

Required Rate of Return

The rate of return required by any supplier of capital will, of course, vary through time. A generic rate of return conceptually includes compensation for five major factors, any one of which can change at any time in a dynamic marketplace:

- The pure "time value of money"

- Inflation (deflation)

- Default

- Untimely/forced liquidation

- Expected taxation

The pure time value of money is simply economic recognition that consumption of goods and services has positive value to human beings and cannot be postponed indefinitely because of the finite lifespan of human beings. Individuals, directly and through the organizations they form, draw satisfaction from consumption[10] and require compensation for anything that delays that consumption. That is, because we prefer to consume sooner rather than later and because supplying capital to others effectively delays the supplier's ability to use those funds for consumption, a "pure rate of interest" is required to compensate for the delay. Empirically, the pure rate of interest as an annual rate has been in the 2 to 2-1/2 percent range.

For example, suppose a bank supplies $36,000 of capital to an organization today and expects the loan to be paid back after one year. The bank may require (expect) $828 (2.3 percent) worth of compensation one year from now in recognition of the fact that the bank's money has been tied up for one year. Thus, a payment to the bank of $36,828 one year hence would provide a full return of and on capital.[11]

The second component of a required rate of return is the additional compensation necessary in an inflationary environment to compensate the capital supplier for expected loss of purchasing power. (In the case of expected deflation, an adjustment reducing the overall required rate of return would occur.) Between the time the capital is initially supplied and the time that returns to capital are made, price increases in the capital supplier's "market basket" of goods and services will have reduced the real value of the supplier's initial investment. The purchasing power adjustment that compensates for this expected loss of value is applied both to the initial capital itself and to the compensation-for-delayed-consumption (pure interest) return.

Continuing the numerical example begun above, if a 4 percent inflation rate is expected (that is, it will take $10.40 one year from now to buy the same quantities of goods and services now costing $10.00), the bank would require payment of $38,301.12 one year hence ($36,828 plus 4 percent of $36,828).

The third component of an overall required rate of return on capital is compensation for the risk of possible nonpayment or delay in payment of some or all of the total return due to the capital supplier.[12] Default arises because of an insufficiency of cash to service capital, reflecting cash flow variability that derives primarily from an organization's basic economic activity (business risk). For each class of capital supplier, the risk can be mitigated or magnified by the relative position (priority or lack thereof) of that class's claim among all capital claims on the organization (financial risk).[13] Financial risk and its implications will be considered in more detail in the next section. Business risk arises from the nature of the economic environment and from operational characteristics of each organization.

One way to think about business risk is to array three categories of elements: systemic risk (inter-and intrasystem phenomena, e.g., political factors such as expropriation or nationalization of assets, fluctuations in exchange rates (monetary and fiscal policy), market risk (e.g., elements of competition, public and/or private regulation, supplier power, third-party purchasing power, technological obsolescence), and organizational risk (e.g., quality of managerial and operating personnel and processes, input/output efficiency). All of these elements interacting will cause some organizations to experience cash flows that fall short of what is required to meet the expectations of some or all of their capital suppliers, with a resultant default.

It is important to recognize the differential roles of management in addressing these three categories of risk. Managers have virtually no control with regard to systemic risk. Managers may be able to exert only some influence on various elements of market risk, through, for example, negotiations with suppliers or purchasers. But managers are largely responsible for the decisions that define the level of organizational risk.

Continuing our numerical example begun above, suppose that the bank expects a one percent rate of complete default (i.e., for every 100 loans of this type made, 99 are paid in full on time, and 1 goes to total default and repay nothing). To cover this contingency, the bank will charge a premium on each loan it makes. To compute the premium, divide the total payment that fully compensates the bank for the pure time value of money and for inflation by one minus the failure rate:

$38,301.12/(1–.01) = $38,301.12/.99 = $38,688.00

This assures the bank of full returns on all of its loans by spreading the risk of failure across all the loans it makes:

100 x $38,301.12 = $3,830,112 = 99 x 38,688.00

Other, slightly more complicated calculations are possible that would take into account partial repayments and late repayments.

The fourth component of a basic rate of return deals with the generic risks associated with an uncertain future. Suppliers of capital, like all managers, attempt to forecast future economic conditions. Good as our crystal balls and computer models may be, no one can have absolute confidence in forecasts of next year's monetary policy, inflation rate, and rates of taxation or of the likelihood of default on a claim. Thus, required rates of return fluctuate daily, as expectations about future events and conditions change. In this fluctuating environment, the capital supplier bears the risks associated with the possible necessity of having to sell the capital claim for an unknown price[14] to someone else prior to its original or expected maturity. The further in the future the expected maturity, the greater is the possibility of having to do this. Not only is there the possibility of sustaining a capital loss, but generally there will also be conversion or transaction costs associated with the untimely or forced liquidation of the claim.

These risks of loss are in part related to the amount of time remaining until all returns to a capital claim are expected to be realized—the longer the time, the greater the risk—but they are also related to the natural degree of volatility in the claim-specific risk factors noted above and to the efficiency or lack thereof in the secondary market for the claim. Typically, an additional premium for bearing such risks, an "illiquidity premium,"[15] is observable in required rates of return as compensation for future interest rate (and capital value) fluctuation. While there is no way to calculate an exact amount for the illiquidity premium, it might be as little as one-half of one percent for a one-year maturity and several percentage points for a 10-year maturity.

In our example, rather than requiring $38,688.00, the bank might ask for an additional $193.44 (a one-half of one percent), or a total of $38,881.44.

The fifth component of marketplace required rates of return is compensation for taxation. Different taxes may be levied simultaneously by several different levels of government, and the nature and rate of taxation levied by each level may depend on the characteristics of both the supplier and the user of the capital.

Suppose, in our example, that the return on the $36,000 in capital (that is, all return in excess of $36,000, or $2,881.44) is considered taxable income. Because that $2,881.44 is seen as what is necessary to fairly compensate the capital supplier for real interest, inflation, the risk of default, and the risk of untimely liquidation, the capital supplier must receive before-tax compensation of sufficient magnitude so that after meeting the tax liability, $2,881.44 will remain. To find the appropriate before-tax amount, simply divide the required after-tax dollar return on capital by one minus the applicable marginal tax rate. If the bank in this example had to pay tax at a marginal rate of 27.5 percent,[16] the required payment would be:

$36,000 + $2,881.44/(1–.275) = $36,000 + $2,881.44/0.725 = $36,000 + 3,974.40 = $39,974.40, or an 11.04 percent required rate of return.

The capital marketplace brings together suppliers and users of capital representing the full spectrum of different tax and inflation environments, all manner of sensitivities to risks, and widely divergent opinions as to future economic conditions and business risks. Hence, market-determined rates of return ultimately represent the relative supplies of and demands for capital from many heterogeneous market participants. Nonetheless, market-clearing rates of return necessarily satisfy capital suppliers in the conceptual dimensions noted. If they did not, the capital would not be supplied.

Classes of Capital Suppliers, Financial Risk, and Required Rates

The discussion above of required rates of return was generic for all suppliers of capital. The simplest capital structure is that of an organization with no debt and a single owner (equity), while complex capital structures may contain several types of debt, a number of categories of equity, and various forms of leasing. For this section we consider only the first level of complexity—an organization having just two kinds of suppliers of capital, both internally homogeneous: suppliers of equity capital and suppliers of debt capital.

Although debt suppliers may not have been the first parties chronologically to provide capital to the organization, they are definitely the parties first in line to receive returns to capital. This is because organizations enter into explicit contracts with suppliers of debt, promising to pay them specific sums of interest and principal at definite future times. These contractual claims take precedence over returns to equity suppliers, who are legally entitled only to whatever is left over after all contractual claims are fully satisfied.

Therefore, debt is always viewed as less risky than equity, because debt has first claim on the organization's cash flows. There is, therefore, a difference in the financial risk faced by suppliers of debt and equity capital.

If an organization were 100 percent equity-financed, equity would bear all of the risks and costs discussed earlier. If the organization approached being

100 percent debt-financed, debt would have assumed almost all of these risks and costs. At points in the middle (say 50 percent debt and 50 percent equity), debt's first claim on the organization's resources makes it less risky than equity, and thus its required rate of return will be less. Indeed, debt's risk is not only less than equity's, but also is less than the average risk of the overall organization.

In a parallel manner, equity's inherent risk would be magnified by the financial risk associated with increasing proportions of debt having a priority claim in the capital structure. As debt claims a greater and greater share of operational cash flows available to service capital, it becomes increasingly likely that variability in those flows might leave little or no funds after debt service to meet the expectations of equity suppliers. Equity suppliers require a higher rate of return to compensate them for bearing this financial risk over and above the other risks and costs. If there is any debt at all, equity's required rate of return will be higher than debt's and higher than the average rate of return for the overall organization. At high levels of debt financing, equity holders might well require annual rates of return in the 30-40 percent range.

The Cost of Capital

Up to this point, required rates of return have been discussed primarily from the perspective of the capital supplier. The other side of the coin, of course, is the cost of capital to the user. In the simplest cases, these are identical. What the capital supplier receives is what it costs the organization. Various circumstances, however, can cause the cost of debt service to the organization to be less than the required rate of return actually received by the capital supplier.

For example, a corporate for-profit provider pays tax on its net income, taxable revenues less deductible expenses. Interest is one such deductible expense. Suppose a for-profit provider paying taxes at a rate of 40 percent decides to borrow $1000 for one year at an interest rate (required rate of return) of 10 percent. The loan will accrue $100 of interest expense at the end of the year. If the borrower would have had $500 of taxable income without the borrowing, taxes due would have been $200 [=40 percent of $500]. With the borrowing, taxable income is now $400 [=$500 - $100 interest expense] and taxes due are now only $160 [=40 percent of 400]. The tax bill has declined by $40 from $200 to $160. Hence, the $100 interest expense has been partially offset by the $40 tax savings, leaving a net cost for the borrowing of $60. That net cost of $60 is 6 percent of the $1,000 borrowed. Even though the lender receives its full required rate of return of 10 percent ($100), the cost to the borrower is only 6 percent ($60). The 4 percent ($40) difference is, in effect, a government subsidy to the borrower. It lowers the cost of debt to the organization because a third party is absorbing a portion of the return actually received by the capital supplier.[17]

The basic point is that the economics of producing returns to capital (the costs of capital) need to be distinguished from the returns themselves (as viewed by the capital suppliers receiving them).

The long-run survival of any private sector organization, for-profit or not-for-profit, depends on its ability to renew existing capital (not assets) and to attract new capital from time to time. This ability to succeed in attracting infusions of capital from an increasingly competitive capital market relates specifically to the organization's demonstrated ability to preserve the real economic value of existing capital. That value is preserved only if each class of capital supplier receives its respective required rate of return. Because parts of that required rate of return may be provided (or reduced) by external parties (e.g., taxation authorities), internal organizational decisions need to focus only on the net cost of capital. Thus, a provider's operational fiscal returns must attain the cost of capital threshold so that, when supplemented (or reduced) by external parties, capital suppliers will receive their required rates of return and be willing to renew or expand their provision of capital to the organization.

Meeting the expectations of some but not all capital suppliers is insufficient. For example, paying all of the contractual interest and principal payments on time is not, by itself, enough to guarantee future access to capital. It is also necessary to preserve the value of equity capital in order to maintain a strong overall capital structure. A weak equity position is just as surely a hindrance to future borrowing as is failure to meet debt service payments.

Selection of Organization Activities

The "bottom line" (both figuratively and literally) of financial analysis is determining whether or not a given organizational activity (e.g., opening a new clinic, adding more physicians, buying a computer, adding a new service) will pay for itself in the long run or be a drain on the organization's resources (i.e., equity). To do this, finance computes the weighted average cost of capital; identifies the incremental operational cash flows associated with the activity; and, from them, determines the net present value of the alternative or activity.

An organization obtains capital from many different sources: bank loans, individual investors or contributors, grants, bond issues, etc. Each source will have an associated cost of capital. One useful statistic for financial analysis, therefore, is the "weighted average cost of capital" (WACC). This is simply the cost of capital for each supplier weighted by its proportion of total capital measured at market value. For example, suppose a provider is financed by (has total capital of) $1,000,000[18]: a $250,000 loan and a tax-exempt bond issue for $500,000 at net (after-tax and after-reimbursement) costs of 10 percent and 7 percent, respectively, and a $250,000 infusion of equity from a parent entity requiring a 12 percent rate of return. The WACC of this organization would be:

(Loan)   (Bond)   (Equity)

$$\frac{250{,}000}{1{,}000{,}000} \times .10 + \frac{500{,}000}{1{,}000{,}000} \times .07 + \frac{250{,}000}{1{,}000{,}000} \times .12 = 0.25 \times 0.10 + 0.50$$

$$\times 0.07 + 0.25 \times 0.12 = 0.025 + 0.035 + 0.030 = 9.00\%$$

Second, the incremental, operational cash flows associated with the activity must be identified. Operational cash flows are nonaccrual measures of all the cash flows in and out of the organization other than cash flows to and from capital suppliers (e.g., interest payments) and cash flows triggered by capital supplier flows (e.g., tax reductions in recognition of interest payments). Operational cash flows, therefore, exclude equity infusions and dividends but include inflows from asset liquidation and outflows for asset acquisition.

In addition to the requirement that cash flows be of the operational rather than the capital type, they also must be strictly incremental. This simply means that we count only those cash flows that will change as a result of the decision regarding the proposal under consideration.[19]

Fiscal evaluation of any proposal begins with an estimate of the expected incremental operational cash flows associated with the proposal, period by period, over an appropriate future time. Once this stream of cash flows is obtained, it must be evaluated in terms of the organization's WACC. This is because organizations should focus on their costs of capital rather than on capital's required rate of return. Specifically, the WACC is used as the "rate of discount" with which to find the value today of a proposal's expected incremental future operational cash flows (including the proposal's expected investment outlays now and henceforth). This value today is called the proposal's net present value (NPV). A positive NPV means that a proposal pays for itself (including the cost of capital to support it) and that there will be funds left over that can be put to other uses. An NPV of zero means that a proposal breaks even in economic terms; it will pay for itself but generate no additional resources beyond the required returns. A negative NPV means that the organization will have to subsidize the proposal, because it cannot be economically self-supporting.[20]

Calculating a proposal's NPV using the WACC as the discount rate involves determining the relative value of each of the incremental operational cash flows.

For all the reasons discussed earlier, as long as there is a positive rate of return, a dollar in hand today is more valuable than a dollar expected tomorrow. If a 20 percent annual rate of return is required (or available), one dollar invested today at that rate will be worth $1.20 one year hence. Similarly, one dollar expected a year from now is worth only 83 1/3 cents today.[21] The discount factor (1.20 in these examples) is equal to one plus the appropriate discount rate expressed as a decimal.

Because the calculation of NPV is largely mechanical,[22] we won't go into great detail here, but a simplified numerical example in Appendix D to this chapter illustrates the application of this concept of value measurement. Net present value is a powerful concept that allows comparison of different courses of action and their consequences in economic terms. However, it is important to remember that financial evaluation is just one input into the overall decision-making process.

Some Normative Considerations

Positive-NPV activities increase an organization's value (i.e., the value of its equity) even after all suppliers of capital, including equity, are satisfied, in the sense of having received exactly their required rate of return. The increase in value in today's dollars is equal to the positive amount of NPV. Negative-NPV activities show the amount by which the value of the organization will decline in today's dollars if all required rates of return are met. (Meeting such requirements is accomplished by drawing down the value of existing equity, a process in which many providers engage, often unknowingly.) In the long term, of course, organizations with negative-NPV portfolios cease to exist through one of two mechanisms. In the most severe case, termination by bankruptcy occurs. In the milder circumstance, future access to the capital markets is denied and a less traumatic liquidation or sale or merger occurs.

For-profit providers have an economic obligation to maximize the wealth of their ownership, subject to all the usual legal and ethical constraints. Hence, for-profit providers should actively seek as many positive-NPV activities in their portfolio of assets and programs as possible.

By contrast, not-for-profit providers should be seen as having an overall neutral-NPV portfolio of activities. This in no way precludes the growth of the organization, for it says nothing about the number or size of activities engaged in. Rather, the "rule" is that not-for-profit organizations should seek an overall portfolio of activities that achieves only a small positive NPV, meeting the required rates of return of all capital suppliers and relevant community constituencies.

For example, consider the example of a hospital or a clinic that is considering a new marketing program that (it is predicted) will have a highly positive NPV. A for-profit organization might choose to increase dividends or distributions to equity as the new income is realized, or it might choose to reinvest the "extra" dollars in activities that increase owners' equity. A not-for-profit organization is faced with the same question: What do we do with the extra dollars? It might choose to add a health education program (return of social value to community); support clinical research or teaching (return to community) and probably an "in-kind" or noncash bonus to workers (increasing the organization's viability); reduce prices to some patients or provide additional charity care (social dividend); or simply retain the money as liquid, short-term assets, such as CDs or Treasury bills (increase organization viability).

A negative-NPV proposal, by definition, is incapable of sustaining itself economically. Assuming all possible cost efficiencies have been incorporated in the proposal, the only way to adjust the value of such a proposal upward is to increase its operational cash inflows by posting higher prices (rates). If, ultimately, such increases are constrained by competition, rate regulation, ordinary price elasticity in the marketplace, or other economic or political factors, and the NPV still remains negative, the proposal must be rejected as a "mainframe" (nondividend)[23] activity. However, this does not necessarily mean that the proposal should be rejected totally. Financial analysis using NPV is only one input into overall decision making. Besides economic factors, there are two other generic concerns that must be examined: long-run strategic payoffs and "social" value.

At this point, the organization's board should review such uneconomic pro-posals (assuming they are of sufficient magnitude to warrant such attention). The substance of the proposal (e.g., the actual service to be delivered) may be viewed by the board as so important to the community that the board will declare the activity a dividend (to the community)[24] or so integrally inter-twined with the organization's mission that it is considered essential. Neither step should be taken lightly (which, of course, is why the matter should be brought to the board in the first place).

Take the case of a social dividend to the community. If the provider is cur-rently meeting the expectations of its equity capital suppliers, does not offset the new dividend by a reduction in an existing dividend, and wishes to main-tain the current value of its capital (i.e., does not wish to partially liquidate through a return of capital), the board, by declaring the dividend, is saying the community expects (requires) the dividend as part of its overall return. This simply means that, unless new inflows of equity capital can be found, main-frame activities will have to bear the additional cost of the new dividend, thereby implying price increases.

If the cash inflows from existing mainframe activities cannot be increased (again assuming cost efficiency has already been attained) and new equity capital is not forthcoming, the dividend that has been declared is, in effect, a partial liquidating dividend. There is absolutely nothing wrong with declaring a partial liquidating dividend, of course, as long as it is done consciously, explicitly. Adopting negative-NPV projects (effective dividends) without being aware of their long-run economic implications, however, can clearly endanger long-run organizational survival.

With respect to strategic decisions to invest in "essential" activities, it is impor-tant that organizational decision making and board policy formulation take a long-run perspective if the organization is to remain viable in a dynamic and competitive environment. On the other hand, the factors cited above (cross-subsidization and partial liquidation of capital) also need to be considered. This approach to explicit, board-level formulation of dividend policy has the major advantage of bringing issues of cross-subsidization out of the shadows and placing them on top of the table for direct deliberation and decision making.

Finally, all organizations should attempt to minimize their WACCs. For a given set of programs and activities, a lower WACC will clearly generate more wealth for for-profit ownership and greater price reductions in the not-for-profit sector. Additionally, more proposals will have NPVs greater than or equal to zero, thereby allowing a broader range of both mainframe services and dividends.

Techniques for minimizing WACC are among a number of advanced fiscal management subjects that cannot be addressed in detail here, but they would include determining and implementing an optimal capital structure, taking a wide variety of possible actions to minimize perceived business risk, and ensuring that the lowest cost sources of capital are being tapped. It is worth noting that the latter technique is one of the stronger economic arguments for retaining tax-exempt debt financing for not-for-profit providers. The lower WACC that results from tax-exempt financing also permits the broader range of mainframe services and dividends noted above.

Further Study of Finance and Accounting

As we have seen above, finance and accounting are important functional areas within the discipline of management.

Finance is primarily concerned with assisting managers in making resource allocation and financing decisions that are consistent with economic value criteria. Finance focuses on forecasting future fiscal events and on evaluating alternative forecasts against value criteria tailored to each organization. For a fuller appreciation of finance as a managerial discipline, see the Ross *et al.* entry in the bibliography.

Exercise caution in assuming a book really deals with finance just because the word "finance" or "financial" is in the title. For example, the Cleverley and Nowicki bibliographic entries are excellent treatments of managerial and cost accounting, but they do not deal with any significant amount of finance, even though one might erroneously assume from their titles that they do.

Financial accounting focuses on *ex post* reporting to internal and external parties. Cost accounting attributes long-run resource costs to individual units of output. These emphases have produced particular processes and formats through which information is generated, reported, and analyzed. For *ex post* reporting, there are income statements, balance sheets, and statements of "cash flow" that are generated by double-entry accounting systems applying generally accepted accounting principles. Cost-attribution involves many complex ways of assigning or allocating categories of resource costs. To be able to appreciate fully such information requires a solid understanding of the rules and processes by which they are produced. That level of understanding is well beyond the scope of this chapter, but excellent starting points for anyone wishing to go more deeply into such material are the Hilton, Horngren *et al.*, and Zelman *et al.* bibliographic entries.

Managerial accounting, like finance, encompasses a variety of analytical techniques that focus on the future, but, unlike finance, focuses more on the day-to-day functioning of the provider and future periods of one to two years. The Zelman bibliographic entry provides a comprehensive survey of managerial accounting tools.

Endnotes

1. The relevant range of activity is typically the maximum capacity of the organization, using existing resources to deliver the service being analyzed within the period of time covered by the analysis. Should the provider decide to meet demand in excess of that capacity, additional capacity costs would have to be incurred. (Such additional costs themselves would almost always be fixed over the additional range of volume those costs would create.) In other words, no fixed cost is absolutely fixed.

2. If the supplies were paid for at an earlier time, finance would have noted the outlay at that time; if the supplies are not yet paid for, a debt (liability) has been incurred, and finance will recognize the future outlay as a reduction of debt.

3. When relatively small amounts of money are involved for relatively short periods of time during which market rates of return—e.g., interest—are relatively low, the quantum of time value is relatively small. It is for this reason that managerial accounting, typically dealing with only a year or so of the future, generally dispenses with incorporating time value into its analyses.

4. Organizations must service their capital to include paying "rent" on the money/resources they use in providing their health care service or product. But how much rent must be paid? Capital suppliers (whether debt or equity) will require a certain rate of return on their funds. In an analogous manner, the organization must also achieve a certain rate of return when it allocates these capital resources to one use or another. Thus, finance has as one of its most basic and important functions ascertaining the appropriate rates of return an organization must (on average) attain from the goods and services it provides in order to achieve long-run economic survival.

5. This is actually a misnomer, because the subject matter in this decision category involves neither capital nor budgeting.

6. To illustrate why a bottom line (net income) that is literally zero is unacceptable, indeed, on an income statement, why a small positive bottom line may also be inadequate, consider the following: If your investment advisor had you invest $100,000 on January 1 for one year and you received a check the following December 31 for $102,000 for the full liquidation of your investment, you would have a $2,000 bottom line, a $2,000 accounting profit (and, if you were a taxable entity, you would owe taxes on that $2,000). You would also be looking for a new investment advisor, because, notwithstanding your "profitable" year, you are less wealthy at December 31 than you were the previous January 1, because, if for no other reason, $102,000 will buy less December 31 than $100,000 would have a year earlier as a result of normal price increases.

7. Having an accounting profit is a necessary but not a sufficient condition to ensure survival. As shown in endnote #20, an organization with a positive bottom line on its income statement may still be failing economically.

8. In addition to direct subsidies, there are indirect subsidies, as, for example, the granting of tax-exempt status and the right to issue tax-exempt securities, both of which tend to raise others' taxes and to make up for the government revenue shortfalls ("tax expenditures") thus created. Another indirect subsidy is the income-tax deductibility of contributions to 501(c)(3) organizations.

9. The accountant embodies this expectation in applying the "ongoing enterprise" principle; the attorney does the same thing in referring to the corporation as "an infinite-life individual" under the law.

10. Consumption is broadly defined here to encompass not only the acquisition of services and material goods but also charitable activity from which the donor derives satisfaction.

11. Return of capital is exactly what it sounds like: the organization pays back money it has been supplied. This is the case when we pay off the principal portion of the loan. Return on capital is the "rent" paid for the use of the money, as, for example, the interest portion of a loan payment. The combination of returns of and on capital is called return to capital.

12. The so-called "risk-free rate," which is the required rate of return on federal government Treasury securities, is a rate that contemplates no risk of default. This is because the federal government literally can't default, because the government could always manufacture the stuff (money) that its securities promise to pay. The risk-free rate, however, recognizes that such securities have all of the other four factors that require compensation.

13. E.g., employees get paid before suppliers, suppliers get paid before bondholders, secured debt gets paid off before unsecured debt, debt gets paid off before equity holders receive any distributions.

14. Or even a known price in the case of a discretionary call or a random mandatory call by the organization to which the capital was supplied.

15. One sometimes hears the term "liquidity premium." This refers to the higher price the market typically (but not always) places on claims with short-term maturities. Because prices and rates of return are inversely related, the terms "illiquidity premium" or "duration premium" refer to the usually higher rates (lower price) on longer time-to-maturity claims.

16. This assumes that there are no offsetting incremental deductions for expenses. If there were, they would lessen the tax burden.

17. It is also possible to have a lower cost of capital in other ways. For example, a not-for-profit provider may also be able to pay interest that is non-taxable to the lender, thereby lowering its cost of capital by choice of financing vehicle. (Tax-free bonds are the most common example of this type of arrangement.) This mechanism, however, does not cause a difference between the organization's cost of capital and the capital supplier's required rate of return, because it simply lowers both.

18. In WACC computations, market values of debt and equity claims are always used rather than "book" or accounting values.

19. One circumstance to be careful of occurs when the adoption of a proposal obviates a future operational cash flow otherwise required in the absence of favorable consideration afforded the proposal under consideration. For

example, suppose a room would need to be repainted next year. A proposal to institute a new service this year calls for the complete renovation of this space now, dispensing with the cost of repainting the room next year. For the purpose of analyzing the proposal, the cost of painting the room next year is treated as a relevant, incremental, operational cash inflow next year associated with the new service proposal. This is because the proposal saves money that would otherwise have been spent.

20. Note that a proposal that generates positive net income as measured by GAAP may have a negative NPV. For example, suppose a provider invests $210,000 for one year and at the end of the year receives back $216,300, a 3 percent rate of return, and an accounting profit of $6,300. [3% of 210,000 = $6,300; $210,000 + $6,300 = $216,300] If the required rate of return on the $210,000 of capital were 5 percent, however, this investment would have an NPV of ($4,000), a negative. [See Appendix D; $216,000/(1.05) = $206,000; $206,000 - $210,000 = ($4,000)] Incidentally, that negative $4,000 is also the present value of the shortfall between what was actually received at the end of the year, $216,000 and what would have been received had the required rate of return been achieved: 5 percent of $210,000 = $10,500; $210,000 + $10,500 = $220,500; $216,300 - $220,500 = ($4,200); ($4,200)/(1.05 = ($4,000). The point here is that although the investment has positive net income under GAAP, it is not sufficiently profitable to provide all capital suppliers their required rates of return. If this proposal were characteristic of the resource allocation decisions being made by the managers of the provider organization, it would be viewed by capital suppliers as unsatisfactory employment of their capital, and they would refuse to make future capital infusions. When that refusal causes the provider to have to forgo investments that are requisite to organizational survival, the provider will disappear, the discipline of the capital markets having prevailed.

21. $0.831/3 return of capital plus $0.162/3 return on capital (20 percent of $0.831/3, equals a $1.00 total return.

22. Many pocket calculators are preprogrammed to perform a number of simple present value calculations, and all basic spreadsheet software for personal computers includes present value functions.

23. A "mainframe" activity is one that is economically self-supporting, a "tub on its own bottom" not requiring external or cross-subsidization to exist. Mainframe activities are those meeting the WACC criterion, thereby providing the cash flows needed to service the organization's capital.

24. Depending on corporate philosophy, for-profit as well as not-for-profit providers may choose widely different approaches to community dividends. The not-for-profit "community-owned" provider, of course, has a much more direct economic tie to its service area and typically must meet higher expectations regarding returns to equity capital in the form of in-kind dividends than the for-profit provider, which also returns cash to the community in the form of taxes.

Bibliography

Books

Bernstein, P. *Against the Gods, The Remarkable Story of Risk.* New York, N.Y.: John Wiley and Sons, 1996. (A very readable review of quantitative approaches to managing risk.)

Cleverly, W. *Essentials of Health Care Finance,* 4th Edition. Rockville, Md.: Aspen Publishers, 1997. (Managerial accounting, some very rudimentary managerial finance.)

Curry, W., Editor. *A Dictionary of Medical Management Terms and Initialisms.* Tampa, Fla.: American College of Physician Executives, 1998. (Incorporates financial management terms.)

Eastaugh, S. *Health Care Finance—Cost Productivity, and Strategic Design.* Rockville, Md.: Aspen Publishers, 1998. (Cost accounting for not-for-profit and for-profit entities, including HMOs; some basic capital access and capital assessment coverage.)

Finkler, S., and Ward, D. *Essentials of Cost Accounting for Health Care Organizations,* 2nd Edition. Rockville, Md.: Aspen Publishers, 1999. (Cost accounting text for health care organizations.)

Finkler, S., and Ward, D. *Issues in Cost Accounting for Health Care Organizations,* 2nd Edition. Rockville, Md.: Aspen Publishers, 1999. (Cost accounting readings for health care organizations.)

Gapenski, L. *Health Care Finance.* Chicago, Ill.: Health Administration Press, 1998. (Another underwhelming effort; see next entry.)

Gapenski, L. *Understanding Health Care Financial Management—Text, Cases, and Models,* Second Edition. Chicago, Ill.: Health Administration Press, 1996. (This is the only managerial finance text focused on health care. Unfortunately, its treatment of finance topics is overly simplistic, even for bachelor-level course work.)

Hilton, R., and others. *Cost Management: Strategies for Business Decisions.* New York, N.Y.: Irwin-McGraw Hill, 2000. (Survey of cost management practices outside health care. Included are examples of process management, financial modeling, performance evaluation, and incentive systems.)

Horngren, C., and others. *Introduction to Management Accounting,* 111th Edition. Upper Saddle River, N.J.: Prentice Hall, 1999. (Good non-health care managerial accounting text; used in many business schools.)

Keown, A., and others. *Foundation of Finance: The Logic and Practice of Financial Management,* Second Edition. Englewood Cliffs, N.J.: Prentice Hall, 1998. (A straightforward non-health finance text.)

McLean, R. *Financial Management in Health Care Organizations.* Albany, N.Y.: Delmar Publishers, 1996. (Introductory treatment of mostly managerial accounting for health care organizations.)

Nowicki, M. *The Financial Management of Hospitals and Healthcare Organizations.* Chicago, Ill.: Health Administration Press, 1998. (Introductory coverage of financial accounting, managerial accounting, and simplified treatment of mostly managerial accounting for health care organizations.)

Ross, S., and others. *Corporate Finance,* Fifth Edition. New York, N.Y.: Irwin-McGraw Hill, 1999. (This is a classic introductory master-level corporate finance textbook. It contains all of the basic financial concepts that have generally been ignored in all "finance" texts written for the health care industry. The only shortfall of the book is that its treatment of cash flow analysis at the beginning of chapter 7 is insufficiently detailed in bridging between the information generated in an accrual accounting system and the generation of incremental operational cash flows required for investment decision making.)

Zelman, W., and others. *Financial Management of Health Care Organizations: An Introduction to Fundamental Tools, Concepts, and Applications.* Malden, Mass.: Blackwell Publishers, Inc., 1998. (This is probably the best existing book on managerial accounting for health care organizations.)

Journals

Healthcare Financial Management. Westchester, Ill.: Healthcare Financial Management Association.

Medical Group Management (MGM) Journal. Englewood, Colo.: Medical Group Management Association.

Hugh W. Long, MBA, PhD, JD, is a Professor of Health Systems Management in Tulane University's School of Public Health and Tropical Medicine and its Institute of Health Services Research. He holds additional appointments at Tulane's School of Law and its Freeman School of Business and is a member of the Graduate School Facility.

Mark D. Covaleski, PhD, CPA, is Professor of Health Care Financial Management and Co-Director of the Administrative Medicine Program at the University of Wisconsin-Madison. He is also adjunct faculty member of the Department of Health Systems Management at Tulane University and teaches in its Master of Medical Management Program.

Appendix A

Financial Statements

The financial statements produced by an accounting system contain information that can be critical in decision-making processes, especially those engaged in by top management and by parties external to the organization. Collectively, the various financial statements present the financial condition of the organization to management, stockholders, lenders, regulators, and other interested parties. Because, typically, the statements are prepared in accordance with generally accepted accounting principles (GAAP), the information can be analyzed and compared with that of previous years and, in some cases, with similar institutions. A thorough and continuing analysis of the financial statements can highlight potential problem areas and aid in determining corrective action.

Basic Financial Statements

The three primary types of financial statements are the balance sheet, the income statement, and the statement of "cash flow." Each of these statements has particular strengths and weaknesses for determining the financial condition of the organization.

The Balance Sheet

The balance sheet shows the financial position of the organization at a point in time. This can be the end of the year, the end of the month, or any other time desired by the administrator. Its reliability is determined by the accuracy of the accounting information and by the appropriateness of generally accepted accounting principles and regulations for the decision being made. The Financial Accounting Standards Board (FASB) and other professional accounting organizations issue guidance through pronouncements and opinions on appropriate accounting practices for presenting fair financial statements. For example, the physical assets of the organization are typically carried at their initial acquisition costs; the amounts carried in inventory and accounts receivable are a function of the accuracy of the record-keeping system and the time selected for the report. Some organizations will use the calendar year as their reporting period. Others may use another fiscal period that is more appropriate in terms of patient services and census. For example, a December 31 cutoff date for the balance sheet may have been selected more as a matter of tradition than because it is a proper time to analyze the financial position. December may typically be a low census month and some other time may be more representative. A typical balance sheet format and types of accounts are shown in figure A-1, page 170.

The components of the balance sheet are typically classified into definite groupings. For example, current assets include assets that are expected to be converted into cash or expenses within the current operating period or within one year. Assets limited as to use are internally restricted funds that have been identified by management for specific uses. The key term is "internally

Figure A1. Typical Balance Sheet

MEDICAL CENTER BALANCE SHEET—JUNE 30, 20x2 and 20x1

Assets	20x2	20x1
CURRENT ASSETS:		
Cash and cash equivalents	$391,767	$1,125,628
Accounts receivable, net of allowance for uncollectible accounts and contractual allowances of $3,393,361 in 19x2 and $2,367,641 in 19x1.	8,399,210	7,524,313
Other accounts receivable	477,274	554,433
Reimbursement settlement receivable	72,601	80,668
Inventory of supplies	356,798	373,901
Prepaid expenses	53,251	80,714
Assets whose use is limited that are required for current liabilities	1,624,400	1,689,400
Total Current Assets	11,375,301	11,429,057
ASSETS WHOSE USE IS LIMITED BY BOARD-DESIGNATION		
Cash and cash equivalents	614,423	1,063,749
Short-term investments	6,348,645	2,966,819
Investment in pooled fund	1,842,483	2,551,979
Accrued interest receivable	31,628	10,079
Total assets whose use is limited	8,837,179	6,592,626
Less- current portion	(1,624,400)	(1,689,400)
Net assets whose use is limited	7,212,779	4,903,226
PROPERTY, PLANT AND EQUIPMENT at cost:		
Hospital operations-		
Land and improvements	1,358,809	1,342,397
Buildings and leasehold improvements	16,607,453	15,556,408
Fixed equipment	14,206,950	14,209,592
Movable equipment	10,401,089	9,769,731
Other		
Construction in progress	80,170	768,910
Total property, plant and equipment	42,654,471	41,647,038
Less accumulated depreciation	(19,645,445)	(17,143,693)
Net property, plant and equipment	23,009,026	24,503,345
DEFERRED PROFESSIONAL LIABILITY COSTS	---	164,000
DEFERRED FINANCING COSTS	533,517	587,313
TOTAL ASSETS	$42,130,623	$41,586,941

Liabilities and Fund Balances	20x2	20x1
CURRENT LIABILITIES		
Accounts payable	$2,326,397	$1,953,484
Accrued payroll, payroll taxes and employee benefits	2,000,348	1,900,659
Accrued interest payable	---	40,895
Other current liabilities	385,821	480,596
Reimbursement settlement payable	665,623	521,561
Payable to related division	630,000	----
Current portion of long-term debt	1,624,400	1,689,400
Total current liabilities	7,632,589	6,586,595
OTHER LIABILITIES AND DEFERRED REVENUE:		
Deferred revenue	70,560	72,240
Reserve for professional liability costs (Note 2)	82,000	164,000
Total other liabilities and deferred revenue	152,560	236,240
LONG-TERM DEBT		
Notes payable	13,949,900	16,354,300
Total long-term debt	13,949,900	16,354,300
Less-current portion	(1,624,400)	(1,689,400)
Net long-term debt	12,325,500	14,664,900
COMMITMENTS AND CONTINGENT LIABILITIES (Note 7)		
FUND BALANCES		
General	21,762,926	20,020,776
Restricted	257,048	78,430
Total fund balances	22,019,974	20,099,206
TOTAL LIABILITIES and FUND BALANCES	$42,130,623	$41,586,941

restricted"; the board can change either the amount or the classification. This can be contrasted to externally restricted funds, which require approval of the donor if changes in use are desired by management. Fixed assets are usually physical plant and equipment, which are expected to benefit more than one period. Fixed assets are converted into current expenses through depreciation techniques. The choice of depreciation methods can have a major impact on reported income and tax liability. Intangible assets are generally listed last because they are the least liquid of the assets and because their actual values depend on the provider's staying in business. Examples include deferred financing costs for debt that has been refinanced or attorney fees for reorganizational costs that have been incurred but must be expended over time because of GAAP.

Offsetting the asset accounts are liabilities and equity accounts of the organization. Liabilities consist of both short-term (current liabilities) and long-term (payable over more than one year) debt. Equity accounts are composed of the initial capital investment of the owners and the earnings retained in the organization from providing services. Equity accounts for not-for-profit organizations are sometimes called fund balances. The amounts reflect what has been retained in the organization after the amounts due to external creditors have been subtracted from total assets (total assets minus total debt equals equity/net worth/fund balances). Balance sheet accounts are usually considered to be permanent accounts; that is, they do not close at the end of each accounting period.

The Income Statement

The income statement measures the results of providing services over a period of time. It, too, is prepared in accordance with generally accepted accounting principles. The accrual method (matching of revenues and expenses), the depreciation method (straight line, accelerated), and the inventory valuation method can have a decided impact on reported income. Under the accrual method of accounting, and where noncash expenses such as depreciation are included, the income reported on the income statement is not the same as cash; in fact, using this method, it is possible to report high income and still experience a serious cash shortage. (This problem will be discussed in greater detail later in this section.) A typical income statement is shown in figure A-2, page 172.

The major components of the income statement are the revenue accounts and the expense accounts. The revenue accounts should be segregated by payer categories. The amounts shown as revenues do not include contractual allowances, discounts, and charity care. Only amounts that have been billed to payers will be included. Bad debts or amounts expected not to be collected are included as an expense account instead of as deduction from revenue. Charity care is only shown as a footnote to the summary statements and is no longer shown as a deduction from revenues. Nonpatient service revenues are shown as operating gains and losses after determination of net income from providing services to patients. Interest earned from investments would not typically be shown as patient care revenues and should be shown after net

Figure A2. Typical Income Statement

Medical Center
Statement of Revenues and Expenses
for the Years Ended June 30, 20x2 and 20x1

	20x2	20x1
Operating Revenues:		
Net patient service revenue	42,547,228	40,075,756
Other operating revenue	1,131,716	1,085,983
Total operating revenues	43,678,944	41,161,739
Operating Expenses:		
Salaries and wages	18,417,626	16,742,397
Payroll taxes and benefits	3,422,329	2,992,994
Professional fees	2,161,173	1,811,640
Supplies and other expenses	12,546,593	12,456,113
Provision for bad debts	1,025,728	230,189
Depreciation and amortization	2,906,091	2,876,525
Interest expense	1,520,809	1,758,331
Total Operating Expenses	42,000,281	38,868,189
Income from Operations	1,678,663	2,293,550
Nonoperating Gains (Losses)		
Investment income, net	693,487	567,292
Other expenses	---	(90,000)
Total Nonoperating Revenues	693,487	477,292
Excess of Revenues over Expenses	$ 2,372,150	$ 2,770,842

patient care income has been determined in order to correctly identify revenues earned from providing service to patients. In health maintenance organizations, interest earned can be shown as operating revenue.

Expenses are typically presented on a functional basis and reflect the amounts expended to provide the services responsible for the revenues shown in the income statement.

Income statement accounts are considered to be temporary accounts, because they are zeroed out at the end of each accounting period to prepare them for the next accounting period.

The Statement of Cash Flows

The balance sheet and the income statement have been required in annual reports for many years. In contrast, the statement of cash flows has only been required since the late 1980s. This relatively new financial statement has been added to the annual report in response to demands for better information about the firm's cash inflows and outflows. While the balance sheet provides a snapshot balance of cash of the final day of the period, it doesn't give the details of how it became that balance. A typed statement of cash flow is shown in figure A-3, page 174. More specifically regarding Medical Center, for example, the unit of analysis for the statement of cash flows would be the difference between the ending cash balance of $391,767 and the beginning cash balance of $1,125,628 (a decrease of $733,861).

The statement of cash flows details how accrual entries on the income statement and changes in the accrual entries on the balance sheet (other than cash itself) relate to change in the cash position. The statement is intended to help the reader understand why and, to some degree, how the cash position decreased by $733,861. This change is not evident in the balance sheet by itself. And the income statement also tells only part of the story, in that net income is a major (but not the only) potential source of cash. That is, the net income of $2,372,150 may account for part of the increase in cash during the year. However, from a cash flow perspective, there are several adjustments to make to this net income figure before we can reach any conclusions as to the amount of cash contributed by operations. For example, as we had discussed earlier, we know that depreciation and amortization expense is a noncash expense. Thus, the cash generated from operations would be the $2,372,150 plus the depreciation expense of $2,906,091. However, there are other adjustments to be made to net income, such as recognizing that all revenue may not have been collected and all expenses may not have been paid. The details surrounding these adjustments are too complicated to cover in this chapter, but they are imbedded in the construction of the statement of cash flows.

Furthermore, cash may be raised by events not captured on the income statement. For example, the Medical Center may have raised cash by borrowing or by selling assets. Such events will be recognized in the statement of cash flows. Finally, even though cash increased from operations (with adjustments) and other sources, cash also went out. We do not see this on the income statement, but cash might have been spent to purchase assets or to pay off some debt. These are essentially transactions within the balance sheet that affect the cash position. These sorts of items would also be in the statement of cash flows.

In short, the statement of cash flows provides more valuable information about liquidity than can be obtained from the balance sheet and the income statement. The statement of cash flows shows where the health care organization generated its cash and how it used it over the entire period covered by the financial statement. This feature is similar to the income statement, which shows revenues and expenses for the entire accounting period. However, the statement of cash flows is more encompassing than the income statement in that it also considers impacts other than from the income statement on cash flow (intra-balance sheet transactions), such as purchasing assets or retiring debt.

Therefore, the statement of cash flows is divided into three major sections:

- Cash from operations.

- Cash from/to investing activities.

- Cash from/to financing activities.

Figure A3. Statements of Cash Flow

Medical Center
Statements of Cash Flow
for the Years Ended June 30, 20x2 and 20x1

	20x2	20x1
Cash Flows from Operating Activities:		
Excess of revenues over expenses	$ 2,372,150	$ 2,770,842
Adjustments to excess of revenues over expenses		
Depreciation and amortization	2,906,091	2,867,525
Bad Debt Expense	1,025,720	230,189
(Gain) Loss on sale of property, plant, and equipment	36,162	(19,346)
Restricted donations and grants	210,180	11,929
Expenditure of restricted donations and grants	31,622	(57,345)
Changes in operating assets and liabilities		
(Increase) decrease in:		
Accounts receivable	(1,900,617)	(1,808,847)
Other accounts receivable	77,159	33,131
Reimbursement settlement receivable	8,067	7,318
Inventory of supplies	17,103	(90,284)
Prepaid expenses	27,463	126,828
Deferred professional liability costs	164,000	(164,000)
Accounts payable	372,913	(303,320)
Accrued payroll, payroll taxes, and employee benefits	99,689	(33,391)
Accrued interest payable	(40,895)	(3,466)
Other current liabilities	(94,775)	(28,864)
Reimbursement settlement payable	144,062	521,561
Other liabilities & deferred revenues	(83,680)	162,320
Net cash provided by operating activities	**$5,309,170**	**$4,222,780**

	20x2	20x1
Cash Flows from Investing Activities:		
Purchase of property, plant, and equipment	$(1,506,819)	$(2,814,626)
Proceeds from sale of property, plant, and equipment	112,741	29,499
Increase in assets whose use is limited	(2,244,553)	(337,626)
Net cash provided by investing activities	(3,638,631)	(3,122,753)
Cash Flows from Financing Activities:		
Principle payments on long-term debt	(2,404,400)	(1,285,400)
Increase in deferred financing costs		(17,550)
Net cash provided by financing activities	(2,404,400)	(1,302,950)
Net Decrease in Cash and Cash Equivalents	(733,861)	(202,923)
Cash and Cash Equivalents at Beginning of Year	1,125,628	1,328,551
Cash and Cash Equivalents at End of Year	$ 391,767	$ 1,125,628

Operating activities are related to revenue- and expense-producing activities of the health care organization as reflected in the income statement. As stated above, these revenue- and expense-producing activities are adjusted by noncash amounts, such as depreciation expense, as well as several other more complicated adjustments. The working capital portion of the balance sheet is also considered among the ordinary activities of the firm, so changes in these amounts are also factored in. The financing activities of the health care organization are concerned with borrowing money (and repaying it), issuance of stock, and payment of dividends. All of these financing activities are potential non-income statement sources of cash (or drains on cash in terms of repaying debt or paying out dividends). Finally, the investing activities of the health care organization are also potential non–income statement uses of cash related to the purchase and sale of fixed assets and securities.

In summary, the income statement focuses on operations of the health care organization. Specifically, what did it cost to provide the service, what did it cost to operate the organization, and how much revenue did the organization get for its services? The statement of cash flows focuses on financial rather than operating aspects of the firm. Where did the money come from, and how did the health care organization spend it? While the major concern of the income statement is profitability, the statement of cash flows is very concerned with cash viability. Is the health care organization generating, and will it generate, enough cash to meet both short-term and long-term obligations?

Financial Statement Analysis

An analysis of financial statements can be accomplished by several methods. Single-point estimates can be obtained for comparison with other institutions or with external standards. A trend line is sometimes useful to identify possible problem areas. Both point and trend analysis are important for management information, but trend analysis has the added benefit of not requiring external comparison data. Because of the dissimilarity of many institutions, point comparisons can be very misleading. The accounts in the balance sheet and the income statement can be analyzed on a percentage basis. Common size and vertical analysis provides information on changes in the structure of the statements in terms of percentages. These composition ratios can indicate when profit margins are shrinking and what is causing the decrease—for example, when certain asset categories are increasing in relationship to the total asset structure. An analysis of two statements is generally more effective than single estimates.

Another commonly used analysis technique is computation and comparison of ratios. Ratios can be grouped into specific management areas to aid in analysis. Four key management areas are:

Liquidity—Can the organization meet its current obligations?

Turnover—Are the organization's assets being used effectively?

Performance—Are the organization's assets being used efficiently?

Capitalization—How are the assets being financed?

A summary of the ratios is included in figure A-4, page 177.

Sample Analysis of the Financial Statements

Using the data from figures A-1, A-2, and A-3 and the ratios from figure A-4, the following analysis could be accomplished for the sample provider:

Liquidity Ratios

Current Ratio = $\dfrac{11,375,301}{7,632,589}$ = 1.49

Daily Cash Outflow = $\dfrac{42,000,281 - (2,906,091 + 1,025,720)}{365}$ = \$104,297

Days of Cash Outflow Available = $\dfrac{391,767}{104,297}$ = 3.76 days

Times Interest Covered = $\dfrac{2,372,150 + 1,520,809}{1,520,809}$ = 2.56

Analysis: The provider has a satisfactory current ratio, but the days of cash outflow are minimal. Collection of accounts receivable or short-term loans will be necessary to meet operating expenses.

Turnover Ratios

Asset Turnover = $\dfrac{43,678,944}{42,130,623}$ = 1.04 times/year

Accounts Receivable Turnover = $\dfrac{43,678,944}{8,399,210}$ = 5.2 times/year

Inventory Turnover = $\dfrac{12,546,593}{356,798}$ = 35.16 days

Average Daily Revenue = $\dfrac{43,678,944}{365}$ = \$119,668

Average Collection Period = $\dfrac{8,399,210}{119,668}$ = 70.19 days

Average Daily Supply Expense = $\dfrac{12,546,593}{365}$ = \$34,374

Figure A4. Summary of Ratios

Liquidity Ratios

Current Ratio = $\dfrac{\text{Current Assets}}{\text{Current Liabilities}}$

Daily Cash Outflow = $\dfrac{\text{Operating Expenses—Noncash Expenses}}{\text{Days in Period}}$

Days of Cash Outflow Available = $\dfrac{\text{Cash}}{\text{Daily Cash Flow}}$

Times Interest Coverage = $\dfrac{\text{Revenues in Excess of Expenses from Operations+ Interest Expense}}{\text{Interest Expense}}$

Debt Service Ratio = $\dfrac{\text{Revenues in Excess of Expenses from Operations + Interest + Depreciation + Annual Debt Service Requirements}}{\text{Annual Debt Service}}$

Working Capital per Bed = $\dfrac{\text{Working Capital}}{\text{Available Beds}}$

Turnover Ratios

Asset Turnover = $\dfrac{\text{Net Operating Revenue}}{\text{Total Assets}}$

Accounts Receivable Turnover = $\dfrac{\text{Net Operating Revenue}}{\text{Net Accounts Receivable}}$

Inventory Turnover = $\dfrac{\text{Supply Expense}}{\text{Inventory}}$

Average Daily Patient Revenue = $\dfrac{\text{Net Operating Revenue}}{\text{Number of Days}}$

Average Collection Period = $\dfrac{\text{Net Accounts Receivable}}{\text{Average Daily Patient Revenue}}$

Average Daily Operating Expenses = $\dfrac{\text{Operating Expenses}}{\text{Number of Days}}$

Accounts Payable Payment Period = $\dfrac{\text{Accounts Payable}}{\text{Number of Days}}$

Performance Ratios

Operating Margin = $\dfrac{\text{Revenues in Excess of Expenses from Operations}}{\text{Net Revenues}}$

Return on Assets = $\dfrac{\text{Revenues in Excess of Expenses from Operations}}{\text{Total Assets}}$

Return on Fund Balance = $\dfrac{\text{Revenues in Excess of Expenses from Operations}}{\text{Fund Balance}}$

Pre-Financing Return on Assets = $\dfrac{\text{Revenues in Excess of Expenses from Operations+ Interest}}{\text{Total Assets}}$

Pre-Financing Return on Fund Balance and Long Term Debt = $\dfrac{\text{Revenues in Excess of Expenses from Operations+ Interest}}{\text{Fund Balance + Long-Term Debt}}$

Capitalization Ratios

Total Debt to Fund Balance = $\dfrac{\text{Total Debt}}{\text{Fund Balance}}$

Long-Term Debt to Total Assets = $\dfrac{\text{Long-Term Debt}}{\text{Total Assets}}$

Total Debt to Total Capitalization = $\dfrac{\text{Total Debt}}{\text{Total Assets}}$

Accounts
Payable   = $\dfrac{2,326,387}{34,374}$ = 67.68 days
Payment Period

Analysis: Utilization of assets is average, as measured by the asset turnover of 1.04. The accounts receivable collection period of 70 days indicates some follow-up in this area would be useful, while the accounts payable cycle of 67.68 days means that bills are not paid promptly.

Performance Ratios

Operating Margin   = $\dfrac{2,372,150}{43,678,944}$ = .054

Return on Assets   = $\dfrac{2,372,150}{42,130,623}$ = .0563

Return on   = $\dfrac{2,372,150}{22,019,974}$ = .1077
Fund Balance

Prefinancing   = $\dfrac{2,372,150 + 1,520,809}{42,130,623}$ = .092
Return on Assets

Analysis: The owner has a reasonable operating margin (.054). The return on fund balance is high (10.77 percent) because of use of short-term credit in current liabilities.

Capitalization Ratios

Total Debt to   = $\dfrac{42,130,623 - 22,019,974}{22,019,974}$ = $\dfrac{20,110,649}{22,019,974}$ = .91
Fund Balances

Long-Term Debt   = $\dfrac{12,325,500}{42,130,623}$ = .29
to Total Assets

Total Debt to   = $\dfrac{42,130,623 - 22,019,974}{42,130,623}$ = $\dfrac{20,110,649}{42,130,623}$ = .48
Total Assets

Analysis: The provider has 50 percent of capital from debt sources, which, in most cases, would be considered high. This may or may not be a problem, depending on the certainty of the payment process. If accounts receivable are sound, there should be no problem in paying off the debt. It might be prudent to add more long-term capital, through either retained earnings or a fund drive from the community.

Appendix B

Cost/Volume/Profit Models

Based on our understanding of cost behavior, a tool can be developed that will enable managers to make better forecasts of volume and better estimates of what the corresponding charge rate should be, or to assess more accurately the effects of changes in variable or fixed costs. To review our understanding of cost behavior, the following definitions are presented:

- Variable costs are assumed to vary directly in proportion to the volume of services provided.

- Fixed costs are assumed not to vary with volume changes.

Given these two basic assumptions, the cost structure for the service can be expressed as follows:

(1)   Total Costs (TC) = Total Fixed Costs (TFC) + Total Variable Costs (TVC); TC = TFC + TVC.

(2)   TVC = Variable Costs per Unit of Service (VCU) x Volume (or number of units) of Service (Q). Therefore, equation (1) can also be expressed as TC = TFC + (VCU x Q).

(3)   Average Total Cost (ATC) = Total Cost per unit x Volume of service = $\dfrac{TC}{Q}$

The first three equations can be expressed in the following model when revenues and profits requirements are introduced:

(4)   Total Revenues (TR)[1] = Rate per Unit of Service (R) x Volume of Service (Q); TR = R x Q.

Desired Profit or Income (I) can be expressed as a dollar requirement or as a percentage of total revenue requirement and on a before- or after-tax basis.[2]

(5a)   After-tax dollar requirement   =   I
        Before-tax dollar requirement =   I/(1 - tax rate)

(5b)   After-tax percentage of total revenue requirement = %TR
        Before-tax percentage of total revenue requirement = %TR/(1 - tax rate)

The summary and complete model can be expressed as:

(6)   TR = TC + I or
        RxQ = TFC + (VCU)(Q) + I (1 - tax rate)

        or, solving for R,

(7) $R = \dfrac{TFC}{Q} + VCU + \dfrac{I}{(1 - \text{tax rate}) \times Q}$

An example of how this equation can be used is to determine the rate that must be charged to obtain a desired level of profit.

Given:

TFC	=	$50,000
VCU	=	$11
Desired I (after taxes)	=	$10,000
Tax rate	=	37.5%
Q	=	5,000

Substituting:

$R = \dfrac{\$50,000}{5,000} + 11 + \dfrac{\$10,000}{(1 - .375) \times 5,000}$

$R = \$10 + 11 + \dfrac{2}{(1 - .375)}$

$R = \$10 + \$11 + \$3.20 = \$24.20$

This answer can be verified by completing a simplified income statement:

Total Revenue	5,000	x	$24.20	=	$121,000	
Variable Costs	5,000	x	$11.00	=	$ 55,000	
Contribution Margin	5,000	x	$13.20	=	$ 66,000	

Total Fixed Costs	$ 50,000
Income Before Taxes	$ 16,000
Taxes at a 37½ % Rate	$ 6,000
Income After Taxes	$ 10,000

The basic cost/volume/profit model of equation (7) can also be used, for example, to compare the effects of buying more equipment (increased fixed costs) with those of switching to outside suppliers on a fee-for-service basis (increased variable costs). Of course, the estimates going into the model do not have to be, indeed cannot be, precise. Few events in the future can be determined precisely. What is needed is an estimate of the reasonableness of the numbers. Is this rate reasonable? Can this quantity realistically be obtained? How sensitive are the results to alternative assumptions? The model allows the input necessary for this type of analysis.

Capitation

The basic cost/volume/profit model of equation (7) can also be used in a cap-itated environment. However, the volume factor (Q) must be expressed in the manner in which we generate revenue—the monthly premium dollar that is referred to as member months (mm). In this case, let us assume that we are considering a contract to cover 125,000 mm. Thus, Q = 125,000 mm. The unit of service expression from the fee-for-service example (5,000) is still relevant. Instead of the volume factor (Q), however, it is a utilization expression. Thus, utilization (U) = 5,000 units ÷ 125,000 = .04 per mm. At this point we can set the price (monthly premium) that we need to achieve the desired income of $10,000 as expressed in the fee-for-service environment. This is done in the following:

Given:

TFC	=	$50,000
VCU	=	$11
Desired Income (after taxes)	=	$10,000
Tax rate	=	37.5%
Q	=	125,000
U	=	.04 mm

Substitutions:

$$R = \frac{\$50,000}{125,000 \text{ mm}} + \$11(.04) + \frac{\$10,000}{(1-,375) \times 125,000 \text{ mm}}$$

$$R = .40 \text{ mm} + .44 \text{ mm} + .128 \text{ mm} = \$.968 \text{ mm}$$

This answer can be verified by completing a simplified income statement:

Total Revenue	125,000 mm	x	.968	=	$121,000
Variable Costs	125,000 mm	x	.44	=	55,000
Contribution Margin	125,000 mm	x	.528	=	66,000

Total Fixed Costs	50,000
Income Before Taxes	16,000
Taxes @ 37.5% Rate	6,000
Income after Taxes	$ 10,000

Following this logic further, notice the positive implications if we are able to control utilization such that it drops from .04 mm to .03 mm. This results in variable costs being expressed as .03 x $11 unit = $.33 mm. These implications are seen in the following simplified income statement.

Total Revenue	125,000 mm	x	.968	=	$121,000
Variable Costs	125,000 mm	x	.33	=	41,250
Contribution Margi	125,000 mm	x	.638	=	79,750
Total Fixed Costs					50,000
Income Before Taxes					29,750
Taxes @ 37.5% Rate					11,156
Income after Taxes					$ 18,594

Note this improvement in income: $18,594 – 10,000 = $ 8,594. This increase results from control of utilization as follows: .01 (decrease in utilization from .04 to .03) x $11 x 125,000 mm = $13,750 less $5,156 (the 37.5 percent tax rate) = $8,594.

Multiple Payers

For many departments, there is no single rate for services provided because of the varying amounts paid by different third-party payers. Each individual rate may reflect third-party regulations; competitive pressures; and/or managerial judgments about future costs, market dynamics, inflation, etc. Once individual rates have been estimated, the same approach described above can be used, but the single rate used in the model above becomes a weighted average of the various payer rates. In the example above, a single rate of $24.20 resulted. But this $24.20 could represent an average rate developed in the following manner:

	Proportion of Total Volume	x	Rate		
Medicare	30%	x	$20.00	=	$ 6.00
Medicaid	50%	x	15.40	=	$ 7.70
Charge-Based	20%	x	52.50	=	$10.50
			Average Revenue		$24.20

The following example shows how the rate for a charge-based payer can be determined where multiple payers exist.

Given:

- 40,000 lab tests are forecast.
- The Medicare rate is $32.00 and Medicare is 40% of all activity.
- The Medicaid rate is $20.00 and Medicaid is 50% of all activity.
- Charge-based activity is 10% of all activity.
- Fixed costs are $600,000.
- Variable costs are $10.00 per lab test.
- The desired profit margin is $100,000 after taxes.
- The tax rate is 37.5%

What rate must be charged to charge-based payers to meet the desired profit margin? Using the model developed above and substituting the new information, the average rate would be:

$$RA = [TFC + (VCU \times Q) + \frac{I}{(1 - tax\ rate)}] \div Q$$

$$RA = [\$600,000 + (\$10 \times 40,000) + \frac{\$100,000}{(1 - .375)}] \div 40,000$$

$$RA = \frac{\$600,000}{40,000} + \$10 + \frac{\$160,000}{40,000} = \$15 + \$10 + \$4 = \$29$$

Using the weighted average approach developed above, the charge for charge-based payers would be:

	Proportion of Total Volume	x	Rate		
Medicare	40%	x	$32.00	=	$10.00
Medicaid	50%	x	20.00	=	$12.80
Charge-Based	10%	x	RChg	=	$?
			Average Revenue		$29.00

RChg = ($29.00 - $10.00 - $12.80) divided by .10 = $6.20 ÷ .10 = $62.00, the required charge for charge-based payers.

These results can be verified using the income statement approach:

Revenues

Medicare	40%	x	40,000	x	$32.00	=	$ 512,000
Medicaid	50%	x	40,000	x	22.00	=	400,000
Charge-Based	10%	x	40,000	x	62.00	=	248,000
			Total Revenue				= $1,160,000

Expenses

Fixed Costs	$ 600,000
Variable Costs (40,000 x $10)	400,000
Total Costs	$1,000,000
Profit before taxes	$ 160,000
Taxes at 37.5%	60,000
Profit after taxes	$ 100,000

If the mix of the various payers changes, the effect on the rate can also be determined and adjustments can be made accordingly.

A Contribution Model

A short-cut approach to the cost/volume/profit model is one that focuses on the contribution margin (CM) or on the difference between the rate (R) and the variable cost per unit (VCU). Through concentration on the contribution margin, answers can rapidly be obtained to the questions posed above. For example, the basic contribution model can be expressed as:

$$(8) \qquad TFC \quad + \quad \frac{I}{1 - \text{tax rate}} \quad = Q \times CM$$

where I is the desired after-tax income and CM is defined as (R - VCU). Given the numbers in the first example above:

R	=	$ 24.20
TFC	=	$50,000
VCU	=	$ 11
I	=	10,000
Tax rate	=	37.5%
Q	=	Unknown

Substituting in the Equation (8):

$$\$50,000 + \frac{\$10,000}{(1 - .375)} = Q \times \$13.20$$

$$Q = \frac{\$50,000 + \$16,000}{\$13.20}$$

$$= \frac{\$66,000}{\$13.20}$$

$$= 5,000$$

The contribution margin approach can also be used effectively to monitor and report on departmental activities. The basic format changes to define margin as the difference between total revenues and direct costs (TR - DC). Direct costs include all costs for which the department supervisor is responsible. For example, the department supervisor is responsible for salaries paid and supplies used. Depreciation on equipment used only in the department, any special maintenance, etc. are considered direct costs. Other costs, such as general administration, utilities, and housekeeping, are considered indirect costs, because they are not under the control of the department supervisor but are generally allocated. An example performance report might be:

Total Revenues	$100,000
Total Direct Costs	70,000
Direct Margin	$30,000
Allocated Indirect Costs	25,000
Departmental Income	$5,000

The direct margin should be the point of emphasis for the control process. The amount of indirect costs can be changed by the choice of allocation methods as well as by third-party payment regulations. Although the bottom line is a proper concern of senior managers, it is questionable whether it should be used to evaluate lower levels of supervisors, whose range of choice and control is limited.

Footnotes

1. Total revenues are defined as the amount expected to be collected from all patients.

2. This works for not-for-profit organizations as well. With a tax rate of zero, the before-tax and after-tax requirements are simply equal.

Appendix C

Basic Budgeting Techniques

Flexible and Static Budgeting

Identification of variable and fixed cost components of cost categories makes it possible to use flexible budgeting techniques. A flexible budget is a budget that is adjusted for volume changes. For example, if nurse staffing is based on patient days, the budget allowance for nurse staffing would change with changes in patient activity level. Nursing administration costs, in comparison, are relatively fixed for reasonable ranges of patient activity.

Suppose 65,700 patient days were budgeted for a hospital's revenue projections. If we required 2.5 RN hours per patient day, our budgeted RN hours would be 65,700 x 2.5 = 164,250. These hours could then be converted to a dollar cost by extending them at the average RN hourly rate. If that were $12 per hour, the total budgeted cost would be $1,971,000. If we did not adjust this budgeted amount for variation in patient days, we would be using a static budget approach. The budget logic is as follows:

	Output	Standards	Input
Budget	65,700 days x	2.5 RN hours = per day	164,250 RN hours $12 $1,971,000

A static budget approach to making judgments about organizational performance would take the planned budget as the basis against which to compare actual RN salary costs during the period. This adherence to a budgeted amount when costs are variable can lead to dysfunctional managerial decisions. For example, if patient days are less than planned, the budget for RN salaries would be too loose, and, even if actual RN costs were equal or slightly less than the budgeted amount, RNs would not have been used efficiently. If patient days are greater than planned, strict adherence to the budgeted RN costs would result in fewer RN hours being available for each patient day, and a reduction in the quality of care could result.

Flexible budgeting adjusts the budget for changes in levels of activity. For example, assume actual nursing costs were $2,203,200. Also assume that the number of patient days was 68,000, compared to the 65,700 that were planned. A static budget suggests an unfavorable variance:

	Output	Standards	Input
Budget	65,700 days x	2.5 RN hours = per day	164,250 RN hours x ____$12 $1,971,000
Actual	68,000 days x	2.7 RN hours = per day	183,600 RN hours x ____$12 $2,203,200

Unfavorable Variance   (1,971,000 – 2,203,200) $(232,200)

However, a flexible budget would first adjust expected cash to the actual value level before determining the variance:

	Output	Standards	Input
Budget	65,700 days x	2.5 RN hours = per day	164,250 RN hours x ____$12 $1,971,000
Flexible Budget	68,000 days x	2.5 RN hours = per day	170,000 RN hours x ____$12 $2,040,000
Actual	68,000 days x	2.7 RN hours = per day	183,600 RN hours x ____$12 $2,203,200

Total Variance   ($1,971,000 – 2,203,200) $(232,200)

Volume (allowable)   ($1,971,000 – 2,040,000) $69,000
(2,300 additional patient days x 2.5 RN hrs/day x $12)

Unfavorable Variance   ($2,040,000 – 2,203,200) $(163,200)

In most organizations, the flexible budget approach offers a more realistic assessment of performance and a better approach to cost control. For many providers, when most costs are relatively fixed, the static budget approach may be adequate. But if variable costs, even if relatively small, can be determined, the flexible approach provides more detailed information and can identify excess as well as insufficient resource utilization.

Appendix D

Net Present Value Calculations

Assume that a proposal to be evaluated requires an initial cash investment of $1,000 and is expected to provide incremental cash inflows of $372 at the end of the first year and $1,296 at the end of the second year. The organization's overall WACC is estimated to be 20 percent during both years. This 20 percent rate means that the $1,000 investment should provide a total return of at least $1,200 if the proposed activity lasts just one year. But this proposal covers two years, and, while it provides only $372 in the first year, it also generates $1,296 in the second year. This means that we must evaluate both of the cash inflows to see if their combined value provides a total return sufficient to meet our 20 percent WACC.

To value flows over two years, we simply do what we already know how to do, but we do it twice:

Present Value at 20%		Incremental Operational Cash Inflows	
		End of Year 1	End of Year 2
$ 900	◀— 2nd year cash inflow ÷ by 1.20 twice ◀—		$1,296
$ 310	◀— 1st year flow ÷ by 1.20 ◀—	$372	
		1,080 ÷1.20	
$1,210	◀— ÷ 1.20 ◀—	$1,452	
Combined value of both cash inflows viewed as of today		Combined value of both cash inflows viewed as of the end of Year 1	

- 1,000 Value of initial outflow
$ 210 Net Present Value

Because the present value of the $1,000 initial cash outflow today is a negative $1,000, the NPV of this proposal is a positive $210. Obviously, this proposal is very desirable from a fiscal viewpoint.

A different way of arriving at the same result is as follows:

1. $1,000 invested at 20 percent for two years yields $1,440 = ($1,000 x 1.20 x 1.20). Therefore, if a proposal returned exactly $1,440 on a $1,000 investment after two years it would exactly meet the organization's WACC and have a net present value of zero.

2. But this proposal returns $372 after one year and $1,296 the second year. Because they're not the "same" kind of dollars, you can't just add $372 and $1,296. But you can adjust the $372 by presuming you could invest it at the same 20 percent rate that was applied above:

$372 x 1.20 = $ 446.40   (value of first year payment
at end of second year)

                1,296.00   (Second year payment)

            $1,742.40   (Total return at end of
second year; also the combined
value of both cash inflows viewed
as of end of year 2)

3. Comparing the $1,742 total return after two years to the $1,440 required return from Step 1, the proposal generates extra return of $302.40. This amount is called the "net future value" of the proposal.

4. To convert net future value to net present value, you have to discount it back for two years. As discussed previously, you simply divide the $302.40 by the discount factor (in this case 1.20) twice, because two years of adjustment have to be made: $302.40 ÷ 1.20 = $252.00; $252.00 ÷ 1.20 = $210.00, the net present value calculated initially.

Chapter  **Planning and Marketing: An External Perspective to Competitive Strategy**

by Eric N. Berkowitz, PhD

Since the mid-1970s, the management of health care organizations has gone through a period of rapid change in response to an increasingly complex environment. One aspect of this change has been the introduction of marketing as a functional area within the management setting. Common to many traditional industries, marketing was considered a novel approach to respond to the increasingly competitive environment being felt by many provider organizations in the mid-1970s. Yet, since the early introduction of marketing, the effectiveness of this functional area within health care has been limited. To a large extent, this lack of contribution of marketing may well be a function of an inappropriate perception of what marketing is and of how it contributes to the management of a health care organization. The purpose of this chapter is to discuss the meaning of marketing and how it affects the planning process of organizations, as well as the key components of marketing strategy formulation.

Marketing is both a process and a philosophy. In integrating marketing into an organization, the hospital or the medical group must view the service offering not from the perspective of the provider, but rather from that of the buyer. To be market-driven is to be customer-responsive. In its simplest form, marketing may be defined as the process by which customer needs are identified and a product (or service) is developed in response to those needs.[1] The service is delivered, priced, and promoted according to the best way to attract the consumer. In this perspective of marketing, there are four components of strategy that will be discussed in greater depth in this chapter. These four components, referred to as the four Ps of marketing, or the marketing mix, are product, price, place, and promotion. All organizations have these four components in their control to some extent. That is, what products or services should be offered and at what price? How should these services be delivered or made accessible (place), and in what manner can the market be informed of the service's existence (promotion)? Later in this chapter, each of these components is discussed in greater depth.

The consumer is at the center of the marketing process. It is the consumer's needs to which the organization responds. For most health care organizations, this definition of the consumer varies and rarely consists of a single constituency. Figure 1, page 191, shows some of the multiple markets that exist for a hospital, a multispecialty group practice, or a single program such as adolescent chemical dependency. The challenge for health care organizations in developing an effective marketing approach is balancing the often varying needs of each market with the respective clinical service quality issues of the provider.

The Market-Driven Planning Sequence

Recognizing that marketing is driven by the consumer has a significant implication for the planning process of the organization. Historically, health care organizations were not market-driven. Rather, planning occurred from an internal perspective. In the typical planning mode, the hospital or group might examine statistics on the market in terms of age or income, along with various epidemiological data of the primary and secondary service areas. The confluence of these factors might lead to a decision that a particular service was or wasn't needed in the community. After committing to the development of the service, it was then left to the administrator or chief financial officer to determine the pricing for the service. No formal strategy was developed for the service beyond the offering of this new program. Scheduling, location of the satellite facility, or determination of how the market would be informed of the service was left to the discretion of the providers of the service.

In a market-driven approach, the introduction of a new service occurs as the result of a very different set of activities. Often, providers within a group or a hospital might suggest a new service, such as rehabilitation medicine or a scoliosis clinic. Before the service is rolled out, an assessment of the market is made. Is there a demand for this new service? Are there other providers in the market? What price are buyers willing to pay for this offering? Where would users like to receive this service and during what hours? In a market-driven sequence, the definition of a service is really provided by the likely buyer or user of the service. The provider's role is to ensure clinical quality and to deliver the offering.

In considering the conditions that existed for most health care organizations up to the mid-1970s, it is easy to understand why a market-based approach was never integrated into typical health care planning. For most of the 1950s, 1960s, and even 1970s, most communities were still underserved with regard to a range of clinical services or providers. In fact, for most hospitals and other medical institutions, this period was not one of great cost or utilization pressure. When a service was offered, the primary problem was typically that of trying to meet demand rather than to stimulate it. In the rare instance in which a medical organization offered a new service that was not successful, it was often viewed by the board of trustees or physicians as a good learning experience. Why is a marketing-based approach now a more common occurrence? Rarely is the problem now facing medical organizations one of meeting demand. It is more likely a situation of trying to generate utilization or volume.

Figure 1. Multiple Markets/Multiple Provider

Provider	Markets
Hospital	Patients
	Physicians
	Corporations
	HMOs
Multispecialty Group	Patients
	Physicians
	Corporations
Adolescent Chemical	Parents
Dependency Program	Judges
	Social Workers
	Third-Party Payers

Additionally, 15 or 20 years ago, most health care organizations were in relatively strong financial positions. A new clinical service that was not successful financially could be seen as a learning experience. Today, there are few health care organizations that can afford very many learning experiences.

The importance of a market-driven approach is being recognized among medical groups that have ventured into extended hour programs or weekend appointment schedules. Often, these programs are tried because a particular physician in the group has gone to a conference and heard that other medical groups are offering weekend hours. After offering these hours, the group finds that the only thing accomplished was to increase the overhead of the organization and make the quality of life for the staff less desirable.

In using the market-based approach to planning, one would consider the offering of weekend hours or any new service by also determining whether it is for an offensive or defensive strategic purpose. For example, the organization should first survey consumers who they would like to get as patients (but do not presently) and ask, "If the XYZ medical group were to offer weekend hours by appointment, how likely would you be to switch to it for your care?" That is, would the weekend hours increase business, an offensive strategy. Or, one might pose the question to existing patients whom the group wishes to maintain by asking, "If another medical group in the community were to offer weekend hours by appointment, how likely would you be to switch?" Is the group developing a market-driven strategy to retain a customer base, a defensive rationale?

It Begins with Research

Essential to effective marketing is the need to conduct marketing research.[2] As discussed previously, marketing involves an external to internal planning perspective. It is marketing research that provides the external perspective. It is not the purpose of this chapter to describe all the intricacies of marketing research methodologies. However, it is important to recognize that it is the rare successful marketing company that does not conduct marketing research on an ongoing basis.

Secondary Data

Marketing research can use either primary or secondary data. Secondary data are collected for purposes beyond the specific problem at hand. In health care, several commercial, secondary data sources are often used:

- *Census data.* Companies such as Urban Decision Systems offer simplified ways of using census data arranged by zip code.

- *Syndicated marketing research.* These are research efforts to which a health care organization can subscribe to receive regular updates on particular topics. The National Research Corporation (NRC) publishes its annual Healthcare Market Guide, an annual survey of 100,000 households in the top 100 markets in the United States. These data provide perceptual information regarding hospitals in a particular market as well as other breakdowns of interest. NRC is just one of several companies now entering the syndicated market research data field in health care.[3]

- *Web-based information.* Increasingly, the Internet has provided a valuable source of secondary data on competitors, trends, and resources for organizations. The number of health-related Web sites is increasing at a dramatic rate. A major concern with much information on the Web is the need to check for accuracy. However, often the data and information obtained from this resource are timelier than those from typical data sources.

With any secondary data, it is important to recognize their major limitation. The data were not collected for the specific institution or issue of concern. In using secondary market research data, one must always be concerned with the quality of the study, the timeliness of the data, the relevance of the sample, and whether the classifications of the data are worthwhile.

Primary Data

Because of the limitations of secondary data, most organizations will collect primary data for a project of importance. Figure 2, page 193, shows common methods used in collecting primary data and the respective tradeoffs with each technique. Increasingly in health care, focus groups are seen as a valuable tool.[4] In focus groups, 10-12 individuals are led through a series of relatively open-ended questions by a trained moderator. While they do not provide empirical numbers, focus groups can often reveal issues and concerns that can be explored further in a mail or phone survey. Focus groups are increasingly used in two different steps in the marketing research process. Many organizations use them at the beginning of the research process to reveal issues, such as the possible reasons a radiology group isn't getting referrals. Or, focus groups can be used at the end of the research process to

Figure 2. Alternative Research Methodologies*

Approach Criteria	Personal Interview	RESEARCH METHODOLOGY Telephone Survey	Mail Survey	Focus Groups
Economy	Most expensive.	Avoids interviewer travel, relatively expensive. Trained interviewers needed.	Potentially lower costs (if response rate sufficient).	Relatively expensive.
Interviewer bias	High likelihood of bias. Trust. Appearance.	Less than personal interviewer. No face-to-face contact. Suspicion of phone call.	Interviewer bias eliminated. Anonymity provided.	Need trained moderator.
Flexibility	Most flexible Responses can be probed. Assistance can be provided in completing forms. Observations can be made.	Cannot make observations. Probing possible to a degree.	Least flexible.	Very flexible.
Sampling and respondent cooperation	Most complete sample possible, with sufficient call back strategy.	Limited to people with telephones. No answers. Refusals are common.	Mailing list. Nonresponse a major problem.	Need close selection.

* Reprinted from Hillestad, S., and Berkowitz, E. *Health Care Marketing Plans: From Strategy to Action*. Second Edition. Rockville, Md.: Aspen Press, 1991, p. 100.

help explain the results in a survey. For example, a focus group might be constructed to better understand why 75 percent of the people indicated they were somewhat dissatisfied with the service of the emergency department.

No doubt all readers of this book have been at the receiving end of phone, mail, and personal interviews, so no definitions of each approach are needed. However, a few comments about each methodology may be helpful. In conducting personal and telephone interviews, it is important to use trained interviewers. The potential for bias with an untrained interviewer can make data collection highly suspect. Phone interviewers are also a very valuable way to collect information quickly.[5] Mail surveys are difficult to conduct because of nonresponse bias. While there are many methods for improving response rates for mail surveys, the ultimate question is always whether the person who responded is in any way different from the individual who did not respond. Except for the cost savings of mail surveys, there is little else to speak to their advantage beyond protection of the identity of the respondent.

Defining the Target Market and Market Segmentation

There is one other aspect of marketing and marketing strategy that must be underscored in order for a market-based approach to planning to be effective—the target market. The term target market may be best defined as one or more specific groups of customers to whom an organization directs its strategy.[6]

Target Markets

Target markets have never been a consideration in health care. When hospital CEOs are asked about their target markets, they respond with data about the primary or the secondary service area, or with a zip code analysis of who has been admitted through the emergency department. When a physician establishes a practice, the office is opened and people who call or walk in are treated. In traditional marketing, the target market is an organizationally determined aspect of strategy. It is more a question of whom does the organization want to attract? Then, the market-based planning approach is aimed at members of this target market. Subsequent strategy is built around attracting this targeted population.

An important ethical comment must be raised around the entire issue of target markets in health care. The definition of a target market does not imply denying care to anyone who walks into the medical organization for treatment, but treating anyone who walks through the door is different from developing a strategy to go after a particular group of consumers. The four Ps discussed in the following pages are directed to a target market that is determined by the organization. Having determined the target market, the organization can begin to formulate a marketing strategy based on the four Ps of product, price, place, and promotion.

Market Segmentation

A central concept drives marketing thinking—market segmentation. Market segmentation is identification of a subgroup of consumers in the population with similar wants and needs and tailoring of the marketing mix to meet that subgroup's needs. The belief is that the closer the organization can tailor the marketing mix to an individual's preferences, the greater the likelihood that the individual will buy the product or service from that provider.

There are two traditional ways to segment the market. The first has been common in health care, sociodemographics. The marketing is segmented by age, gender, income, or ethnicity. In health care, programs have been established in pediatrics, geriatrics, and women's health. Even income has been a form of segmentation in health care. The Washington Hospital Center has developed its Pavilion, a well-decorated area of the hospital with amenities such as heated towel racks, carpeting, specially prepared meals, and even a concierge service targeted to the upscale patient.

A second way to segment has interesting implications for marketing strategy in a fee-for-service world and dramatic implications in a managed care world. This approach is referred to as heavy half segmentation. Heavy half segmentation is based on the principle that a small group of consumers tend to account for a disproportionate amount of a product's sales. For example, 17 percent of all households account for 88 percent of all the beer sold; 39 percent of all households account for 90 percent of all soft drinks sold. A middle group of consumers account for the remaining percentage of the product sales, and a large percentage of consumers do not buy the product at all.

The heavy half phenomenon applies and has important marketing implications in health care. For example, in a fee-for-service world, a primary care practice will find that a large percentage of its patient revenue is generated from a relatively small number of charts. The important marketing goal for this segment in a fee-for-service environment is to maintain these consumers. Prior to making any operational changes within the practice or a program, it is imperative to pretest the change with loyal consumers to ensure that they will not become alienated or dissatisfied. The key objective with the consumers who use the practice but are not heavy users is to identify what can be done to make them loyal users. Is their use limited because they are healthy, or is it that they are splitting their care among providers? Finally, within any practice or health care organization's service area, there are a large number of consumer who do not use the facility or practice at all. The major marketing question is to determine whether they do not use it because they have heard negative things about the facility or because they are loyal to other providers. Or, is their lack of use because of no knowledge of what the organization can offer them in terms of meeting their health care needs? This latter issue becomes a promotional challenge for marketing.

The heavy half segmentation perspective has some interesting implications in a managed care world. Most managed care organizations would recognize that this segmentation scheme exists. A large percentage of the organization's utilization tends to come from a small percent of subscribers. A middle group of subscribers account for the balance of the remaining utilization, which is not significant but is within the norms of health utilization statistics. Some subscribers join the plan but never use the practice during the contract period. From a marketing perspective, the objectives shift from a fee-for-service world. The heavy users are a group who must be served. And to deny care to this group because they are a financial drain on the organization would be unethical and illegal. Yet, from a marketing perspective, the key challenge is to maintain the subscriber base of medium and nonusers. With the middle segment of subscribers, the goal is to ensure that they experience no service delivery failures when they interact with the organization. Because these occasional users have limited experience with the managed care plan, any service delivery failure may give them justification for switching to another plan when their contract renewal period occurs. The nonuser segment must be targeted in the last quarter prior to re-enrollment. These individuals should be contacted and should have some direct, personal interaction with the managed care entity. This interaction might consist of a health assessment or a brief health status discussion with a doctor. The reason is that, within 90 days, that person will be faced with a re-enrollment decision. That valued subscriber must have some sense of identity with the organization to ensure that he or she will not shift to a lower cost plan.

Product: The Foundation of Strategy

The focus of marketing strategy revolves around the product or service. In marketing, a central concept to developing the product or service strategy is the product life cycle. The product life cycle concept assumes that all products (or services) go through four distinct stages; introduction, growth, maturity, and decline. Figure 3, page 197, shows a generalized product life cycle curve. On the x-axis is time, and the y-axis represents sales or gross revenues. In each stage, market conditions change, which requires a change in organizational strategy. At the introduction stage, sales rise slowly. At growth, significant increases in sales occur, which level off during maturity. Ultimately, revenue drops during decline.

Introduction

In the introduction stage, the new service enters the market. For example, the first HMO opens in the community. With regard to marketing strategy, there is one overriding objective in the introduction stage: to generate awareness for the new service. At this stage, promotion becomes important. Either advertising announcing the new service or strong personal sales efforts, such as informational lectures by physicians or others, are required to inform potential users of the service.

In terms of pricing decisions, there are two typical options at the introduction stage—skimming or penetration. In rolling out a new product or service, there are some distinct advantages to a low or penetration pricing strategy. Typically, this approach makes acceptance of the new service easier, because the buyer's financial risk is reduced. Also, it has the effect of delaying competitors from entering the market. Any new competitor must attempt to price lower, which is often difficult when facing a penetration pricing strategy. For many service businesses, however, this pricing approach is risky. When estimation of demand for a new service is somewhat difficult to accurately gauge, a penetration pricing strategy may lead to some capacity problems in the organization. That is, as often happens for a medical service, demand can be greater than can be met through the staffing of the clinical service. While the organization is pleased at the market response, the delay in access to the new service can create ill will in the marketplace.

When capacity is an issue, it may be wise to price high (skimming). In this way, buyers who truly value the service will purchase it. The provider can gradually meet a larger potential demand by lowering prices as facility capacity expands. Skimming also allows the organization to recoup its often high investment costs in setting up a new program before more aggressive price cutting occurs as other competitors enter the market. In a service business such as health care, a high price also plays an important role in terms of image. For many buyers, there is often a perceived price/quality relationship that is enhanced by a higher price. This positioning aspect of price is discussed in greater detail later in this section. The major disadvantage of a high price is that it encourages competition to enter the market. Other providers, seeing the high price being charged for a particular service, may feel that they could enter the market, offer a program of similar quality, and

Figure 3. The Product Life Cycle

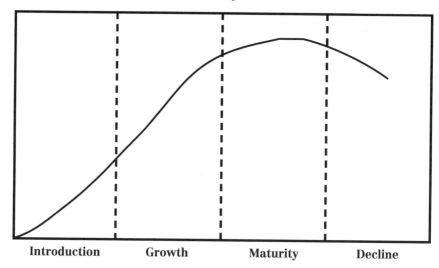

| Introduction | Growth | Maturity | Decline |

be more attractive to the market by undercutting the higher priced alternative. This type of market condition has been seen among HMOs that are competing in a particular city. As new competitors enter the market, they are accompanied by drastic cutting of premiums.

One other aspect of the introduction stage is essential from a marketing perspective. Product quality must meet customers' expectations. The quickest way to kill a new product is to offer it to the market before internal problems are worked out. For example, aggressive promoting of an industrial medicine program is essential in the introduction stage of the life cycle. Yet, if there are staffing problems or physical plant constraints or logistics that have not been worked out, a market disaster is sure to occur. Corporations are attracted by the promotion of the new industrial medicine program. Salespeople sign contracts. Workers begin to show up for physicals, rehabilitation, or treatment for job-related injuries, and the health care organization does not have the resources or the capacity to meet the demand in a timely, efficient fashion. It is very unlikely that these dissatisfied buyers will be willing to sign contracts in the second year on the basis of assurances from the provider that the "kinks" have been worked out.

Being the first entrant into the market has the marketing advantage of being able to establish the market's expectation with regard to the product or service. The first entrant can set the price/value relationship of the particular program in the minds of the buyers.

Growth

The second stage of the product life cycle is the period of the most rapid increases in sales. It is in this stage that competitors enter the market. At the growth stage, the focus of attention becomes locking up the referral flow for patients. In the HMO market, for example, when new competitors entered the scene, the early HMOs tried to lock up existing providers with favorable terms conditional on the providers signing exclusive contracts. For the new entrants at the growth stage, the key is to develop a differential advantage relative to the first provider. Typically, the source of the differential advantage is some aspect of the marketing mix. The second or third medical group to enter might offer extended hours or more satellite locations, or the new HMO might require a lower premium.

The issue of a differential advantage is a key concern once a competitor enters the market. The first entrant (the firm that began in the introduction stage) has the differential advantage of being first. The price that the first entrant pays in being first is primarily a promotional or an educational cost. That is, the first entrant must educate the market as to what is the value of a behavioral medicine program integrated within a primary care clinic or of a new approach to management or treatment of a particular disease. Each successive entrant must establish a differential advantage relative to the first. The four Ps are the place to turn, along with the target market selection, for a differential advantage. A later entrant could enter with a broader service line (the product component), more satellite facilities or extended hours (place), a lower premium per covered life (price), or better or more extensive advertising or public relations (promotion). Experience shows that it is often difficult to enter the market as a second or third entrant with a higher price. Additionally, promotion is a weak form of differential advantage, because the benefits are often temporal and transitory. Ideally, in terms of the four Ps, one might turn to the product or to distribution to establish a differential advantage of value to the market.

In addition to the four Ps, an organization can turn to the target market for a differential advantage. That is, the organization can tailor its program or services to a particular market segment, such as the high-income consumer or women. Women's health programs have been implemented by many facilities to establish a differential advantage with a comprehensive bundle of services for a particular market. As mentioned earlier, the Pavilion at the Washington Hospital Center is an attempt to establish a differential advantage with a specific set of upscale consumers.

Maturity

The third phase of the life cycle is when sales begin to level off. At this point, marginal competitors often will begin to leave the market. In many communities, the HMO business is in this stage. In some parts of the country, plans have disappeared, and there is consolidation among the remaining plans. The focus of attention at this stage is to maintain market share. Because the market is mature, any lost customers will not be easily replaced. Customer retention is the key. At this point of the life cycle, it is important to look for new opportunities or service alternatives to get back up on the growth curve.

Decline

The final stage is the period of declining sales. At this stage, the organization typically must make the decision to drop the product or determine another efficient way of providing the service. In the past few years in certain markets, some hospitals have dropped obstetrics or pediatrics. Other hospitals, in an attempt to offer a service, have signed agreements to have the service provided by a third party. This stage is often the most difficult for companies to manage. In traditional industries, it is often believed that a disproportionate amount of management time and attention is spent in dealing with declining products.

Price: The Key to Revenue

As previously discussed, price plays an important role for an organization in setting the strategy for the introduction of a new service. Yet it is important to recognize the difference between the marketing and the finance perspectives regarding price. In most health care settings, the issue of price is decided internally. That is, what are internal costs, the overhead allocation, and the margin? It is on the basis of these determinations, in conjunction with reimbursement constraints, that pricing decisions are made.

From a marketing perspective, these internal pricing concerns are important. But, in consideration of the external to internal perspective of marketing, it is the market's willingness to pay a determined price that dictates strategy. That is, how much does the market want to pay for an industrial medicine program? Does the market want the package of services delivered at a bundled or an unbundled price? How price-sensitive is the buyer? The difference between marketing and finance with regard to price is the difference between the floor and the ceiling.

In an internal perspective, the administrator or the chief financial officer is always concerned about cost and overhead. This is the floor. Pricing below this level leads to a loss. From a marketing perspective, the focus of concern is external, on the ceiling. How high would the market go for a particular service if it saw a value added to it? The difference between the ceiling and the floor represents the margin.

To a large extent, changes in the computer industry reflect the difficulty of premium pricing in health care. Twenty years ago, as an emerging industry, computer companies, such as IBM, followed a premium pricing strategy. For a new product with a lot of risk for the buyer, the value added to an IBM computer was the brand name of the organization. IBM was the industry standard. Early buyers of computers can remember the term IBM-compatible as the risk factor when one of these name brand alternatives wasn't purchased. In recent years, however, the products of the computer industry have become commodity goods. It is difficult to premium price a commodity product. IBM, along with manufacturers of other well-known brand names, has seen a precipitate decline in its margins, because consumers are no longer willing to pay a premium. The value added of the brand name is gone.

In health care, the pricing challenge is the same. Ideally, an organization would always prefer to price high. A larger margin is more profitable and allows more room for error. As health care moves to more of a commodity position, however, obtaining a price differential from the buyer is increasingly difficult.

In developing a pricing decision for a service, an important financial concern is break-even analysis. The formula used to calculate a break-even point, the point at which revenue exactly covers fixed and variable costs is:

$$\text{Break-Even Point} = \text{Fixed Cost}/(\text{Price} - \text{Variable Cost})$$

The break-even formula also plays an important role in marketing strategy in that it conveys the hurdle rate, which an organization must achieve competitively to cover its costs, when this amount is related to market share. Specifically, there are three elements to the formula: fixed costs, price, and variable costs. Managerially, one might assume that fixed costs are easily quantified, whether it be to build an outpatient surgery center or to roll out a new health fitness program for executives in which space must be redesigned, equipment purchased, and personnel hired. The more interesting part of the formula is in terms of price and variable costs. These two aspects of break even are judgmental—that is, these variables depend on the organization's strategy.

However, when it comes to marketing costs, a major issue is whether they should be viewed as fixed or variable. For example in rolling out a new service, advertising is often viewed as a necessary budget item. From a marketing person's perspective, then, advertising should be viewed as a fixed cost of the project (i.e., the new service roll-out). However, marketing expenses such as advertising are often considered discretionary items and are not calculated within the cost component of a break-even point. This approach provides an unrealistic estimate of the costs of breaking even in a new project decision.

The amount of sales (or revenue) needed to reach the break-even point can be decreased by increasing the price or by reducing the fixed costs. Yet, the realities of the market must come into play. For example, a health care organization might try to price high as mentioned previously to reduce break-even requirements. The reality check, however, is whether the market will accept the price. Or, the organization could try to reduce variable costs, such as advertising for the new program. The concern here is whether a low-cost strategy will help get market acceptance?

In either case, the break-even formula is an important tool to consider the sensitivity of strategies around price and variable costs (salespeople, promotion, etc.) when tied to market share. It is the representation of the cost of break even relative to the size of the market that indicates the challenge and inherent risk in the new service roll-out. That is, an organization, in developing its marketing strategy, never wants to calculate a single break-even point. Rather, several alternative break-even points that relate to different options regarding price and variable costs should be calculated. These break-even points should then be converted to indicate what market shares are required to meet them. This insight provides some perspective on the sensitivity of marketing strategy to marketplace realities.

In marketing, pricing is also a consideration in positioning the product or service in customers' minds.[7] An organization must decide whether it prefers the price to be high or low relative to the competition and whether price will play an active or a passive part in the positioning of the service. In an active pricing strategy, the price is a dominant part of positioning the product or service, and it is prominently displayed in communications. In a passive strategy, attributes other than price are focused on in communication of value to the customer.

Figure 4, page 202, shows the four quadrants with regard to price positioning. In the high price/active position, the organization makes no excuses that the product costs more. This was the long-standing claim of Curtis Mathes television sets when they touted "the most expensive television set that money can buy." This position is often used by organizations in which the objective quality of the product is hard to discern or evaluate. Price then becomes a cue for quality.

In the low price/active position, Wal-Mart proudly shows advertisements that highlight that its prices are falling daily. This position is being staked out by some Medicare HMO plans. In the passive price position, one could be like Maytag. The company does not focus on the fact that it is a premium priced product, but rather touts the reliability of its appliances. This position is one many health care organizations strive to achieve by highlighting their unique areas of clinical expertise or the level of clinical quality that they are perceived as delivering.

The final price position may be viewed in some ways as an odd alternative, in that the organization has a low price but does not talk about it. In fact, this is a position taken by many hospitals obligated to provide free care. These institutions, however, would never solicit such business. To some extent, the sliding scale pricing strategy of Community Health Centers sponsored by the U.S. Public Health Service uses the low price/passive position.

Place: Getting the Service

The third component of marketing strategy is often called place, or distribution. In the traditional product setting, it involves all the decisions of moving a product from producer to consumer. In developing marketing strategies around this component, the organization is concerned with where a service is offered, what hours it might be available, and how it will be accessed. In health care, place or distribution issues focus on decisions regarding the flow of patients through the system. Figure 5, page 203, shows several alternative patient flows through the system, called in marketing the channel of distribution. As can been in column A, the simplest flow of patients is to the primary care doctor. As one moves from B through D, other intermediaries often intervene, be they specialists, hospitals, tertiary hospitals, or HMO companies.

In terms of dealing with patient flow, the goal is to always control this channel of distribution. Two common strategies, referred to as either push or pull, are often used in marketing. In a push strategy, the organization develops an approach to work through the intermediaries in the channel. For example, in channel C, the hospital wants to get patients from physicians. Often, these intermediaries, the doctors, have privileges at more than one hospital. One

Figure 4. Price Positioning Matrix

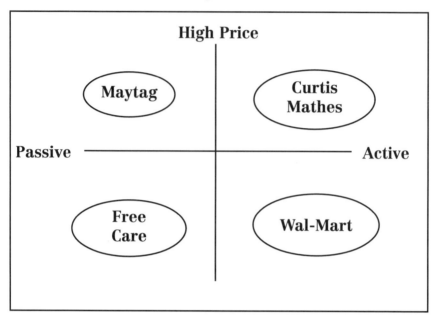

approach might consist of developing a medical office building and giving discounted rent to the doctors. In this way, the physician located next to a particular hospital might encourage patients to be admitted to that facility. Another approach, less cost intensive, might consist of programs to make doctors feel positively toward a particular facility. Weekend retreats, valet parking for physicians, and good lunches in the doctors lounge are all relatively low-cost ways of encouraging intermediaries in the channel to direct patient flow.

The alternative to push approaches is pull strategies. In a pull strategy, the organization bypasses the intermediaries and goes directly to the user, in this case the patient. An HMO, for example, occasionally faces resistance when trying to have its plan offered in a particular company. If the company (figure 5, column D) does not offer the HMO, employees can never access the plan. In this case, the intermediary must be bypassed. The HMO might run an advertisement that says, "If your company does not offer the XYZ HMO, you cannot pick one of the better plans available. Ask your boss why not?" The goal of such an approach is to encourage potential patients to approach the company and demand that the plan be offered. A similar pull strategy is being seen by many hospitals that advertise a particular center of excellence The purpose is to get the patient to ask the doctor about being admitted to that institution if the problem is relevant. Or, if the doctor does not have privileges at the facility, the patient can bypass the intermediary and go directly to the facility. In order for a pull strategy to work effectively, the organization or service must have very strong brand name recognition. Mayo, for example, can benefit from a pull strategy. A patient told of a major problem might

Figure 5. Alternative Patient Flows

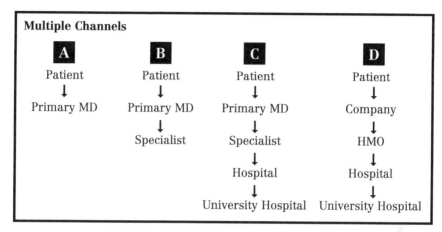

say, "I'm not staying locally. I'm going to the Mayo Clinic." In essence, the reputation of the Mayo Clinic pulls patients around the local physician and specialty referral network.

In recent years in health care, pharmaceutical companies have been most aggressive in their use of a pull strategy. The direct marketing to consumers of prescription drugs has become commonplace as these companies became restricted in the type of incentive programs they could use in trying to direct physicians to prescribe their particular product. The dramatic rise in Internet use has resulted in a new distribution channel for services. While medical service cannot be delivered over this medium, supplies, pharmaceuticals, and even diagnosis of patient illnesses portends significant new channel opportunities for health care organizations.

In reality, most organizations use a combination of push and pull strategies to control the channel of distribution. But it is essential in the development of marketing strategy to identify the intermediaries in the channel and to develop programs to control the flow of patients.

Promotion

The final element of marketing strategy is promotion. The promotional mix consists of four approaches: public relations, advertising, personal selling, and sales promotions.

In health care, reliance has traditionally been placed on public relations. Public relations can be defined as any nondirectly paid presentation or activity for an organization. Public relations activities consist of working with the media for the placement of favorable stories about health care facilities or of sponsoring community programs to create a favorable image of the group within the community. Health fairs, fun runs, and free blood pressure screening are all common activities that are designed to create a favorable impression.

A major function of public relations is to work to have favorable stories placed in the media about the health care group. Because the attention paid by the media is not directly paid for, a favorable story reported in the press about a doctor, a hospital, or an HMO is of great value. Most people view these stories as having a great deal of credibility. They are viewed differently from an advertisement. Yet it is in trying to obtain favorable press that the weakness of this approach is revealed. It is the rare physician who has not been interviewed by the media at some length. As most readers of this book can attest, reading an article in which you were interviewed often leads to a reaction such as, "I didn't say that," Because publicity is a function of the media deciding to run the story, there is little control over the message. If the health care organization tries to get the story repeated on a second day, it is unlikely to be successful, because the media no longer view the story as newsworthy. It is because of these limitations that most health care organizations have turned to advertising.

Advertising can be defined as a directly paid form of presentation of a service, product, or organization. Because a health care organization pays the media to run its advertisement, the organization has control over several important elements. The health care organization can control to whom the message is sent, when the message is sent, how often the message is sent, and how the message is sent. The health care provider can decide what newspaper is best, what day of the week the ad should run, how large the ad should be, and how frequently the message should be told. None of these elements can be controlled in a story generated through public relations activities. A major limitation of advertising relative to public relations, however, involves credibility. Consumers understand an advertisement is a form of self-promotion and often process the information more critically.

While the purpose of this chapter is not to explain all the components of creating a successful advertising program, it is important to outline a few key ingredients. A well-run advertising campaign begins with a definition of the target audience. The organization should have a fairly well-defined profile of whom it wants to attract. This aspect was discussed earlier in this chapter and underscores the importance of the organization's clearly defining the target market. In this way, appropriate media can be selected to reach the target audience. Second, a well-run advertising campaign is centered on advertisements that are pretested with the intended audience. A major difference to date between many of the advertisements developed in health care and those of more traditional companies has been the lack of pretesting. Often, in health care organizations, an advertisement is developed internally and then placed with the media. The doctors in the group often review the ad and give approval or suggest some minor changes. In a well-run advertising campaign, the pretest should be conducted with a sample of people for whom the ad is intended. Do these people like the ad? Do they understand what is being said? Is there any additional information that they would like to see in the ad? Finally, in a well-run ad campaign, there is a measurable set of objectives that guide the copy and the media strategy of the campaign.

The third component of promotional strategy is the use of personal selling. Traditionally, salespeople were rare in health care organizations other than HMOs, which had representatives who presented the respective plans within a company. Increasingly, however, the use of personal sales forces for contact with intermediaries in the channel of distribution has grown. Hospitals have used sales representatives to contact physicians; radiology departments have used salespeople to contact referral sources; and adolescent chemical dependency programs have salespeople contacting judges, social workers, and probation officers.[8]

Salespeople can perform multiple roles.[9] The common role is selling or obtaining new business. But salespeople are also useful in conducting field research on the competition or on prospective user needs. Salespeople also play an important missionary role of maintaining goodwill and of dealing with any user complaints or problems. For medical organizations that depend on referrals, this last role is particularly valuable.

The final component of promotional strategy involves the use of sales promotions, the common form being coupons. While a regular strategy for most consumer goods marketers, coupons have infrequently been used in health care. Some reported uses have been the offering of a free health screen for first-time users of a new service, or a small price reduction on the first office visit of a new patient. To a large extent, the value of sales promotions is the ability to track the response to an advertisement. Coupons allow the organization to track whether individuals are reading an ad and finding the offer of sufficient interest to act. In general, the response rate to direct mail coupons is one and one-half to three percent.

Summary

Marketing is a process that focuses on the buyers of a service. Essential to the development of any effective marketing strategy is the need to understand buyers' requirements and demands. Contrary to traditional health care planning, which is motivated by the requirements of those internal to the organization, marketing is an external to internal approach. After fully understanding buyers' requirements, the organization develops a strategy based on the four components of the marketing mix: product, price, place, and promotion.

References

1. For a comprehensive perspective on the nature of marketing and the role of consumer input, see Berkowitz, E., and others. *Marketing,* Fourth Edition. Homewood, Ill.: Richard D. Irwin, Inc., 1994, chap. 1.

2. An interesting article that displays the contribution of the marketing research approach is Tucker, L., and others. "The Role of Marketing Research in Securing a Certificate of Need for a New Renal Transplant Facility." *Journal of Health Care Marketing* 11(2):63-9, June 1991.

3. A detailed discussion of secondary data sources in health care is provided in Hillestad, S., and Berkowitz, E. *Health Care Marketing Plans: From Strategy to Action.* Second Edition. Rockville, Md.: Aspen Publishers, 1991, pp. 90-6.

4. A useful reference on focus groups is Kreuger, R. *Focus Groups: A Practical Guide for Applied Research.* Newbury Park, Calif.: Sage Press, 1988.

5. A useful article to see the application of telephone interviewing is Gombeski, W., and others. "Overnight Assessment of Marketing crises." *Journal of Health Care Marketing* 11(1):51-4, March 1991.

6. Berkowitz, E., and others. *Marketing,* Fourth Edition. Homewood, Ill.: Richard D. Irwin, Inc., 1994.

7. Tellis, G. "Creative Pricing Strategies for Medical Services." *Journal of Medical Practice Management* 3(2):120-4, Fall 1987.

8. Bates, B., and McSurley, H. "The Sales Function in Radiology Departments." *Administrative Radiology* 8(9):16-9, Sept. 1989.

9. Mack, K., and Newbold, P. *Health Care Sales.* San Francisco, Calif.: Jossey-Bass Publishers, 1991, chap. 1.

Eric N. Berkowitz is Professor, Department of Marketing, University of Massachusetts, Amherst.

Chapter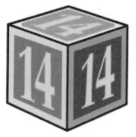

An Overview of Legal Issues

by Mark E. Lutes, David J. Weader, Jeffrey Bennett, and Neil S. Olderman

T his chapter identifies certain legal concerns facing clinical department managers (CDMs). It is not intended to be a comprehensive or exhaustive discussion of all the potentially relevant issues. Rather, it is intended to familiarize CDMs with a number of the issues that may arise in the performance of their duties.

Some of the topics discussed below may not be applicable to all CDMs. This would largely depend on the scope of the CDM's duties and the CDM's relationship with the health care organization. The chapter is divided into seven parts:

- Corporate Law

- Medical Staff Credentialing and Peer Review

- Employment Law

- Fraud and Abuse Laws

- Antitrust

- Physician Contracting

- Patient Care

These parts identify legal issues related to roles typically assumed by CDMs within a health care organization—corporate director, peer reviewer, manager, participant in strategic decision-making processes, physician contract negotiator, and patient care/quality assurance monitor.

Corporate Law: The Corporate Director's Duties of Care and Loyalty

In some instances, a member of a health care organization's clinical staff, oftentimes a medical staff officer or a CDM, is elected to the organization's board of directors or is an ex officio member of the board. One purpose for including a member of the clinical staff on the board of directors is to have clinical staff representation and input in the organization's formulation of policy. In such cases, a CDM's duties extend beyond merely representing the interests of fellow clinicians.

Board members of a health care organization, like the members of any corporate board, are charged with the exercise of the duty of care and the duty of loyalty in performing their organizational functions. The functions of a board member are, among other things, to protect and preserve the corporation's financial solvency and stability; establish corporate governing policy; manage, supervise, and direct the affairs of the corporation; select competent officers; select competent and qualified clinical staff members; ensure the provision of care in accordance with prevailing quality standards; and avoid self-dealing or profiting unjustly from the relationship with the corporation. Each board function must be undertaken with that level of care that would be exercised by a reasonably prudent person with similar knowledge and experience under the circumstances. Moreover, such functions must be undertaken by the board member solely in the best interests of the corporation and not out of an interest in personal gain.

Until 1985, judicial interpretation of the duties of care and loyalty were characterized by the "business judgment rule." Under the business judgment rule, courts found liability for breach of the duty of care only in cases of gross or willful negligence. Therefore, directors (or trustees in the case of a not-for-profit corporation) who took actions in good faith, after a reasonable effort had been made to become informed of the relevant issues, and who did not act in contravention of the organization's interests, were not saddled with liability for the unintended effects of their errors in judgment.

Some courts have begun to create a higher standard for directors in exercising their responsibilities. This new judicial thinking began with the Delaware Supreme Court's decision in *Smith v. Van Gorkom*.[1] Since the *Van Gorkom* decision, a line of cases has developed that stands for the proposition that directors will be held to a higher standard in determining whether they have met their fiduciary duties and hence are able to shield themselves from liability under the business judgment rule. One court has interpreted the duties of care and loyalty as requiring directors to take affirmative steps to defend and protect the interests with which they are entrusted.[2]

Some state legislatures have passed laws designed to offset the effects of these cases. These statutes essentially codify the business judgment rule and set forth minimum standards directors must meet to shield themselves from liability. In these jurisdictions, liability is only imposed if it is shown that the director was willfully or grossly negligent. As a CDM, it would be prudent to become familiar with the expectations placed on directors by the law in your jurisdiction.

A breach of a director's duty of loyalty to the corporation occurs when the director's personal interests and the best interests of the corporation are conflicting. Conflicts of interest typically arise where a director has some personal interest, usually economic, in the full board's taking certain actions. Transactions tainted by self-dealing may result in litigation against not only the organization and the interested director or trustee, but also the corporation's shareholders (or members in the case of a not-for-profit organization).

In cases in which a conflict exists, the interested director must fully disclose his or her interest in the transaction, and the decision must be made after fair and reasonable consideration, in an open manner, and without fraud or imposition.[3] The interested director bears the burden of demonstrating that the transaction was fair from the corporation's perspective. Still, some state courts have held that in no case may a director or trustee profit from a transaction with the corporation that he or she serves, even if the corporation is provided beneficial terms.[4]

Medical Staff Credentialing and Peer Review

It is not unlikely that, as an expert in a particular medical specialty or through familiarity with a particular case, a CDM will become part of a peer review program or a credentialing process. Therefore, knowledge of legal issues relating to credentialing and peer review could avoid potential liability on the part of the CDM and the health care organization.

Due Process

The principal grounds for judicial reversal of a health care organization's credentialing decision is whether the process was procedurally fair. The precise legal question asks whether adequate "due process" was afforded.

In the hospital setting, analysis of the due process issue is broken down into two major categories: due process afforded new applicants for staff privileges and due process afforded members of the medical staff whose privileges are under review. Traditionally, new applicants for staff privileges are deemed to have fewer due process rights, because, technically, nothing is being taken from them except an opportunity that the law considers a privilege as opposed to a right. A sub-issue is whether the practitioner is seeking or has privileges at a public as opposed to a private institution. The answer to this question is similarly crucial in determining how much process is due.

Public institutions are considered agents of the state and must meet a higher standard of due process. The higher standard is imposed through the constitutional right to due process contained in the Fifth Amendment to the U.S. Constitution and is made applicable to the states through the Fourteenth Amendment. Where a public institution is conducting the credentialing process, a more stringent standard will be applied in evaluating the due process afforded membership applicants and staff members. The courts in a majority of jurisdictions have been reluctant, however, to extend constitutional due process protections in the context of private hospital credentialing decisions.[5] Thus, for private hospitals, judicial review of credentialing decisions is generally confined to an inquiry as to whether the hospital followed its own bylaws.[6] Some courts go so far as to deem the medical staff bylaws to be a contract between the hospital and the medical staff's members.[7]

In a few jurisdictions, the courts have looked beyond the procedure used by a private hospital and reviewed the substance of the hospital's decision. New Jersey courts, for instance, have reasoned that the public interest in quality of care permits courts to determine if medical staff selections are "arbitrary, capricious, or unreasonable." This approach was first enunciated in *Greisman v. Newcomb Hosp.*[8] and was based on findings that even private hospitals receive a substantial portion of their revenues from public funds, receive tax benefits, and often constitute virtual monopolies in their areas. California courts have applied common law fair process theory out of a concern that denial of medical staff membership would effectively impair the applicant's right to fully practice his or her profession.[9]

Immunity from Liability for Actions Taken Incidentally to the Credentialing and Peer Review Process Under the Health Care Quality Improvement Act

A principal concern among individuals taking part in the credentialing and peer review processes is whether they will be personally subject to civil claims brought by plaintiffs alleging harm as a result of decisions or process. A number of states have statutes protecting participants in peer review actions. These state laws vary as to activities and persons protected and therefore cannot be effectively discussed in this chapter. The immunity created by these statutes is limited to certain peer review bodies and to individuals defined in the statute as having assisted those bodies. Generally, peer review bodies engaged in the process of evaluating physician competence and quality of care or in any other activity delineated in the statute are granted immunity from suit if they adhere to appropriate standards or criteria in performing the review function.[10]

In 1986, Congress supplemented state peer review immunity schemes with the Health Care Quality Improvement Act (HCQIA).[11] HCQIA provides a uniform federal scheme for immunity from most state and federal civil damages to persons providing information to or performing credentialing or peer review functions.

More specifically, HCQIA immunity protects persons who provide information to a health care entity,[12] its governing body, or any committee established by the health care entity to conduct professional review activities regarding the competence or professional conduct of a physician unless the person providing the information knowingly provides false information to the body performing professional review. However, for individuals on a professional review body to avail themselves of protection from civil liability, the body's decisions must be supported by the following conditions:

- A reasonable belief that taking such action would further the provision of high-quality health care.

- A reasonable effort to obtain the facts of the matter.

- Adequate notice and hearing.

- A reasonable belief that the action taken was warranted in light of the facts presented.

The immunity provided professional review activities under HCQIA does not apply to actions brought under the federal civil rights laws, injunctive or declaratory judgment actions, actions brought by government agencies, or criminal suits. Similarly, actions brought by nonphysician practitioners or chiropractors do not fall within the scope of HCQIA's immunity protections.

In addition, states were given the option to prohibit the use of HCQIA immunity for actions brought under state law. Some states have elected to "opt out" and expand due process rights for physicians. California was one state that selected this alternative course. The effect of a state "opting out" is to force professional review bodies to offer a panoply of fair process protections as part of their decision-making process. Moreover, immunity would not be guaranteed even in cases in which all due process requirements imposed by state law were met.

HCQIA requires reporting of certain adverse actions taken against the clinical privileges of physicians to the medical licensing board.[13] Adverse actions that must be reported include:

- Any action taken by the health care entity that adversely affects the clinical privileges of a physician for longer than 30 days.

- An action that results in the physician's surrender of his or her clinical privileges while the physician's competence or professional conduct is being investigated by the health care entity's professional review body.

- The surrender of clinical privileges in return for an investigation's not taking place.

By law, the report must be filed with the state licensing board within 15 days of the date on which the adverse action is taken. The state licensing board then has 15 days to file a report with the federal Department of Health and Human Services (HHS), the agency charged with the development of the National Practitioner Data Bank (NPDB). Further, the state licensing board must inform HHS of a health care entity's failure to file a required report. HCQIA also provides protection to persons and entities making the required reports without knowledge of their falsity.

Furthermore, HCQIA requires hospitals to request information from NPDB when screening applicants for a medical staff position or granting clinical privileges and every two years for the entire medical staff. Other health care entities, such as HMOs, may request information from NPDB when screening applicants for medical staff positions or granting clinical privileges. Failure to inquire into a practitioner's file could expose the health care entity to the risk of having such a failure used as prima facie evidence of negligence in an action for negligent hiring or retention of a clinical staff member, because HCQIA provides that the health care facility is presumed to know all relevant information in NPDB. To reduce exposure to liability, CDMs should be aware of their roles in the credentialing and peer review processes and, where appropriate, make efforts to ensure that proper NPDB reporting and inquiry are a regular practice of the health care organization.

Employment Law

Depending on the circumstances involved, a CDM may participate in interviewing job applicants, in making hiring decisions, and in other activities involving the employment relationship between an individual and the health care organization. Accordingly, a CDM should be aware of the body of law that applies to employers and their interactions with employees or prospective employees. The following discussion identifies and describes some of the issues that a CDM should recognize. For more detailed information or for specific guidance, a CDM should consult with counsel or other appropriate individuals, such as human resources personnel.

The Americans with Disabilities Act

The Americans with Disabilities Act (ADA) provides protection against discrimination to disabled individuals. As applied to the workplace, ADA "seeks to ensure access [for disabled individuals] to equal employment opportunities based on merit."[14] Toward that end, Title I of ADA prohibits employers from discriminating against any "qualified individual with a disability" with respect to all aspects of the employment relationship, including recruitment, job applications, interviews, hiring, discharge, compensation, benefits, promotions, and transfers.[15]

What Employers Are Subject to ADA Requirements?

ADA provides that an employer subject to its provisions is an entity or person "engaged in an industry affecting commerce who has 15 or more employees for each working day in each of 20 or more calendar weeks in the current or preceding calendar year, and any agent of such person [or entity]."[16] The exception to this general definition provides that an employer does not include the United States government, a corporation wholly owned by the United States, an Indian tribe, or a bona fide private membership club that is exempt from taxation under Section 501(c)(3) of the Internal Revenue Code. Based on the broad scope of this definition of employer, a CDM generally will be working for an entity subject to the provisions of ADA.

What Are an Employer's Obligations?

An employer subject to ADA has an affirmative obligation to make "reasonable accommodations for the known disabilities of an otherwise qualified job applicant or employee, unless such reasonable accommodation would impose an undue economic hardship on the employer."[17] A reasonable accommodation means any modification or adjustment that would allow a qualified individual with a disability to enjoy equal employment opportunities in the application process; the performance of the essential functions of the job; or the enjoyment of equal benefits and privileges of employment.[18] ADA regulations provide that a "reasonable accommodation" includes, but is not limited to:

- Making existing facilities accessible to and usable by a qualified individual with a disability.

- Job restructuring.

- Part-time or modified work schedules.

- Reassignment to a vacant position.

- Appropriate adjustments or modifications to examinations, training materials, or policies.

- Providing qualified readers or interpreters.[19]

Numerous other options for job restructuring exist, depending on the circumstances surrounding an individual employer.

In addition to its duty to provide reasonable accommodations, an employer cannot otherwise discriminate against a qualified individual with a disability in the workplace. Such discrimination includes:

Limiting, segregating, or classifying a job applicant or employee in a way that adversely affects that individual's job opportunities or status because of a disability of the individual.

- Entering into contracts that have the effect of subjecting the employer's qualified individual with a disability to discrimination based on that disability.

- Utilizing standards, criteria, or methods of administration that have the effect of discrimination on the basis of disability or that perpetuate the discrimination of others, even if such standards, criteria, or methods of administration are not intended to produce such results.

- Excluding or otherwise denying equal jobs or benefits to an employee or an applicant because of the person's relationship or association with an individual known to have a disability.[20]

Who Is a Qualified Individual?

According to ADA, a "qualified individual with a disability" is "an individual with a disability who, with or without reasonable accommodation, can perform the essential functions of the employment position that such individual holds or desires."[21]

ADA defines "disability" with respect to an individual as "(i) a physical or mental impairment that substantially limits one or more major life activities of the individual; (ii) a past record of such impairment; or (iii) being regarded as having such an impairment."[22] The regulations promulgated under ADA define "physical impairment" to include any physiological disorder or condition, cosmetic disfigurement, or anatomical loss affecting one or more body systems, including, but not limited to, cardiovascular, neurological, musculoskeletal, respiratory, and special sensory organs.[23] In addition, ADA regulations define "mental impairment" to include any mental or psychological disorder, including, but not limited to, mental retardation, emotional or mental illness, and specific learning disabilities.[24]

The result of these provisions is a legal definition of "disability" that is broader than conventional understanding. The definition covers not only individuals who are confined to a wheelchair or are blind but also individuals with impairments such as cancer, diabetes, AIDS or HIV, bad backs, colon resections, major mental depression, and sensitivity to cigarette smoke.[25] However, several recent Supreme Court decisions appear to have narrowed the scope of conditions covered by the term "disability." These decisions indicate that, in judging whether an individual has a "disability," mitigating or corrective measures must be considered, including medications, devices, and the body's own systems' acting to correct a condition.[25a] In *Sutton v. United Airlines*, for example, the Supreme Court determined that severely myopic sisters who had applied for employment as commercial airline pilots, and whose uncorrected visual acuity was worse than 20/200, were not "disabled" under ADA. The Supreme Court reasoned that a "disability," as intended by ADA, did not exist because corrective measures made the sisters' visual acuity 20/20 or better, which enabled the sisters to function identically to individuals without similar impairments.

Although an individual may be determined to be "disabled" in order to benefit from ADA's protection, such individual must be qualified and therefore able to perform the essential job functions (with or without reasonable accommodations) of the job.

What Functions Are Essential?

ADA regulations indicate that determinations of whether a function is essential to the job may be based on, but not be limited to, the following factors:

- Whether a position exists to perform a particular function.

- Whether removing the function would fundamentally alter the job.

- Whether there are a limited number of employees among whom the performance of that job function can be distributed.

- The amount of time or degree of skill required to perform the function.

- Whether written job descriptions including this function were prepared before advertising or interviewing applicants for the job.

- The terms of a collective bargaining agreement.

- An employer's business judgment as to which functions are essential.[26]

What Should a CDM Be Aware of?

As an individual involved in the employment relationship, a CDM should, at the very least, be aware of basic ADA issues discussed in this section and their application to the workplace. In particular, a CDM should understand how the requirements of ADA affect the interviewing, examination, and hiring of job applicants and when the employer's duty to provide reasonable accommodations is triggered.

With respect to the hiring process, a CDM should know that ADA specifically prohibits employers from inquiring into the existence, nature, or severity of a disability of a job applicant and from conducting medical examinations of job applicants.[27] Examples of inquiries an employer cannot make include:

- Are you disabled?

- Are you healthy?

- Do you have any physical or mental impairments that might limit your ability to do your job?

- Would you need reasonable accommodations to perform this job?

- Any indirect inquiries that would likely disclose a disability of the applicant, such as: Have you ever filed a workers' compensation claim? How many sick days did you take at your last job? Will you need certain accommodations to perform this job?[28]

- Completion of an application form that includes a list of disabilities and asks the applicant to indicate any that he or she has or may have had in the past.

An employer may, however, inquire into the ability of a job applicant, whose known disability may interfere with or prevent the performance of job-related functions, to perform such functions.[29] This inquiry may be made of such job applicants regardless of whether the employer routinely makes such a request of all applicants in that job category.[30] Examples of inquiries that an employer may make include the following.

- Do you have a license to act as an occupational therapist?

- Can you transport and lift 50-pound canisters of oxygen, with or without reasonable accommodation (if the job requires the transporting and lifting of 50-pound canisters of oxygen)?

- How do you handle stress, or Do you work better or worse in stressful situations? (But not the follow-up questions, "Have you sought treatment for your inability to handle stress?" or "Do you get ill as a result of stress?" as these questions may cause disclosure of a mental impairment.[31])

- An employer can require an applicant to perform a physical agility test in order to gather information regarding the applicant's ability to perform the job.[32]

- If it reasonably appears to the employer that a known disability would interfere with the performance of a job function, the employer can inquire as to how the applicant would perform such functions. For example, if an applicant with one leg is seeking a job repairing furnaces, the employer could ask the applicant to explain or demonstrate how the applicant would be able to get down the basement stairs of a house with the required tools, with or without reasonable accommodation.

The distinction between permissible and impermissible questions can often be difficult to discern. Accordingly, it is important for a CDM involved in hiring to carefully consider how to pose interview questions and to review the hiring process with counsel or the human resources department of the health care organization.[33]

With respect to the duty to provide reasonable accommodations, a CDM should be aware that the employee or the prospective employee carries the burden of requesting a reasonable accommodation.[34] In other words, in order to trigger the employer's duty, the qualified individual with a disability must let the employer know that a modification in the job is needed because of his or her medical condition.

When a qualified individual with a disability has made a request for a reasonable accommodation, the employer must make a reasonable effort to ascertain the appropriate accommodation for the individual. In determining the appropriate accommodations, the employer should consult with the individual to consider job-related limitations and the potential effectiveness of the accommodations. If there are two or more effective accommodations available, the employer may select the least expensive option, provided that the individual receives employment benefits commensurate with those furnished by more expensive accommodations.

Other Applicable Laws

There are other employment laws that a CDM may need to be aware of, such as Title VII of the Civil Rights Act of 1964 (as amended by the Employment Opportunity Act of 1972 and the Civil Rights Act of 1991), the Family and Medical Leave Act (FMLA) of 1993, and workers' compensation laws.

Title VII prohibits employment discrimination, in both the public and the private sectors, on the basis of race, color, religion, sex, and national origin.[35] Title VII claims against employers tend to be based on one of the following theories: disparate treatment (intentional discrimination by the employer based on race, sex, etc.); disparate impact (the employer's use of a test that is not discriminatory on its face but results in discrimination against members of a protected group); retaliatory discharge for the filing of a discrimination claim by an employee; and constructive discharge by the employer on the basis of an employee's race, sex, etc.[36]

FMLA entitles eligible employees, both male and female, to take up to 12 weeks of unpaid, job-protected leave for the birth or the adoption of a child or the beginning of a child's foster care; for the care of a parent, spouse, or child with a serious health condition; and for the employee's own serious health condition.[37] Employees who have been employed by the current employer for 12 or more months and have worked for a minimum of 1,250 hours during the 12-month period immediately preceding the leave request are eligible for FMLA benefits.[38] FMLA covers employers that employ 50 or more employees for each working day during each of 20 or more calendar work weeks in the current or preceding calendar year and that are engaged in commerce or in an industry affecting commerce.[39]

Workers' compensation laws vary from state to state but generally require an employer to cover the costs of job-related injuries or illnesses to its employees through insurance or self-insurance.

If familiarity with these or other employment laws, including ADA, becomes necessary, a CDM should consult with counsel or other appropriate individuals, such as human resources personnel.

Fraud and Abuse Laws

Given the current focus on health care fraud and a CDM's dual role as a health care manager and a health care professional, a CDM must have a working knowledge of fraud and abuse laws that govern the health care industry. The following federal laws are particularly applicable:

- The Federal Anti-Kickback Statute.

- The Federal Self-Referral (Stark) Statute.

- The Federal False Claims Statute.

- The Health Insurance Portability and Accountability Act.

A CDM should be aware that, in addition to these federal laws, states have their own fraud and abuse laws. As it is beyond the scope of this section to discuss the fraud and abuse laws of each state, a CDM should look to in-house or local counsel for information regarding applicable state law. The discussion of fraud and abuse laws in this section should serve as an adequate introduction to the relevant issues. For an in-depth review of these laws and government enforcement actions, a CDM should refer to a book devoted to fraud and abuse issues, such as *Legal Issues in Healthcare Fraud and Abuse: Navigating the Uncertainties* by the authors' colleagues, Carrie Valiant and David Matyas. Much of the following section is drawn from this book.

The Anti-Kickback Statute

The federal Anti-Kickback Statute covers more than simple bribes and kick-backs; it also covers remuneration generally where referrals may take place. The requirements of the Anti-Kickback Statute affect many health care business transactions. For example, a CDM should be aware that joint ventures, space and equipment leases, discounts on goods and services, physician recruitment incentives, management and personal services contracts, physician practice acquisitions, and employment arrangements all present Anti-Kickback Statute issues.[40]

Prohibited Inducements

The Anti-Kickback Statute imposes criminal penalties on individuals and entities that knowingly and willfully solicit or receive remuneration "in return for referring an individual to a person for the furnishing or arranging for the furnishing of any item or service" or "in return for purchasing, leasing, ordering, or arranging for or recommending purchasing, leasing, or ordering any good, facility, service, or item for which payment may be made in whole or in part under..." a federal health care program.[41] The types of remuneration prohibited by the Anti-Kickback Statute include, but are not limited to, kickbacks, bribes, and rebates. Additionally, the statute expressly prohibits both direct and indirect remuneration.

Penalties

A person convicted of knowingly and willfully violating the Anti-Kickback Statute may be found guilty of a felony and fined not more than $25,000 or imprisoned for not more than 5 years, or both, for each violation. Violators of the Anti-Kickback Statute also are subject to exclusion from federal health care programs upon a determination of a violation by HHS, regardless of whether a criminal conviction has been obtained. In addition, the Balanced Budget Act of 1997 grants the Secretary of HHS authority to impose civil monetary penalties up to $50,000 and three times the amount of the remuneration in question for each violation of the Anti-Kickback Statute.

Exceptions and Safe Harbors

The Anti-Kickback Statute includes limited statutory exceptions for certain financial arrangements:

- Discounts that are properly disclosed and appropriately reflected in the costs claimed or charges made by the provider or entity.

- Payments made by an employer to an employee, who has a bona fide employment relationship with such employer, for employment in the provision of covered items and services.

- Amounts paid by providers to group purchasing organizations in certain circumstances.

- Waivers of coinsurance with respect to certain federally qualified health centers.

In addition, HHS has promulgated regulations, termed "safe harbors," specifying certain payment practices that are excepted from the prohibitions of the Anti-Kickback Statute.[42] However, the protection afforded by the safe harbor regulations is limited to very narrow circumstances. Safe harbors include, but are not limited to:

- Space and equipment rentals, personal services contracts, and management contracts. In order to fall within these safe harbors, there must be, among other requirements, a written contract for a term of at least one year that specifies the total payment amount (at fair market value and not variable based on volume) and the space, equipment, or services covered.

- The sale of a practice, but only between practitioners.

- Payments to referral services.

- Payments or exchanges of value under certain manufacturer or supplier warranties.

Compliance with the terms of each criterion in a safe harbor regulation is voluntary. Although compliance with these safe harbor regulations assures an entity or an individual that a particular practice does not violate the Anti-Kickback Statute, an action or arrangement that does not satisfy each criterion of a safe harbor does not necessarily violate the Anti-Kickback Statute. Rather, that financial arrangement merely lacks the assurance that it is protected from liability under the Anti-Kickback Statute.

The Self-Referral Statute (Stark Law)

Prohibited Referrals

The federal Self-Referral Statute (the so-called Stark Law) prohibits a physician who has a financial relationship with an entity (or whose immediate family member has a financial relationship with an entity) from making a "referral" of a Medicare or a Medicaid patient to that entity for the furnishing of "designated health services" for which payment may be made under the Medicare or Medicaid programs unless the relationship or service qualifies under a Stark Law statutory exception.[43] The Stark Law also prohibits an entity from billing the Medicare or the Medicaid program for items and services ordered by a physician who has a financial relationship with that entity. The following are key definitions under the Stark Law:

Financial relationship is defined in the Stark Law to include compensation arrangements as well as ownership and investment interests.

- *Designated health services* include, among other services, clinical laboratory services, physical therapy services, occupational therapy services, radiology and radiation therapy services, home health services, and inpatient and outpatient hospital services.

- *Physician* means a doctor of medicine or osteopathy legally authorized to practice medicine and surgery; a doctor of dental surgery or dental medicine legally licensed to practice dentistry; a doctor of optometry; and a chiropractor.

- *Immediate family members* include spouse, natural or adoptive parent, child or sibling; stepparent, stepchild, stepbrother, or stepsister; father-in-law, mother-in-law, son-in-law, daughter-in-law, brother-in-law, sister-in-law, grandparent, grandchild, and spouse of a grandparent or grandchild.

The CDM will need to consult counsel on these definitions. The statutes and proposed regulations create many complex issues as to their applicability.

Penalties

The Stark Law provides for civil penalties of up to $15,000 for each service for those who present or cause to be presented bills or claims for such services that the person knows or should know violate the self-referral ban. A violation also may result in denials of payments or refunds of amounts collected in violation of the law. Violators also may be excluded from the Medicare and Medicaid programs. Circumvention schemes are subject to a separate civil money penalty of up to $100,000 for each such arrangement or scheme.

Exceptions

The Stark Law contains a number of exceptions to the general self-referral proscriptions, including, but not limited to:

- Physician services provided by or under the supervision of another physician in the same group practice as the referring physician.

- Certain designated health services furnished by a physician, or another physician in the same group practice as the referring physician, in the physician's office.

- Compensation paid to a physician or an immediate family member (at fair market value and without regard to volume or value of referrals) in a commercially reasonable bona fide employment agreement for identifiable services.

- Certain payments for rentals of office space or equipment not considered compensation arrangements.

- Compensation under a personal services arrangements between a physician and an entity where the physician is an independent contractor and not an employee of the entity.

- Certain payments made by a hospital to a physician in the course of physician recruitment.[44]

Unlike the exceptions and safe harbors for the Anti-Kickback Statute, the Stark exceptions are not optional. Consequently, the failure of a physician to meet a Stark exception if the physician has a financial relationship with an entity to which that physician refers means that such referrals are prohibited. When considering financial arrangements involving physicians, a CDM should remember that, once a referral is prohibited under the Stark law, it does not matter if the arrangement would conform to an Anti-Kickback Statute exception or safe harbor.

The Federal False Claims Statute

The federal False Claims Act prohibits anyone from knowingly presenting, or causing to be presented, a false or fraudulent claim in order to secure payment from the federal government.[45] A person found to have violated this statute is liable for fines of not less than $5,000 and not more than $10,000 for each claim, plus three times the amount of damages sustained by the federal government.[45] The False Claims Act defines "knowing" and "knowingly" as actual knowledge, deliberate ignorance of the truth, or reckless disregard of the truth or falsity.[46] Therefore, no proof of specific intent to defraud is required to demonstrate a violation of the False Claims Act.

The Anti-Kickback Statute does not provide for a private right of action. As a result, anti-kickback claims have been "bootstrapped" to (or included with) claims made under the False Claims Act, which does include a private right of action. In addition, the government has attempted to "bootstrap" anti-kickback claims to claims under the False Claims Act because the False Claims Act provides for civil monetary penalties and the Anti-Kickback Statute did not until enactment of the Balanced Budget Act of 1997.

False claims cases involving health care providers often include the following issues:

- Billing for items or services not actually rendered.

- Providing and billing for services that are not medically necessary.

- Upcoding, employing "DRG creep," or miscalculating capitation rates.

- Waiver of coinsurance and deductibles.

- Unbundling and fragmenting claims.

- Filing false cost reports.[47]

The Health Insurance Portability and Accountability Act

The Health Insurance Portability and Accountability Act of 1996 (HIPAA) specifically created a new provision that authorizes the imposition of civil monetary penalties for offering inducements to individuals eligible for Medicare or Medicaid if the individual or entity offering the inducement knows or should know that it will influence the patient to order or receive items or services from a particular provider, practitioner, or supplier. Significantly, the statute defines remuneration as including the waiver of coinsurance and deductibles and transfers of items or services for free or for other than fair market value. However, limited exceptions are provided in the statute. For instance, coinsurance waivers that are based on financial need and meet other requirements are protected. Additionally, in light of the potential application of this provision to managed care arrangements, the statute excepts from the scope of illegal remuneration differentials in coinsurance and deductible amounts that are part of a benefit plan design—e.g., as part of a PPO or similar managed care product—and that are disclosed and meet other standards to be defined by HHS. There also is an exception for incentives given to individuals to promote the delivery of preventive care as determined by HHS in regulations.

Antitrust Issues

In the current era of managed health care, payers demand high-quality health care services and tightly controlled costs. Providers have responded by consolidating the provision of health care service through numerous mergers and joint ventures and by fielding partially integrated managed care contracting networks. These types of activities raise potential antitrust concerns, and any CDM participating in the restructuring of provider operations or in negotiation of provider contracts should be versed in the basics of antitrust law.

The main purpose of the antitrust laws is to promote free commercial competition. The antitrust laws were designed to protect the consumer by maximizing the consumer's economic welfare through the efficient use and allocation of resources.[48] In the federal arena, antitrust law is primarily defined by the following statutes:

- The Sherman Act

- The Clayton Act

- The Robinson Patman Act

- The Federal Trade Commission Act.

Most states have passed antitrust laws that generally follow the federal laws.

Section 1 of the Sherman Antitrust Act

The most important federal antitrust statute is the Sherman Antitrust Act of 1890.[49] Section 1 of the Sherman Act prohibits "every contract, combination in the form of trust or otherwise, or conspiracy, in restraint of trade or commerce among the several States, or with foreign nations."[50] In short, Section 1 prohibits an agreement between two or more economic entities that is designed to, or actually does, unreasonably restrain competition.

For purposes of Section 1, a conspiracy has been defined as a "unity of purpose or a common understanding, or a meeting of minds in an unlawful arrangement."[51] Proof of such an agreement may be established either by direct proof[52] or by circumstantial evidence of concerted action.[53] In order to establish a Section 1 violation, a plaintiff must demonstrate an agreement between two or more separate entities.

Traditionally, a corporation and its officers, directors, and agents are considered a single entity and are incapable of conspiring with one another.[54] However, there is an important exception to this general rule. If an employee officer or director has an independent economic interest that goes above and beyond the desire to enhance the corporation's welfare, the individuals may be seen as separate entities capable of conspiring with one another and with the corporation.[55] This exception is particularly important for CDMs in the context of hospitals and medical staffs and in the context of provider-sponsored managed care networks.

It is well settled that independent physicians can conspire among themselves in violation of Section 1.[56] However, courts are split on the question of whether a hospital and its medical staff are a single entity. Some courts have held that a hospital and its medical staff cannot conspire.[57] Others have reasoned that medical staffs or individual members of medical staffs have independent economic interests that make the hospital and the medical staff separate entities capable of conspiring with each other.[58]

Section 2 of the Sherman Antitrust Act

Section 2 of the Sherman Act prohibits monopolization, attempted monopolization, and conspiracies to monopolize.[59] Unlike Section 1, Section 2 covers the unilateral conduct of a single actor with market power. To have an illegal monopoly under Section 2, an entity must possess monopoly power in the relevant market and willfully acquire or maintain that monopoly power, rather than acquire it through growth, the development of a superior product, business savvy, or historical accident.[60]

Typically, monopoly power is defined as the power to control prices or exclude competition within a properly defined relevant market.[61] Market power is said to exist "whenever prices can be raised above the levels that would be charged in a competitive market."[62] A firm's market share within the relevant market is the starting point for analyzing monopoly power.[63] Other relevant factors include technological superiority, relative size of other competitors, barriers to entry, pricing practices, homogeneity of the products, and stability of market shares over time.[64]

Illegal attempted monopolization may be established by proof of a specific intent to monopolize the relevant market, predatory or anticompetitive conduct directed to accomplishing that unlawful conduct, and a "dangerous possibility" of success.[65] If an entity already possesses monopoly power, it may not refuse to deal with another entity in order to gain a competitive advantage, destroy a competitor, or preserve or extend its monopoly.[66] Similarly, a firm that lawfully possesses monopoly power in one market cannot use such power to gain an unwarranted competitive advantage in another market.[67]

Finally, under Section 2 of the Sherman Act, if an entity owns or controls a facility that is essential to participation in the market and that cannot practically or reasonably be duplicated, the entity must provide access to the facility on a fair and nondiscriminatory basis.[68] In the health care industry, an argument under this essential facility doctrine typically arises when a hospital denies a practitioner access to hospital facilities. In this situation, the practitioner would have to show that access to the hospital is essential to the physician's practice, that the hospital facility cannot be practicably duplicated, and that access to this facility was denied on an unreasonable or discriminatory basis. Typically, such claims are not established because access to the facility is not essential to the physician's practice or because there are other facilities at which the physician could practice.[69]

Section 7 of the Clayton Act

Section 7 of the Clayton Act prohibits mergers, acquisitions, and joint ventures that may substantially lessen competition or tend to create a monopoly in any line of commerce in any section of the country.[70] A merger does not actually have to unreasonably restrain competition; rather, it only needs to present the "reasonable probability" of substantially lessening competition. Therefore, Section 7 focuses on probabilities rather than certainties or speculative possibilities.[71]

The U. S. Department of Justice and the Federal Trade Commission jointly issued Horizontal Merger Guidelines in 1992, and they were updated in 1996.[72] The Guidelines set forth the circumstances under which a merger or acquisition will be challenged. The Guidelines basically analyze the change in market concentration that will result from the transaction. If the transaction results in too much market concentration, the agencies will attempt to block the transaction, unless offsetting factors are present. The Guidelines also recognize other factors that aggravate or mitigate the concern raised by high concentration, such as ease of entry into the relevant market, changing market conditions, financial condition of competitors in the market, and economic efficiencies that will result from the transaction.

Under Section 7A of the Clayton Act, certain proposed mergers, acquisitions, and joint ventures may not be consummated until 30 days after the Federal Trade Commission and the Department of Justice are notified of the transaction.[73] The "file and wait" requirements are commonly known as the premerger notification Hart Scott Rodino program. Generally, such notification is required if one of the entities involved in the transaction has "annual net sales" (a term generally comparable to revenues) or total assets in excess of $100 million and the other has "annual net sales" or total assets in excess of $10 million, and the acquisition price or the value of the acquired stocks or assets exceeds $15 million.

However, there are numerous attribution rules requiring consolidation of companies under common control for purposes of determining the Act's applicability. Thus, counsel should be consulted, because the penalty for not filing, where the Act requires a filing, is $10,000 a day.

Section 2(a) of the Clayton Act, as amended by the Robinson Patman Act

Section 2(a) of the Clayton Act, as amended by the Robinson Patman Act, prohibits a seller from selling commodities of like grade and quality at different prices where the effect may substantially lessen competition or tend to create a monopoly.[74] In general, this provision was intended to "level the playing field" for customers who are competing with one another by preventing sellers from discriminating in the prices, services, and facilities they give them.[75] However, it has turned out to be the most criticized and complex of the federal antitrust laws.[76] Most critics argue that this provision has been interpreted in ways that restrict price and service competition, because it tends to preclude sellers from offering different prices and terms of sale to different purchasers, irrespective of competitive conditions. Some courts have even reasoned that the statute promotes competitors over competition.[77]

The Act does contain a number of defenses for sellers who offer different buyers different prices. Under Section 2(a), the cost-justification defense permits price discrimination when it is based on differences in the cost that the seller incurs in serving different customers, and the changed condition defense is applicable when market conditions change.[78] Finally, Section 2(b) provides the meeting competition defense, under which otherwise illegal price discrimination is permissible if the seller acts in good faith (relying on a reasonable factual basis) to meet an equally low price of a competitor.[79]

The Federal Trade Commission Act

The Federal Trade Commission Act was passed in 1914 to supplement the provisions of the Sherman Act.[80] Section 1 creates the Federal Trade Commission (FTC) and provides for five commissioners appointed by the President for seven-year terms.[81] Section 5 of the Federal Trade Commission Act is the most important substantive section. Section 5(a)(1) states that "unfair methods of competition in or affecting commerce...are hereby declared unlawful."[82] This section has been held to extend beyond practices that would violate the other antitrust laws, but it is typically construed to be in harmony with the Sherman and Clayton Acts. Section (5)(a)(2) gives the FTC broad power to "prevent persons, partnerships, or corporations from using unfair methods of competition in or affecting commerce."[83] This language has enabled the FTC to protect consumers from a variety of unfair or deceptive marketing techniques, including false advertising and misleading product promotion.

Defining the "Relevant Market"

As noted above, the antitrust laws are designed to promote commercial competition. This is a very broad concept, and definition of the relevant market is the first issue that must be resolved when conducting an antitrust assessment under Sections 1 and 2 of the Sherman Act and Section 7 of the Clayton Act. Definition of the relative market establishes a framework for assessing the amount of relative control a party exercises and the severity of the anticompetitive threat posed by the party's actions or proposed actions.

The relevant market comprises the geographic market and the product market. The relevant product market includes all products or services that consumers consider reasonable substitutes for one another. In the hospital setting, for example, the relevant product market is generally defined as the cluster of services associated with acute inpatient care, although there is considerable debate as to whether ambulatory surgery centers, for instance, also compete in the market.[84]

The relevant geographic market, on the other hand, is typically defined as the physical area in which sellers of the particular product or service operate plus the area to which purchasers could practicably turn for the product if sellers in the area were to attempt to exercise market power by increasing price or decreasing quality.[85] In antitrust cases involving hospitals, the geographic market is typically defined by the distance patients would be willing to travel to obtain a particular service provided by the hospital if price increased or quality decreased.[86] Differences in geographic markets might depend on the nature of the service (e.g., primary care versus tertiary care) or the business class (commercial versus Medicare). After the geographic market and the product market are determined, the market power of parties who are merging, otherwise affiliating, or reaching an agreement that might restrain trade can be accurately assessed.

Penalties for Violating the Antitrust Laws

The federal antitrust laws are generally enforced by both the FTC and the Antitrust Division of the U. S. Department of Justice (DOJ). Many states also have antitrust laws that are enforced by the states' attorneys general. Each agency can sue to enjoin transactions or to obtain various civil remedies. However, only DOJ can enforce the criminal provisions contained in Sections 1 and 2 of the Sherman Act, Section 3 of the Robinson Patman Act, and Section 14 of the Clayton Act, and only the FTC can enforce the Federal Trade Commission Act.

Violations of the Sherman Act are felonies. For individuals, the maximum penalty for each violation is three years imprisonment and/or a fine of up to $350,000. For corporations, the maximum fine is $10 million.

Additionally, persons or firms injured by violations of the Sherman, Clayton, or Robinson Patman Acts may bring civil suits and recover three times the amount of actual damages resulting from the offense plus attorneys' fees and other costs of litigation.

Physician Contracting

A CDM may occasionally assist the health care organization in negotiating and entering into contracts with physicians or physician groups. Consequently, a CDM should be familiar with certain provisions that are usually found in such contracts when entering into negotiations and producing the initial draft of a contract. This section discusses a number of these standard provisions and, in some cases, includes typical language for such provisions. Although this section provides only a brief review of some standard provisions, knowledge of these provisions can help a CDM to expedite the contracting process.

In reviewing this section, a CDM should be aware of the difference between employment agreements and independent contractor agreements. There may be differences in how certain provisions are used in employment agreements as opposed to independent contractor agreements. Where appropriate, these differences will be noted.

It is important for a CDM to be aware of the need to draft physician contracts in light of federal and state fraud and abuse law, state law regarding the corporate practice of medicine, and federal and state law regarding the tax-exempt status of the health care organization, if applicable. Of course, counsel should be involved to review and approve the final contract between the health care organization and the physician or physician group.

Specific Provisions

Assignment

Because a physician provides personal services, a health care organization will want to ensure that the physician or the physician group will not assign the rights and obligations contained in the agreement to someone else. However, given the prevalence of consolidation and other similar transactions in the health care industry, the health care organization will often want to retain the flexibility to assign its rights and obligations to affiliated or successor corporations. Accordingly, an assignment provision may contain language similar to the following:

> This Agreement may not be assigned by any party without prior written consent of the other party, except that Health Care Organization may assign this Agreement to a successor corporation that carries on its business or to a legal entity controlled by or under common control with Health Care Organization. Subject to the foregoing limitation upon assignment, this Agreement shall be binding upon and inure to the benefit of the successors and assigns of the parties.

Billing

In an employment agreement, a health care organization should include a provision that indicates that the health care organization, not the physician, will bill for, and be entitled to receive payment for, all professional services, as the health care organization will be paying the physician a salary.

In an independent contractor agreement, the physician or physician group is generally responsible for billing for professional services. A standard billing provision in an independent contractor agreement might be drafted as follows:

> Physician shall be solely responsible for all billing for services rendered by Physician and Physician's employees in accordance with this Agreement and shall be solely responsible for all of Physician's contractual allowances, free care, bad debts, collections, etc. Any costs or expenses involved in billing or collection shall be the sole responsibility of Physician, and amounts collected shall be the sole property of Physician. Health Care Organization shall perform appropriate billing and collection functions for all services furnished by Health Care Organization and shall not be responsible for any of Physician's billing and collection costs and expenses.

Alternatively, the health care organization could provide billing services for the physician in an independent contractor agreement at a fair market value price.

Medical Staff Bylaws

A health care organization with a medical staff, such as a hospital, should include a clause that addresses interpretation of the agreement in light of its medical staff bylaws. Because some state courts have concluded that medical staff bylaws are a contract, this type of clause is important to include in order to avoid a conflict over whether the bylaws supersede the agreement in certain circumstances. A typical interpretation provision might state the following:

> To the extent that any provisions of this Agreement are inconsistent with the provisions of the Medical Staff Bylaws and Rules and Regulations, the provisions of this Agreement shall prevail and shall be deemed to have superseded the inconsistent provisions of said Bylaws and Rules and Regulations. These provisions of said Bylaws and Rules and Regulations, and the Health Care Organization's policies and standards, with respect to hearings, appellate review, grievances, etc. shall not apply to the expiration, termination, or possible renewal of this Agreement.

Choice of Law

A health care organization should include a choice of law provision that indicates which state's laws will govern the agreement and the rights, powers, and liabilities of the parties to the agreement. Although it is usually obvious which state's laws govern, this issue should not be neglected in drafting the contract, because it would be particularly wasteful to end up litigating it.

Duties/Responsibilities

The set of duties and responsibilities of the physician or physician group constitutes the most fundamental element of a physician contract. Accordingly, it is very important for a health care organization to clearly stipulate these duties and responsibilities in the physician contract. As a full description of a physician's duties and responsibilities can often cover several pages, this section will simply list issues that are often addressed in this aspect of the contract. These areas generally include a requirement regarding the maintenance of proper practice qualifications, such as licensure and board certification; a requirement to maintain membership on the health care organization's medical staff; specific clinical requirements, such as the scope of clinical services to be provided by the physician or physician group, on-call and coverage times, and education of support and professional staff; a requirement regarding participation in the quality improvement/quality assurance process of the health care organization; and a requirement to act in a manner consistent with federal and state law, the health care organization's policies and procedures, and the medical staff bylaws, rules, and regulations. These requirements may be set forth as separate contractual provisions.

Status of Physician

A health care organization should include a provision that designates the status of the physician (i.e., employee or independent contractor). A typical status provision may state the following:

> It is expressly acknowledged by the parties to this Agreement that Physician is an independent contractor and that nothing in this Agreement is intended nor shall be construed to create an employer/employee relationship, a joint venture relationship, or a lease or landlord/tenant relationship between Physician and Health Care Organization.

Managed Care Contracts

Because health care organizations have become dependent on managed care business, it is common to find a provision that requires the physician or the physician group to participate in certain managed care contracts. Such a provision may consist of language similar to the following:

Physician Group shall procure and maintain participation contracts in any health maintenance organization, preferred provider organization, or third-party payer program in which Health Care Organization is a member and requests the Physician Group to participate. Physician Group shall require all Physicians that it employs to enter into such contracts.

Liability Insurance

In an employment agreement, the health care organization often procures malpractice insurance for the physician. In providing for this coverage in an employment agreement, the health care organization should be sure to require the physician to remain insurable.

In an independent contractor agreement, or in an employment agreement in which the physician is responsible for obtaining malpractice insurance, a liability insurance provision may often look like the following:

> Physician shall at all times maintain insurance for professional (malpractice) and general liability for Physician and Physician's Employees in an amount that is reasonable and acceptable to Health Care Organization and any pertinent bylaw requirements. At all times, Physician shall cause a current certificate of insurance to be furnished by Physician's insurance company to Health Care Organization. In the event of termination of this Agreement, this obligation to be insured shall be binding on Physician and shall survive the termination of this Agreement. If necessary, tail insurance shall be procured by the Physician.
>
> (a) Physician shall obtain and maintain throughout the term of this Agreement, at Physician's expense, from a carrier acceptable to Health Care Organization, comprehensive general liability insurance

covering Physician and Physician's personnel, appropriate workers' compensation coverage for Physician's employed personnel, and professional liability coverage, each with customary retentions and exclusions and with limits customary in the community.

(b)   The foregoing notwithstanding, the limits on Physician's professional liability insurance shall be no less than $_____ per occurrence and $_____ aggregate.

(c)   Physician shall request in writing that its insurance carrier furnish Health Care Organization with at least 10 days' notice prior to the effective date of any reduction, cancellation, or termination of any professional or general liability insurance policy carried under sections (a) or (b) above. Physician shall also provide immediate written notice to Health Care Organization of any adverse change to any such coverage as well as any claim filed against Physician.

(d)   Physician shall promptly furnish to Health Care Organization an annual certificate from the liability carrier evidencing maintenance of the required minimum amount of professional liability insurance as stated above.

Restrictive Covenants

Health care organizations generally include noncompetition clauses (restrictive covenants) in physician contracts. While specific state requirements differ, generally speaking, noncompetition clauses must be appropriately limited in scope, as to both geographic area and duration, in order to be enforceable. In addition, noncompetition clauses may heighten antitrust concerns and may suggest that the health care organization is more interested in market share than in community benefit. Accordingly, great care should be taken to tightly draft such clauses in order to ensure that they are enforceable and that they do not result in unwanted legal consequences for the health care organization. A typical noncompetition clause may look like the following:

> Physician agrees that, during the term hereof and for a period of one year after the termination of this Agreement, such Physician shall not establish, operate, or provide physician or other medical services (whether as an employee, shareholder, partner, independent contractor, manager, consultant, or otherwise) at any medical office, clinic, or other health care facility providing services similar to those provided by Health Care Organization within 15 miles of the main premises at which Physician practiced at the time of such termination of employment, as set forth in Exhibit __ (the "Practice Area").

Term and Termination

It is important for a health care organization to devote sufficient time to term and termination provisions in drafting a physician agreement. In some cases, contracts will be drawn to meet a safe harbor under the anti-kickback laws, in which case the term of a physician contract should be at least one year. A well-drafted termination provision can enable a health care organization to easily exit from a relationship in which the other party is not performing. Term and termination provisions generally look like the following:

(a)   Term. The term of this Agreement shall be for   year(s),   commencing on _____ (the "Commencement Date") and expiring on _____. The Agreement shall not be automatically renewed for any additional terms.

(b)   Termination with Cause. Health Care Organization shall have the right to terminate this Agreement immediately for breach of [insert relevant sections] of this Agreement, or in the event that Physician fails to meet the requirements [insert relevant sections or requirements, such as failure to provide adequate patient care, loss of licensure or clinical privileges, failure to follow hospital policies and procedures, etc.]. In addition, either party may terminate this Agreement in the event of material breach by giving the breaching party written notice of the breach and the opportunity to cure the breach within days. If the breach is not cured within the _____ - day period, the non-breaching party may terminate this Agreement immediately.

(c)   [Optional effectively reduces the term to the length of the notice period] Termination without Cause. The Agreement may be terminated, without cause or penalty, by either party upon providing the other party with at least _____ days' prior written notice of its intention to terminate this Agreement.

Termination and Staff Privileges

A health care organization with a medical staff may want to include in a contract relating to an exclusive service a provision that provides for termination of the medical staff privileges of the physician upon termination of the agreement. This type of provision may consist of language similar to the following:

Notwithstanding any provision of this Agreement, or of the Medical Staff Bylaws, its Rules and Regulations, and policies of Health Care Organization, or of the standards of any accrediting body or professional organization, Medical Staff membership and clinical privileges of the Physician at the Health Care Organization shall terminate simultaneously with expiration or termination of this Agreement. Provisions of the Bylaws, Rules and Regulations, and policies of Health Care Organization or of accrediting bodies or professional organizations, with respect to hearings, appellate reviews, etc., shall not apply.

If the agreement involves a physician group, this type of provision should also indicate that medical staff membership and clinical privileges of a group physician will terminate simultaneously if the physician is no longer employed by, or associated with, the group.

Patient Care Issues

Nondiscrimination in the Provision of Care

Federal Law

There are a number of federal statutes that require certain health care institutions to provide health care services on a nondiscriminatory basis. Further, the Constitution, as well as state and local laws, impose a similar legal mandate. More specifically, the Civil Rights Act of 1964[87] prohibits discrimination based on race in designated places of "public accommodation" and by publicly owned facilities. The provisions contained in Titles II and IV have been applied by the courts to public hospitals. Additionally, Title VI of the Civil Rights Act prohibits discrimination on the basis of race, color, or national origin by an institution receiving "federal financial assistance." Hospitals receiving Medicare and/or Medicaid funds are deemed to be recipients of federal financial assistance. Accordingly, the nondiscrimination requirement is applied to the hospital's admission policies, the availability of services, and the assignment of rooms.

A second federal statute, the Hill-Burton Act,[88] requires that hospitals receiving assistance under the Hill-Burton program make their facilities available to all persons within the community. This community service requirement is agreed to by the hospital as a condition of its receiving federal funds. Hospitals receiving Hill-Burton funds are required to participate in the Medicare/Medicaid programs; to provide emergency care to persons residing or employed in the service area without regard to their ability to pay; and to make hospital services available to persons within the community without regard to race, creed, color, or national origin or to whether the treating physician is a physician on staff at the hospital. Under the Hill-Burton Act, it is also the hospital's duty to ensure that physicians on its medical staff agree to accept Medicaid patients.

A Hill-Burton hospital must not only agree to make services available to the community, but also guarantee a specified volume of free care. The "uncompensated care" assurance is calculated as an amount of free care equal to 10 percent of the Hill-Burton assistance granted under the Act or 3 percent of the hospital's Medicare/Medicaid operating costs. This free care assurance must be upheld for a period of 20 years. In the event a hospital is unable to meet its free care obligation for a given year, the amount of free care is carried forward to the following year. In cases in which a hospital is unable to meet its free-care obligations, it must establish out-reach programs to satisfy the terms of the Hill-Burton Act grant. The Department of Health and Human Services, Public Health Service, Office of Facilities Compliance, enforces the Hill-Burton Act.

The courts have held that a patient may bring a private right of action to enforce a hospital's free-care obligation under the Act.[89] Nevertheless, hospitals are not required to render free care in cases in which they do not have the necessary facilities or in which they reject a patient's transfer absent knowledge of the existence of emergency circumstances.[90]

A third federal statute, the Rehabilitation Act of 1973, prohibits discrimination in federally assisted programs against persons who have a handicap condition or a record of such impairment or are perceived as having a handicap impairment. The U. S. Supreme Court has interpreted the term "handicap" to include a communicable disease such as tuberculosis.[91] Commentators suggest that this rationale is likely to be construed by the courts as including AIDS and AIDS-Related Conditions (ARC) within the scope of the term handicap for purposes of the Rehabilitation Act of 1973.

Several states have adopted analogous statutes. Some jurisdictions have gone so far as to expressly hold AIDS as being a handicap under local law.[92] The Rehabilitation Act of 1973 provides for a private right of action to enforce the nondiscrimination provision contained in Section 504 of the Act.

From a constitutional perspective, the due process and equal protection clauses of the Fourteenth Amendment to the U. S. Constitution are applicable to public hospitals. The Fourteenth Amendment provides that "no state shall deprive any person of life, liberty, or property without due process of law, nor deny any person within its jurisdiction the equal protection of the laws." In the public hospital setting, the Fourteenth Amendment has been used successfully by individuals seeking care at a particular hospital.

Nevertheless, the definition of public hospital has taken on a life of its own. The public/private question is at issue, because the Fourteenth Amendment is only applicable to "state action" as opposed to private actions. This gives rise to a question as to whether a private hospital can ever be engaged in action sufficient to constitute state action. On the one hand, there is the argument that, if a private facility accepts state or federal funds, it is in fact engaged in state action. In general, however, a hospital's participation in the Medicare/Medicaid program, the granting of a federal or state tax exemption, and the acceptance of government financial aid have been found to be insufficient to convert a private hospital's actions or policies into actions of the state.

There are, however, limited circumstances in which private hospitals may be so intertwined with a public or government responsibility that the courts will find the presence of state action for purposes of applying the Constitution. For example, the Fourth Circuit has held that private hospitals participating in the Hill-Burton program are engaged in state action based on the fact that they cooperated in a federal-state planning function and were receiving funds as a result.[93] Furthermore, a hospital which was located on land in which a local government had a future interest conditioned on the hospital's ceasing its operations and which received local government financial assistance was held to be engaged in state action for purposes of the Fourteenth Amendment.[94]

State Law

Both state and local law may require nondiscrimination in the provision of services. Such laws are generally applied to business entities serving the public or providing public accommodations. Depending on a particular statute, such nondiscrimination provisions may be applicable to private hospitals. Typically, these nondiscrimination requirements will appear in the hospital licensure statutes. Such nondiscrimination requirements may also appear in state tax-exemption laws, as is the case in Oklahoma. Some of these state or local laws impose atypical nondiscrimination provisions, in that they are applicable to categories other than race, religion, color, national origin, sex, age, or handicap. These nondiscrimination provisions prohibit hospitals from discriminating in providing services to or admitting patients of physicians who do not have staff privileges at the particular hospital.

Montana has such a nondiscrimination requirement. The language in the statute is broader than the typical nondiscrimination provision in that it cuts across racial lines and is not limited to classifications set forth in the statute. From the patient's perspective, the Montana statute is easier to litigate under. Instead of having to prove that there was some racial, ethnic, or sex-based rationale for not being admitted or treated properly, a patient is able to make the same charges based primarily on the fact that he or she was not referred to the facility by a member of its medical staff.

Patient "Antidumping" Requirements

Beginning in 1986, Congress required hospitals participating in the Medicare program to provide examinations and treatment to individuals with emergency medical conditions in an effort to prevent refusal of treatment or transfer of individuals to other facilities before institution of emergency medical treatment because the individual lacked the financial resources to pay for the emergency services. This federal law is commonly referred to as COBRA or patient "antidumping" legislation.[95,96] The antidumping law is of particular interest to CDMs in the emergency medicine area. However, it is prudent for every CDM, no matter what the area of specialty, to be familiar with the rules regarding treatment and transfer of emergency patients, because a variety of clinical departments may be involved in the treatment of emergency patients.

Basic Screening Requirement

The patient antidumping law is applicable to any hospital that participates in the Medicare program.[97] Further, such provisions apply to any physician who provides services at a hospital that is required to comply with COBRA and who is in a position to examine, treat, or transfer individuals presenting themselves at the hospital who would otherwise be entitled to the protections of the antidumping laws.

The basic requirements of COBRA are that the Medicare-participating hospital screen the condition of any person who seeks treatment in its emergency department to determine whether an emergency medical condition exists.[97,98]

The duty to screen the condition of any person applies to individuals seeking services from a Medicare-participating hospital whether or not the individual is covered by Medicare or has the ability to pay for such services. As a practical matter, a screening examination may not be delayed in order to determine the individual's method of payment or type of insurance.[99]

If an emergency medical condition exists, the individual must be given treatment in order to stabilize the condition prior to being transferred to another facility.[100] In the event the hospital is unable to stabilize the emergency medical condition, the statute imposes specific requirements before a transfer may be made.

In order to fulfill the hospital's duties under the statute, persons in an emergency department must conduct an appropriate screening examination within the capabilities of the department to determine whether an emergency medical condition exists.[97] This means that all resources routinely available to the emergency department, including ancillary services, must be accessible and usable in the initial screening process.[97]

If an emergency medical condition exists, the hospital must provide either further examination and treatment within its capabilities to stabilize the medical condition or an appropriate transfer to another health care facility. COBRA does not require that treatment be provided if the individual or surrogate refuses to consent to treatment or refuses to be transferred to another facility where treatment could be provided, assuming that transfer would be appropriate.[101] Nevertheless, a hospital is required to take all reasonable steps to secure the individual's written and informed consent on refusing an examination and treatment or refusing a transfer.

Consent Rule and Certification of Transfer

If the hospital is unable to obtain informed consent from the individual refusing an examination and/or treatment, it should carefully document the specific events leading up to such refusal and the ultimate failure to examine or treat the individual. This is important because, under COBRA, it is presumed that the individual presenting him- or herself at an emergency department is requesting examination and treatment for a medical condition. The burden is on the hospital to establish by a preponderance of the evidence that the request for such examination for treatment was withdrawn.[102]

An individual whose emergency medical condition has not been stabilized may be transferred from the hospital under certain conditions, including whether the transfer is both "authorized" and "appropriate." The transfer is authorized only if it is made with the individual's informed consent or with a physician's certification.

COBRA requires that the hospital take all reasonable steps to obtain evidence of informed consent. Emergency department physicians must be prepared to inform the individual or a surrogate of the risks and/or benefits of a transfer or a lack of transfer in order to obtain written informed consent.[103] In the event the individual or his or her surrogate is unable to provide informed consent, the transfer of an individual whose medical condition has not been stabilized may be based on a physician's certification.

The physician certification essentially states that, based on the information available at the time, the medical benefits reasonably expected from medical treatment at the transferee facility outweigh the increased risks to the individual due to the transfer.[104] Under COBRA, only a physician may currently certify a transfer. Effective July 1, 1990, hospitals were required to designate on-call physicians to be responsible for making a risk/benefit determination regarding whether a transfer is appropriate.

In the event no physician is physically present at the hospital, the hospital must ensure that a physician is available for consultation and that the physician is the person who determines that the transfer is appropriate. Designated physicians who fail to respond to a request for certification of transfer are potentially subject to civil action and statutory penalties.

Physician certification of a transfer must always include the physician's signature and should be obtained at the earliest possible time. COBRA permits, under certain emergency circumstances, communication of a physician certification via telephone. However, a physician's signature is always required and must be obtained at the earliest possible time.

Other Transfer Prerequisites

In order for a patient transfer to be appropriate, certain conditions must be met in addition to obtaining either a patient consent or physician certification, whichever is applicable.[105] The requisite conditions are that:

- Medical treatment, within the capabilities of the emergency department of the transferring facility, has been provided in order to minimize health risks to the individual.

- The transferee facility must have consented to receive the individual and must have available space and qualified personnel to treat the individual.

- All available medical records that relate to the individual's emergency medical condition and that include observations of the individual's condition, preliminary diagnosis, treatment provided, results of tests administered, and the informed written consent for the transfer or physician certification if applicable must be presented to the transferee hospital upon transfer.

- The transfer must be conducted by qualified personnel and through the use of transportation equipment that is most appropriate in light of the individual's medical condition.

The Health Care Financing Administration (HCFA) has taken the position in the past that transferring hospitals must complete the transfer of patients to transferee facilities even in cases where the transferee facility refuses to accept the transfer because of lack of capacity. HCFA staff members have found in the past that the receiving facility will make space available somehow upon transfer of the individual. This policy statement may be indicative of HCFA's lack of tolerance for institutions that refuse transfers on the basis of capacity.

Enforcement

The requirements of the patient antidumping statute may be enforced by HCFA, a transferee facility, or the individual suffering harm because of a violation of the antidumping law. In cases in which HCFA enforces the provisions of the antidumping law, it will typically order the state agency responsible for ensuring that the hospital complies with Medicare requirements to conduct an investigation. Assuming the state agency's investigation determines there is a violation, HCFA may recommend termination of the Medicare provider agreement at the end of a 90-day waiting period. The decision regarding the determination and timing of the Medicare provider agreement is made by the HCFA regional office with jurisdiction over the facility.

In the event HCFA determines that a violation of COBRA has occurred, it may seek to assess civil monetary penalties through an action filed by the Office of the Inspector General (OIG). The law is unclear as to whether the civil penalties contemplated by COBRA would be available to a party other than the Secretary of Health and Human Services. At least one federal court has held that it has jurisdiction to hear a claim for civil penalties brought by an individual against a physician for allegedly violating COBRA.[106]

Civil monetary penalties may be imposed against the hospital or the physician. OIG may impose civil penalties of up to $50,000 per violation.[107] However, the civil monetary penalty assessable against a hospital with fewer than 100 beds is limited to $25,000. The civil monetary penalties are in addition to suspension or termination of the participation agreement with Medicare.

A physician who is responsible for the screening examination and other necessary treatment may be assessed civil monetary penalties if he or she negligently violates a requirement of COBRA.[108] The penalties are capped at $50,000 per violation. The penalties apply to physicians who sign a certification to transfer an individual if the physician knew or should have known that the benefits of the transfer did not outweigh its risks. Moreover, civil penalties may be assessed against a physician who misrepresents an individual's conditions or the obligations of the health care facility. In addition, the physician may be excluded from participation under Medicare if it is found that his or her violation of COBRA was gross and flagrant or repeated.

A hospital as well as an on-call physician may be subject to liability for a violation of COBRA in the event the on-call physician refuses to or fails to appear to provide stabilizing treatment to the patient.[109] The penalties would not apply to a physician who orders the transfer of an individual because the physician determines that, without the services of an on-call physician, the benefits of a transfer outweigh the apparent risks.[109] Therefore, even where a hospital does not knowingly violate the provisions of COBRA, it still may be subject to liability for the acts of its agents and the physician through whom it looks to satisfy its COBRA responsibilities. Furthermore, a facility that suffers economic loss as a result of an individual who is improperly transferred is entitled to seek restitution from the hospital transferring the individual.[110]

Finally, COBRA provides a private right of action to individuals suffering personal harm as a direct result of a hospital's violation of COBRA. Such individuals are permitted to pursue damages available under state law for such injuries or such other equitable relief as is appropriate.[111] The statutory private right of action and claims are against the hospital and not the physician. However, the physician may be subject to medical malpractice claims brought by the individual injured by the physician's negligence in treatment.

Administrative Requirements for Facilities

COBRA imposes on the hospital several administrative requirements. First, the hospital must adopt a policy to ensure compliance with the antidumping provisions of COBRA. This is also a requirement of the Joint Commission on Accreditation of Healthcare Organizations (JCAHO). JCAHO requires that, as a condition of accreditation, the hospital have an established policy regarding the treatment of individuals in its emergency department. Generally, a hospital's antidumping policy includes a statement of intent; the pertinent statutory definitions; the hospital's method for coordinating the services of the various hospital departments that may be required to comply with the terms of the policy, including the emergency department, the labor and delivery department, and those ancillary service departments that render services to the emergency department; the responsibilities of on-call physicians and the consequences of failing to respond; the requirements of transferring an individual; the procedures or requirements necessary to determine if the facility lacks the capacity to accept a transfer; the identification of persons responsible for making any necessary decisions; the requirement that the treating physicians obtain and document the individual's consent to transfer; and the hospital's policy with regard to retention of the records of patients treated and/or transferred under the COBRA requirements.

Hospitals are required to maintain medical records and other records related to individuals who are transferred to or from a facility prior to stabilizing an emergency medical condition. The records are to be kept for a period of five years from the date of the transfer. COBRA also specifies the required contents of the medical records. One key aspect of the patient transfer record is the patient consent form or, in the alternative, the physician certification form.

COBRA requires a hospital to maintain a list of physicians who are on-call to provide medical treatment required to stabilize individuals with emergency medical conditions. The hospital must also post signs conspicuously throughout the emergency department that specify the rights of an individual to receive medical treatment. In addition, hospitals are required to post signs indicating whether or not the hospital participates in the Medicaid program under a state plan approved under Medicare. HCFA has issued detailed and specific instructions regarding the posting of the notice and the form of the notice.

Analogous State Law

Over the past several years, various states have begun to enact antidumping legislation. Numerous states, including California, New York, Florida, and Texas, have enacted laws to guarantee access to emergency care and to prohibit denial of services. As is the case in Florida, several state antidumping laws allow for denial, revocation, or suspension of a license for hospitals found to violate the emergency services requirements. A patient dumping incident, in many states, could threaten both a hospital's state licensure and its Medicare participation. Further, because the federal statute does not preempt state law, HCFA and the state department of health could arguably proceed concurrently, and sanctions could be triggered at both levels.

Detention of Patients

CDMs may encounter situations in which a patient is admitted to a facility against his or her wishes. In some cases, a CDM may be given oversight responsibilities in this area that would include monitoring of staff compliance with a hospital's or health care organization's patient detention policy.

Patients admitted and treated in facilities against their wishes have traditionally sued the facilities on the basis of false imprisonment. In short, any patient held against his or her will and without legal authority has a cause of action against the party causing the nonconsensual detention. In false imprisonment cases, actual restraint does not have to be proven. The courts have held that threats by medical or hospital staff that would lead a reasonable person to fear harm provide sufficient restraint to maintain an action based on false imprisonment. Similarly, detaining a patient for failure to pay an outstanding hospital bill has been deemed to constitute false imprisonment.

State statutes may be instructive in delineating explicit conditions under which detention of patients is permitted and procedures for instituting such detentions. For example, New York's Patient Bill of Rights statute[112] explicitly states the conditions under which a patient may be restrained either physically or through the use of chemicals. All states have laws providing specific procedures for committing an individual who is mentally ill or a dangerous substance abuser to a mental health or substance abuse treatment facility. Generally, hospitals are permitted to detain these individuals in the course of treatment upon notifying the appropriate authorities and obtaining commitment or custody orders from such authority.

Discharge Planning

Assuming a patient has been admitted to a hospital, has been treated without being unlawfully detained, and is medically ready for discharge, the hospital must then satisfy its posthospital care obligations. Generally, the hospital is not legally obligated to provide posthospital care or to ensure that the plan of posthospital care is actually implemented. The hospital is merely required to assess the patient's medical status at the time of discharge, identify posthospital services that may benefit the patient, and make a reasonable effort to make those services available to the patient. In cases in which the hospital demonstrates a lack of due care in performing the discharge planning function, liability will be imposed. In cases in which there was a clear failure to inform the patient of a reasonably foreseeable outcome of discharge or in which the hospital failed to ascertain the patient's circumstances relative to planning post-discharge care, courts have found negligence on the part of the hospital.

In certain cases, patients will refuse to leave the hospital upon notification from a physician that they are ready for discharge. Depending on his or her specific authority, a CDM could find him- or herself in the middle of a dispute between the patient and the treating physician. In some states, the statutes are instructive as to the ramifications of a patient's failure to leave a hospital. For example, North Carolina law makes it a misdemeanor for a patient to fail to leave a hospital upon the discharge order of two physicians. In the event that state law is silent on the issue, the hospital may resort to an action to evict the patient as a trespasser. At least one court has suggested that a hospital has a duty to take such action in the interests of other members of the community desirous of using the hospital's limited resources.[113]

Patient Consent to Treatment

In recent years, the issues surrounding a patient's consent to treatment have taken on new importance. The right of the patient to control the course of his or her medical treatment, including the right to terminate care, has become a prevalent issue in hospitals around the country. The requirements for patient consent are now being imposed through statutory/regulatory mandates rather than through common law. It is important that a CDM, and the providers under his or her charge, understand the rules for communicating and decision making present in every patient/physician relationship, not only for purposes of reducing the risk of potential liability but also as a means of improving patient satisfaction.

Consent and Informed Consent Compared

Consent encompasses two separate doctrines, consent and informed consent. Under the doctrine of consent, a physician is required to obtain the patient's permission prior to beginning treatment. The failure of the physician to obtain consent constitutes the tort of battery.[114] Battery, in tort law, is nonconsensual touching. Therefore, motive, including a desire to protect the patient, is irrelevant, as is the fact that the treatment may have been administered appropriately.

Civil actions for battery based on a failure to obtain consent are most likely to be brought as a result of a physician's providing treatment other than that described to the patient or altering the method of delivery of particular treatment without informing the patient.[115] Consent need not always be expressed.

It can be implied from the patient's conduct, as is often the case with routine medical procedures.

Informed consent doctrine was developed by the courts in cases brought against providers under negligence law and is not applicable in cases involving the intentional tort of battery. In order to establish a prima facie case of negligence, the plaintiff must establish that a duty was owed by the allegedly negligent defendant; that such duty was breached; and that such breach caused actual injury to the plaintiff. The theory of informed consent is based on the principle that a physician stands in a special relationship of trust toward a patient. The physician owes the patient the duty not to withhold any facts that are necessary to form the basis of an intelligent decision by the patient to undergo the proposed treatment.[116]

During the 1970s, many states adopted informed consent statutes that generally codified the common law consent requirements, often adopting the professional practice standards for disclosure.

Scope of Disclosure

The principal issue in informed consent cases is the scope of the physician's explanation. Generally, the courts have required that a patient be told the nature and purpose of the procedure; the risks and consequences; the alternatives to the proposed course of treatment; and, most recently, the risks of no treatment at all.

In recognition of the fact that certain information must be provided, it appears that at least two standards have emerged with respect to how much information need be disclosed to the patient. One standard is the "professional practice standard," which requires the physician to make such disclosure as a reasonable medical practitioner in similar circumstances would make.[117] In practical terms, the professional practice standard is proved in court through the use of expert testimony as to the applicable standard in the community.

An alternative standard is the "reasonable patient" or "materiality rule," which requires the physician to disclose the information that a reasonable person in the patient's position would consider material in deciding whether to undergo the proposed treatment.[118] Under the reasonable patient rule, the determination as to whether the detail of the disclosure was sufficient is made by a jury as opposed to an expert witness. As a general rule, however, the disclosure of a particular risk in large part depends on the frequency and the severity of the risk. Very severe risks, such as death, damage to physical appearance or sexual functioning, and likelihood of incapacitation are considered material and subject to disclosure even if they are rare.

Patients alleging a lack of informed consent must prove not only that the physician breached his or her duty to provide adequate information to make a decision, but also that the patient would not have consented if he or she had known the risks and that the patient was injured by a risk that was not disclosed.

Exceptions to the Consent Requirement

Several exceptions to the general rule that consent must be obtained prior to performing certain medical procedures have been created by the courts. One exception is in the case of an emergency. Generally, this is found to mean that, if the delay in treatment necessary to obtain the patient consent would result in significant harm to the patient, the physician may proceed with treatment without consent.[119] At least one court has held that the treatment being provided without consent need not be life-saving as long as time is critical and the potential harm to the patient is more than trivial. However, where it is possible to obtain consent from a patient's appropriate surrogate, such consent should be obtained, even in an emergency.[120]

Another exception to the general rule of consent appears in cases in which a patient is under general anesthesia in surgery and an unanticipated condition arises that the physician determines requires attention in order to protect the patient from the risk and the discomfort of a second surgical procedure.[121] The condition must truly be unanticipated in order to fall within the exception. The courts have not been quick to find a condition to be unanticipated if it results in a procedure to remove an organ or alter reproductive capacity or that significantly increases the risks associated with a particular surgery. However, in cases in which a physician discusses the possibility that an unanticipated condition might arise during surgery prior to actually performing the surgery, courts are more likely to find in favor of the physician under the exception.[122]

A third exception to the general rule of consent arises in cases involving a therapeutic privilege. The therapeutic privilege may be invoked if a physician reasonably believes that the patient's mental or physical well-being would suffer as a result of the physician's disclosure of certain information in order to obtain the patient's consent.

Finally, the patient may request that he or she not be informed. This is more commonly known as waiver of informed consent.

Hospital Policy Development

The consent issue is particularly important to CDMs, because hospitals have been held liable in cases in which physicians fail to obtain consent, even when the physician is not an employee. Additionally, JCAHO requires hospitals to develop and implement informed consent policies. State hospital licensing departments may also regulate informed consent policies and practices. At least one court has suggested that hospitals may have an affirmative duty to require physicians to make proper disclosure to their patients.[123] Furthermore, studies have shown that consent policies enhance communication between staff and patients and may improve patient satisfaction.

An effective consent policy should contain a requirement that the physician obtain the patient's consent. Responsibility for obtaining patient consent should not be delegated by the physician to nurses, interns, or residents. Consent should be obtained through a conversation between the physician and the patient. The physician's explanation of the risks and the procedures should be in language that a layman can understand. Further, in the case of non-English speaking patients, translations should be provided.

The physician should inform the patient of the nature and the purpose of the procedure or treatment, the risks, the alternatives, and the risks of no treatment at all. Most important, the patient should be given an opportunity to ask questions. Finally, the patient should be informed about the individual performing the procedure or surgery.

Consent should be obtained prior to the proposed treatment to provide the patient with adequate time to deliberate. However, consent should not be sought so far in advance as to allow the patient's physical condition to change. If possible, consent should be obtained under circumstances in which the patient's ability to absorb the information and make a rational decision is not affected, as might be the case in which the patient is in severe pain or under sedation.

Moreover, the informed consent policy should define mental capacity and specify the surrogates authorized to act in the event the patient is found to lack mental capacity. A psychiatric evaluation should be recommended if a patient's mental capacity is unclear. Finally, the policy should include a procedure to obtain patient consent when the patient has no surrogate.

Some states have enacted statutory requirements for disclosure that mandate that certain risks be disclosed by the physician and that certain procedures be followed in informing patients. Generally, the courts seem to strictly adhere to the standards set out in the statute when hearing cases alleging failure to properly disclose.

Patient Refusal of Treatment

The law governing the right to refuse or discontinue medical treatment is predominantly a creature of the states. The judicial opinions in this area reveal the presence of two conflicting principles. The first principle is the notion that a mentally competent adult patient has the right to refuse treatment. This principle is grounded in the notion that each man is considered to be the master of his own body and, assuming he is mentally capable to make such a decision, may expressly prohibit the performance of life-saving surgery or other medical treatment.[124] The second principle is that medical care necessary to preserve life must be provided, absent some recognized legal exception. The courts have derived this rule from the emergency exception to the informed consent rule and from the traditional paternalistic role the courts play with respect to medical treatment for incompetent persons.[125]

Competent Adults

Competent adults have been held to have a qualified right to refuse medical treatment, including life-sustaining treatment, based on a right to privacy and on religious grounds.[126] Furthermore, the courts have recognized a patient's right to refuse medical treatment based on a common law right of self-determination and on public policy grounds.[127] However, the competent adult patient's right to self-determination is limited. The courts have recognized four countervailing interests relative to the patient's right of self-determination: preservation of life, protection of the interests of innocent third parties, prevention of suicide, and protection of the ethical integrity of the medical profession.

Previous judicial determinations have been based primarily on preservation of life and/or protection of the interests of innocent third parties. Typically, the state's interest in preservation of life is offset in cases in which a terminally ill patient is receiving prolonged medical care that is determined to result in extending the patient's suffering. However, in *Cruzan v. Director*,[128] the U.S. Supreme Court concluded that the state's interest in preservation of life requires a greater level of proof of a patient's desire to terminate life-sustaining treatment. Along these lines, various states have begun to enact living will statutes in an attempt to create a legal avenue for proof of a patient's wishes in the event of terminal illness that could be used as evidence probative of the patient's intent.

In cases involving refusal of treatment based on religious beliefs, the courts generally apply more restrictive standards, particularly if there are third-party interests involved, such as unborn or minor children. For example, the courts have routinely ordered blood transfusions for pregnant women or mothers of small children despite contrary religious beliefs.[129] However, there is a minority of cases that reject the majority view.[130]

Incompetent Adults

Some courts have upheld the incompetent patient's right to self-determination in cases in which there is a medical consensus that the patient is terminally ill and without hope of recovery.[131] Generally speaking, however, in cases involving legally or mentally incompetent patients, the issue comes down to whether a decision as to the patient's well-being can be made by some other party, who is called the surrogate decision maker. There is a rebuttable presumption that the family of a legally or mentally incompetent patient is an appropriate surrogate for purposes of exercising the patient's rights.

However, the U.S. Supreme Court added another wrinkle to the rebuttable presumption standard. In *Cruzan*,[128] the Court recognized the state's interest in preserving life. Specifically, the Court concluded that the state's interest in preserving life can supersede the patient's interest in privacy or self-determination, as well as the presumptive guardianship rights of the patient's family. The Court concluded further that there is no constitutional requirement for a state to recognize family relationships when the family intends to act contrary to the interests of the state and there is no other probative evidence supporting the patient's desire to refuse treatment. The five-member majority of the Supreme Court ultimately held that the state can require "clear and convincing" evidence of the patient's desire to refuse treatment based on the court's rationale that incompetent persons do not possess the same rights as competent persons because they are unable to make an informed and voluntary choice to exercise those rights.

Parents as Surrogates for Minors

The law is slightly different with regard to the rights of parents acting as surrogate decision makers on behalf of their minor children. A majority of the courts have prohibited parents and legal guardians from refusing life-sustaining care for their minor children, especially in cases in which there is a consensus that the prognosis with treatment is favorable.[132] Some state legislatures have mandated that parents of minors provide medically necessary care for their children even if such care is contrary to the parents' religious beliefs.[133]

Further, several courts have ordered parents to provide medically necessary care for their children where the court determines that the failure to do so poses an unreasonable risk of harm to the child, even in cases in which such care is contrary to the parents' religious beliefs.[134] However, parents and legal guardians have been permitted by the courts to decline certain conventional medical treatments in favor of unorthodox approaches.[135] Where there is medical consensus that a minor is terminally ill or in a persistent vegetative state and that treatment would be futile or inadvisable, the withholding of such treatment has been permitted.[136] In cases involving mature minors, the courts have occasionally permitted the minor to refuse certain treatments on religious grounds.[137] For newborn children with severe disabilities that would cause death if left untreated, the courts have gone both ways.[138]

The decision to withdraw or withhold nutrition or hydration by artificial means has been held to be governed by the same principles applied in cases involving the withdrawal of medical treatment. For example, the Supreme Court, in Cruzan,[128] espoused this view, although the issue was not directly before the Court. Additionally, the California Court of Appeals quashed an attempted criminal indictment of two physicians who withdrew an artificial feeding tube from a vegetative patient in accordance with the wishes of the patient's family.[139] The Court's reasoning in this case was based on the grounds that artificial nutrition was indistinguishable from other medical treatments.

Confidentiality of Medical Records and Patient Information

The right of physical possession and control of a patient's medical record is vested in the provider. Possession and control of documents related to the patient's treatment, such as x-rays, laboratory reports, and consultants' reports, are similarly vested in the provider. Neither the patient nor his or her authorized representative has a right to physical possession of the medical record. However, the right to possess and control the physical record is distinguished in the law from the right to control access to the information contained in the record. Generally, patients and legitimately interested third parties have the right, under certain circumstances, to inspect and copy the record and/or to receive certain information contained in the record.

Technically, there is no constitutional right of privacy. However, the U.S. Supreme Court has inferred the right to privacy from the Fifth and Fourteenth

Amendments to the Constitution.[140] Generally, the right has not been extended specifically to confidentiality of information. However, the Supreme Court has suggested the existence of a constitutional right to preserve confidentiality relative to medical treatment that is vested in every patient.[141] In addition, some lower federal courts and state courts have found a constitutional right to privacy in cases involving disclosure of medical information.[142] Nonetheless, the patient's constitutional right to privacy with respect to disclosure of information in his or her medical records has not been recognized in all situations. For example, one court has held that the disclosure of the names of abortion clinic patients was not violative of the patients' constitutional right to privacy.[143]

Several federal and state statutes protect the confidentiality of Medicare records, alcohol and drug abuse records of patients treated in a federally assisted program or activity relating to alcoholism/drug abuse, medical records maintained by federal agencies, confidential information contained in peer review organization records, and information contained in mental health research records that identifies research subjects. Further, the confidentiality of medical records has been established by statute and regulation in several states. However, a majority of states continue to rely on common law, ethical standards, and professional norms to protect the confidentiality of patient information. In states in which statutory protection is provided, the laws generally require that the disclosing party obtain the patient's consent prior to releasing or transferring patient medical records.[144]

In addition to record protection statutes and case law, many states have physician/patient privilege statutes that apply to physician testimony as opposed to the disclosure of confidential medical information contained in a record. The courts have generally construed the statutory privilege narrowly to apply to in-court testimony of a physician because patient privilege did not exist at common law but was developed by statute. Physicians and hospitals are not permitted to waive the privilege, nor are they permitted to assert the privilege on their own behalf. The privilege is asserted solely on the patient's behalf. Some courts have held that a hospital or a physician has a duty to assert the physician/patient privilege when records are sought in a court proceeding.

In cases in which a patient brings a personal injury suit against a provider, the physician/patient privilege is waived.[145] In addition, various state legislatures have adopted statutes protecting communications between certain providers—i.e., psychotherapists-patient privilege statutes—and confidentiality of information contained in records such as those prepared as a result of treatment in a mental health facility or in an alcohol and drug abuse program.

As for professional standards governing the confidentiality of medical records, JCAHO medical record standards require written consent of the patient or an authorized representative as a condition to the release of medical information to persons not otherwise authorized to receive the information.[146] Similarly, the "Underlying Principles of Medical Ethics" of the American Medical Association[147] and the "Patient's Bill of Rights" of the American Hospital Association[148] require that patient confidences be safeguarded in accordance with relevant law.

Patient Access

Many states have enacted statutes and regulations that grant patients and/or their authorized representatives access to their medical records. Generally, these statutes include a provision permitting a patient to inspect the record itself, as well as to know the information contained in it. Some states have enacted statutes that limit patients' access to their own psychiatric records. These statutes typically do not address access to records by minors. Minors have been permitted access to their medical records in cases in which they are legally recognized as being capable of consenting to treatment.

Several courts have recognized a patient's common law right to access to his or her medical records. However, such access is limited in cases in which the information contained in the medical record would be detrimental to the interests of the patient, a third party, or the custodian of the records. A patient's right to access to his or her medical records is not without restriction. There is no constitutional property right to one's medical record information. In fact, courts generally have required that the information requested must fulfill a legitimate need for the patient. Generally, such a need has been characterized as being necessary to facilitate further health care or to evaluate a legal action. The request for such information must be specific. Courts have upheld denials of requests to inspect medical records when such a request was for no specific purpose and was not narrowed to a type of information.

Some courts have upheld provider denials of patient requests for access to medical information on the grounds that the release of such information might adversely affect the patient's health and well-being. However, courts have upheld denials by providers only in cases in which the denial is based on the professional judgment of a physician and is properly documented.

Third-Party Access

In certain instances, third parties are permitted access to medical information contained in a patient's medical record. The law generally permits medical personnel to have access to a patient's record when there is a legitimate purpose for such access. In addition, a patient may authorize the release of medical information (e.g., to commercial insurers) through the execution of a valid consent. Absent a statutory provision to the contrary or a legal guardian contesting such release, a parent of a minor may gain access to the minor's records upon request.

Certain federal laws may permit access to patient medical records by federal agencies without consent by the patient. For example, intermediaries acting on behalf of HHS under the Medicare program may examine medical records in connection with a hospital's annual Medicare audit. Similarly, state agencies that require mandatory reporting of certain patient information, such as birth, death, certain types of procedures (abortions), sexually transmitted diseases or other communicable diseases, child abuse, prescription of certain drugs that are subject to abuse, and gunshot or other wounds often seen as a result of violent crimes, are statutorily granted access to patient-specific medical information. Finally, state medical disciplinary boards responsible for investigating physician misconduct are typically granted access to patient records through court orders. Some courts have required the removal of patient-identifying information absent a special showing of a compelling state interest in the release of the medical information contained in the patient's record.

Conclusion

Legal considerations will continue to be of significant concern to CDMs in a variety of operational situations. While obtaining legal input may be perceived as a cost in the short term, a CDM is likely to experience long-term operational benefits and efficiencies as a result of seeking legal assistance in instances in which uncertainty exists.

References and Endnotes

1. *Smith v. Van Gorkom,* 488 A.2d 858 (Del. 1985).

2. *Mills Acquisition Co. v. Macmillan, Inc.,* 559 A2d 1261 (Del 1989).

3. *Stearn v. Lucy Webb Hays Sch.,* 381 F. Supp. 1003 (D.D.C. 1974).

4. *Warren v. Wheatly,* 331 S.W.2d 843 (Ark. 1960).

5. *Mahmoodian v. United Hosp. Ctr., Inc.,* 404 S.E.2d 750 (W.Va. 1991); Stiller v. LaPorte Hosp., Inc., 570 N.E.2d 99 (Ind. Ct. App. 1991).

6. *Gianetti v. Norwalk Hosp.,* 557 A.2d 1249 (Conn. 1989); Gates v. Holy Cross Hosp., 529 N.E. 2d 1014 (Ill. App. Ct. 1988).

7. *Anne Arundel Gen. Hosp. v. O'Brien,* 432 A.2d 483 (Md. Ct. Spec. App. 1981). Contra Weary v. Baylor Univ. Hosp., 360 S.W.2d 895 (Tex. 1962).

8. *Greisman v. Newcomb Hosp.,* 192 A.2d 817 (N.J. 1963).

9. *Rosenblit v. Superior Court,* 231 Cal. App.3d 1434 (Ct. App. 1991); Ascherman v. Saint Francis Memorial Hosp., 45 Cal. App. 3d 507 (Ct. App. 1975).

10. AHA Peer Review Immunity Task Force, American Academy of Hospital Attorneys. *Immunity for Peer Review Participants in Hospitals: What is it? Where Does It Come From? How Do You Protect It?* Chicago, Ill.: American Hospital Association, 1989, p. 6.

11. Health Care Quality Improvement Act, 42 U.S.C. §§ 11101 et seq.

12. Health care entities include hospitals, medical groups, health mainte- nance organizations, and other entities that conduct peer review and provide health care services.

13. There is some debate as to whether the failure to report a particular adverse action against a physician will result in immunity not being available for that action. Despite some ambiguity on the issue in case law, a strict reading of the statute and regulations suggests that the immunity should continue in effect until the Secretary of Health and Human Services notifies the institution and gives it an opportunity to correct alleged deficiencies. Only if noncompliance continues would the immunity be lifted, after publication of the entity's name in the *Federal Register.*

14. 29 C.F.R. pt. 1630 App.

15. 42 U.S.C.A. § 12112(a).

16. 42 U.S.C.A. § 12111(5).

17. 42 U.S.C.A. § 12112 (b).

18. 29 C.F.R. § 1630.2(o)(1).

19. 29 C.F.R. § 1630.2(o)(2).

20. 42 U.S.C.A. § 12112(b).

21. 42 U.S.C.A. § 12111(8).

22. 42 U.S.C.A. § 12102(2).

23. 29 C.F.R. § 1630.2(h)(1).

24. 29 C.F.R. § 1630.2(h)(2).

25. Frierson, J. *Employer's Guide to the Americans with Disabilities Act.* Washington, D.C.: Bureau of National Affairs, 1995, p. 6. Although the terms "disability" and "impairments" encompass many conditions, employers should recognize that traits or behaviors are not impairments, even though they may be linked to impairments. Appendix to 29 C.F.R. § 1630.2(h)

25a. *Sutton et. al. v. United Airlines, Inc.,* ___ U.S. ___ (June 22, 1999); *Albertsons, Inc. v. Kirkingburg,* ___ U.S. ___ (June 22, 1999); Murphy v. *United Parcel Service, Inc.,* ___ U.S. ___ (June 22, 1999).

26. 29 C.F.R. § 1630.2(n).

27. 42 U.S.C.A. § 12112(d)(2). However, an employer "may require a medical examination after an offer of employment has been made to a job applicant and prior to the commencement of the employment duties of such applicant, and may condition an offer of employment on the results of such examination," provided that all entering employees are subjected to such an examination and that such information is treated as a confidential medical record (subject to certain exceptions). 42 U.S.C.A. § 12112(d)(3).

28. Frierson, J. *op. cit.,* p. 44.

29. 29 C.F.R. § 1630.14(a).

30. 29 C.F.R. pr. 1630.14(a) App.

31. Frierson, J., *op. cit.,* p. 45.

32. 29 C.F.R. pt. 1630.14(a) App.

33. An employer may ask health questions and require a medical examination once an offer of employment has been made to an applicant, provided that all entering employees are subject to such an examination and that the information obtained from the examination is used only for

purposes permitted by the ADA. 42 U.S.C.A. § 12112(d)(3). Again, a CDM should review such questions or examinations with the human resources department or counsel.

34. Appendix to 29 C.F.R. § 1630.9.

35. 42 U.S.C.A. § 2000e *et. seq.*

36. Richey, C. *Manual on Employment Discrimination Law and Civil Rights Actions in the Federal Courts.* New York, N.Y.: Clark Boardman Callaghan, 1997.

37. 29 U.S.C.A. § 2612. The requirements of FMLA apply to any employer that employs 50 or more employees for each working day during each of 20 or more calendar workweeks in the current or preceding calendar year and that is engaged in commerce.

38. 29 U.S.C.A. § 2611(2).

39. 29 U.S.C.A. § 2611(4).

40. Valiant, C., and Matyas, D. *Legal Issues in Healthcare Fraud and Abuse: Navigating the Uncertainties,* Second Edition. Washington, D.C.: American Health Lawyers Association, 1997, p. 13. 42 U.S.C.A. § 1320a-7b(b).

41. 42 C.F.R. § 1001.952, *et. seq.*

42. 42 U.S.C.A. § 1395nn.

43. 42 U.S.C.A. § 1395nn(b)-(e).

44. 31 U.S.C.A. § 3729.

45. 31 U.S.C.A. § 3729(b).

46. Valiant and Matyas, *op. cit.,* pp. 171-7.

47. *Jefferson Parrish Hospital District No. 2 v. Hyde,* 466 U.S. 2 (1984).

48. 15 U.S.C. §§ 1-7.

49. 15 U.S.C. § 1.

50. *American Tobacco v. United States,* 328 U.S. 781, 810 (1946).

51. *Dr. Miles Medical Co. v, John D. Park & Sons Co.,* 220 U.S. 373, 394 (1911).

52. *Eastern States Retail Lumber Dealers' Ass'n v. United States,* 234 U.S. 600, 612 (1914).

53. *Copperweld Corp. v. Independent Tube Corp.,* 467 U.S. 752, 770 (1984).

54 *Oltz v. St. Peter's Community Hospital* 861 F.2d 1440 (9th Cir. 1988); Weiss v. York Hospital, 745 F.2d 786 (3rd Cir. 1984), cert. denied, 470 U.S. 1060 (1985).

55. *Weiss v. York Hospital,* 745 F.2d 786 (3rd Cir. 1984), cert. denied, 470 U.S. 1060 (1985).

56. *Oksanen v. Page Memorial Hospital,* 945 F.2d 696, 703-04 (4th Cir. 1991) (en banc), cert. denied, 112 S.Ct. 973 (1992).

57. *Todorov v. DCH Healthcare Auth.,* 921 F.2d 1438, 1455 (11th Cir. 1991)

58. 15 U.S.C. § 2.

59. *United States v. Grinnell Corp.,* 384 U.S. 563, 570-71 (1966).

60. *United States v. E.I. duPont de Nemours & Co.,* 351 U.S. 377 (1956).

61. *Jefferson Parrish Hospital District No. 2 v. Hyde,* 466 U.S. 2, 27 (1984).

62. *United States v. Aluminum Co. of America,* 148 F.2d 416, 424 (2d Cir. 1945).

63. *See e.g., American Standard, Inc. v. Bendix Corp.,* 487 F. Supp. 265, 269 (W.D. Mo. 1980).

64. *Times Picayune Publishing Co. v. United States,* 345 U.S. 594 (1953).

65. *Aspen Skiing Co. v. Aspen Highlands Skiing Corp.,* 472 U.S. 585 (1982).

66. *Otter Tail Power Co. v. United States,* 410 U.S. 366 (1973); *Berkey Photo, Inc. v. Eastman Kodak Co.,* 603 F2d. 263 (2d Cir. 1979), cert. denied, 444 U.S. 1093 (1980).

67. *United States v. Terminal Railroad Association of St. Louis,* 224 U.S. 383 (1912).

68. *McKenzie v. Mercy Hospital,* 854 F.2d 365 (10th Cir. 1988); *Konik v. Champlain Valley Physicians Hosp. Medical Center,* 561 F.Supp 700, 719-24 (N.D. N.Y. 1983) aff'd, 733 F2d 1007 (2d Cir. 1984), cert denied, 469 U.S. 884 (1984).

69. 15 U.S.C. § 18.

70. *United States v. Marine Bancorp,* 418 U.S. 602 (1974).

71. U.S. Department of Justice & Federal Trade Commission, "Horizontal Merger Guidelines." *Federal Register,* p. 41552, Sept. 10, 1992.

72. 15 U.S.C. § 18a.

73. 15 U.S.C. § 13(a).

74. *Alan's of Atlanta, Inc. v. Minolta Corp,* 903 F.2d 1414 (11th Cir. 1990).

75. *FTC v. Fred Meyer, Inc.,* 390 U.S. 341, 349 (1968).

76 *J.F. Feeser, Inc. v. Serv-A-Portion, Inc.,* 909 F.2d 1524 (3rd Cir. 1990).

77. 15 U.S.C. § 13(a).

78. 15 U.S.C. § 13(b).

79. *FTC v. Motion Picture Advertising Serv. Co,* 344 U.S. 392 (1953).

80. 15 U.S.C. § 41.

81. 15 U.S.C. § 45(a)(1).

82. 15 U.S.C. § 45(a)(2).

83. *F.T.C. v. Freeman Hospital,* 69 F.3d 260 (8th Cir. 1995).

84. *Tampa Electric Co. v. Nashville Coal Co.,* 365 U.S. 320, 327 (1961).

85. *FTC v. University Health, Inc.,* 938 F.2d 1206 (11th Cir. 1991).

86. Civil Rights Act of 1964, 42 U.S.C. §§ 2000a et seq.

87. Hill-Burton Act, 42 U.S.C. §§ 291 et seq.

88. *Cook v. Ochsner Found. Hosp.,* 319 F. Supp. 603 (E.D. La. 1970).

89. *Ritter v. Wayne County Gen. Hosp.,* 436 N.W.2d 673 (Mich. Ct. App. 1988).

90. *Arline v. School Bd. of Nassau County,* 480 U.S. 273 (1987).

91. Opinion of the General Counsel, District of Columbia (Oct. 15, 1985).

92. *Simkins v. Moses H. Cone Memorial Hosp.,* 323 F.2d 959 (4th Cir. 1963), cert. denied, 376 U.S. 938 (1964).

93. *Eaton v. Grubbs,* 329 F.2d 710 (4th Cir. 1964).

94. 42 U.S.C. § 1395dd.

95. The COBRA designation derives from the fact that the antidumping provisions were part of the Consolidated Omnibus Reconciliation Act.

96. 42 U.S.C. § 1395dd-(a).

97. The definition of emergency medical conditions now encompasses women experiencing contractions. Formerly, the definition of emergency medical condition involved whether the patient was experiencing active labor.

98. 42 U.S.C. § 1395dd-(h).

99. 42 U.S.C. § 1395dd-(b).

100. 42 U.S.C. § 1395dd-(b)(3).

101. *Stevison v. Enid Health Sys., Inc.*, 920 F.2d 710 (10th Cir. 1990).

102. 42 U.S.C. § 1395dd-(c)(1).

103. 42 U.S.C. § 1395dd-(c)(1)(A)(ii).

104. 42 U.S.C. § 1395dd-(c)(2).

105. *Sorrells v. Babcock*, 733 F. Supp. 1189 (N.D.Ill. 1990).

106. 42 U.S.C. § 1395dd-(d)(1)(A).

107. 42 U.S.C. § 1395dd-(d)(1)(B).

108. 42 U.S.C. § 1395dd-(d)(1)(c).

109. 42 U.S.C. § 1395dd-(d)(2)(B).

110. 42 U.S.C. § 1395dd-(d)(2)(A).

111. N.Y. Pub. Health Law § 2803-c(h).

112. *Lucy Webb Hayes Nat'l Training School v. Geoghegan*, 281 F. Supp. 116 (D.D.C. 1967).

113. *Schloendorff v. Society of New York Hosp.*, 105 N.E. 92 (N.Y. 1914).

114. *Sanders v. Nouri*, 688 S.W.2d 24 (Mo. App. 1985); Kohoutek v. Hafner, 366 N.W.2d 633 (Minn. Ct. App. 1985).

115. *Salgo v. Leland Stanford, Jr. University Board of Trustees*, 317 P.2d 170, 181 (Cal. Ct. App. 1957).

116. *Hook v. Rothstein*, 316 S.E.2d 690 (S.C. Ct. App. 1984).

117. *Paige v. Manuzak*, 471 A.2d 758 (Md. Ct. Spec. App. 1984).

118. *Stafford v. Louisiana State Univ.*, 448 So.2d 852 (La. Ct. App. 1984).

119. *Dewes v. Indian Health Serv.*, 504 F. Supp. 203 (D.S.D. 1980).

120. *Karlsbeck v. Westview Clinic*, 375 N.W.2d 861 (Minn. Ct. App. 1985).

121. *Davidson v. Shirley,* 616 F.2d 224 (5th Cir. 1980).

122. *Magana v. Elie,* 439 N.E.2d 1319 (Ill. Ct. App. 1982).

123. *Natanson v. Kline,* 350 P.2d 1093 (Kan. 1960).

124. *Hawaii v. Standard Oil Co.,* 405 U.S. 251 (1972).

125. *In the matter of Kathleen Farrell,* 529 A2d 404 (N.J. 1987) (refusal of mechanical ventilation upheld on basis of right to privacy); St. Mary's Hosp. v. Ramsey, 465 So. 2d 666 (Fla. Dist. Ct. App. 1985) (refusal of treatment based on religious grounds upheld).

126. Farrell (court recognized common law right to self-determination); *Bouvia v. Superior Court,* 225 Cal. Rptr. 297 (Ct. App. 1986) (discontinuation of nasogastric feeding upheld in part based on public policy codified in California's "Natural Death Act").

127. *Cruzan v. Director, Missouri Dept. of Health,* 110 S. Ct. 2841 (1990).

128. *Crouse Irving Memorial Hospital, Inc. v. Paddock,* 485 N.Y.S.2d 443 (Sup. Ct. 1985); Application of Winthrop University Hospital, 490 N.Y.S.2d 996 (Sup. Ct. 1985).

129. *Fosmire v. Nicoleau,* Civ. Act. No. 267 (N.Y. Ct. App. January 18, 1990) (pregnant Jehovah's Witness permitted to refuse a blood transfusion on religious grounds).

130. *In re Quinlan,* 355 A.2d 647 (N.J. 1976) (incompetent patient's right to self-determination based on constitutional right of privacy).

131. *In re Custody of a Minor,* 379 N.E. 2d 1053 (Mass. 1978).

132. Md. Family Law Code Ann. § 5-203b.

133. *In re Eric B.,* 235 Cal. Rptr. 22 (Ct. App. 1987) (Christian Scientist parents ordered to submit their child to periodic medical evaluation, even though the child's cancer was in remission, because of the court's finding that failure to do so would pose an unreasonable risk of harm to the child).

134. *In re Hofbauer,* 393 N.E.2d 1009 (N.Y. 1979).

135. *In re Phillip B.,* 156 Cal. Rptr. 48 (Ct. App. 1979). In addition, while not directly permitting the withholding of medical treatment in such cases, federal law indicates that such action may sometimes be warranted. The Child Abuse Prevention and Treatment and Adoption Reform statute conditions the receipt of federal grant money by states under the statute on, *inter alia,* assurances that the state has procedures in place to respond to the reporting of medical neglect, including instances of the withholding of medically indicated treatment from dis-

abled infants with life-threatening conditions. 42 U.S.C. § 5106a(b)(2)(B). However, the statute specifically excludes from the definition of the term *withholding of medically indicated treatment* "the failure to provide treatment (other than appropriate nutrition, hydration, or medication) to an infant when, in the treating physician's or physicians' medical judgment: (A) the infant is chronically and irreversibly comatose; (B) the provision of such treatment would (i) merely prolong dying, (ii) not be effective in ameliorating or correcting all of the infant's life-threatening conditions or (iii) otherwise be futile in terms of the survival of the infant; or (C) the provision of such treatment would be virtually futile in terms of the survival of the infant and the treatment itself under such circumstances would be inhumane." 42 U.S.C. § 5106g(6).

136. *In the interest of E.G.,* 515 N.E.2d 286 (Ill. App. Ct. 1987) (Seventeen-year-old minor permitted to refuse blood transfusion on basis of his expressed religious beliefs).

137. *Application of Cicero,* 421 N.Y.S.2d 965 (Sup. Ct. 1979) (court ordered life-sustaining treatment against parents' objections); *Weber v. Stony Brook Hosp.,* 456 N.E.2d 1186 (N.Y. 1983) (court upheld parents' choic of nonsurgical treatment for severely disabled newborn).

138. *Barber v. Superior Court,* 147 Cal.App.3d 1006 (Ct. App. 1983).

139. *Roe v. Wade,* 410 U.S. 113 (1973).

140. *Whalen v. Roe,* 429 U.S. 589 (1977).

141. *In re B,* 394 A.2d 419 (Pa. 1978).

142. *Illinois v. Florendo,* 447 N.E.2d 282 (Ill. 1983).

143. Md. Health Gen. Code § 4-301.

144. *Sklagen v. Greater Southeast Community Hosp.,* 625 F. Supp. 991 (D.D.C. 1984).

145. *Accreditation Manual for Hospitals.* Oakbrook Terrace, Ill.: Joint Commission on Accreditation of Healthcare Organizations, §§ MR.3 to MR.3.4., 1998.

146. *Underlying Principles of Medical Ethics.* Chicago, Ill.: American Medical Association, 1980.

147. *Patient Bill of Rights.* Chicago, Ill.: American Hospital Association, 1992.

Mark E. Lutes is a member of the firm Epstein Becker & Green, P.C., in the firm's Washington, D.C., office. David J. Weader and Jeffrey Bennett are attorneys in the Washington, D.C., office of Epstein Becker & Green, P.C. Neil S. Olderman, who authored sections of the previous version of this chapter, is an attorney in the Chicago, Illinois, office of the firm of Green, Stewart & Farber, P.C. The authors wish to thank Tina Batra for her contributions to this article.

Chapter

The Elements of Medical Quality Management

by David B. Nash, MD, MBA, FACPE

Managing medical quality in today's health care environment is a complex function that interrelates concerns not only about quality, but also about the costs and outcomes of health care interventions. New roles are emerging for physician executives to act as agents of change as more organizations undertake new quality improvement initiatives and establish priorities for measuring performance and assessing outcomes of care.

Seemingly endless demands for data on quality of care are arising from numerous sources—managed care organizations, regulatory agencies, and purchasers and consumers of health care. External organizations are increasingly asking doctors and hospitals to explain what they do and why they do it. Several forces are behind this drive to measure quality of care. After focusing their attention primarily on cost reductions in the 1980s and 1990s, purchasers are now realizing the importance of obtaining health care services not only at a reasonable price but also on the basis of quality. The public and those who pay for medical care are now interested in knowing whether they are getting a good value for their health care dollars. As a result, an increasing number of health care contracts are being awarded on the basis of both cost and quality measurements.

Physicians have long recognized that new approaches and applications to improving quality must be continually sought. But they have viewed traditional quality assessment efforts as intrusive and largely ineffectual. This opinion has developed primarily because these programs relied on case-by-case inspections of patients' medical records and used indicators and thresholds developed with little significant input from physicians. Thus, they are often seen as arbitrary measures subject to erroneous conclusions when used to assess quality of care. In addition, while this method of inspecting physician and hospital performance allows quality assurance staff to track problems and look for trends, it detects problems only after they have occurred and does little to prevent their recurrence. This traditional approach fails to recognize health care delivery as a series of linked process-es requiring the coordinated efforts of many health care professionals. It also does not facilitate systematic analysis and subsequent improvement in patient outcomes.

Avedis Donabedian, often referred to as the founder of health care quality assurance, established a framework for assessing quality that stresses that quality can be measured not only in terms of the structure and process of care but also in terms of the outcomes of care.[1] Structure comprises the physical, human, and organizational properties of the setting in which care is provid-ed. These properties include things such as equipment and the number of licensed doctors and nurses on staff. Process consists of the technical aspects of providing care and the procedures used to ensure that patients receive nec-essary care. For instance, adherence to widely accepted practices and regula-tory requirements are process measures. Outcome encompasses changes in patient health status that can be attributed to the medical care provided. Examples include mortality rates, adverse event rates, and changes in an indi-vidual's health-related well-being. While information about structure and processes of care provide valuable information and are related to the proba-bility of obtaining good patient outcomes, they do not necessarily measure the quality of patient outcomes. In the past, health care regulatory agencies have concentrated on measuring the structure and process of care, with little atten-tion given to outcomes.

Although there have been many attempts to define quality, there is no single comprehensive definition of medical quality, most likely because quality encompasses several different elements and aspects of care. Donabedian recently provided an in-depth review of the various aspects of medical quali-ty.[2] Some of the quality components he described are effectiveness, efficiency, optimality, and acceptability of medical care. Two of the more familiar dimen-sions of medical quality are the technical aspects of care and the interperson-al aspects of care.[3] Technical quality relates to how well patients are diag-nosed and clinically managed, while interpersonal quality depends on how well patients' personal needs are met. Other descriptions of quality incorpo-rate evaluations of patient preferences and considerations for the cost of care. Two such examples are:

- "Quality is the degree to which the process of care increases the probabil-ity of outcomes desired by patients and decreases the probability of unde-sired outcomes, given the state of medical knowledge."[4]

- "Quality health care consists of necessary medical processes that result in cure, significant measured improvement in the patient's condition, allevi-ation of pain or other desired outcomes, and provides real value for the dollars spent."[5]

New research confirms that we now have the tools to classify quality-related problems as underuse, overuse, or misuse and that large numbers of Americans are harmed as a direct result of these issues.[6]

Determining the aspects of medical care that should be used to measure quality has been the focus of intensive research efforts by health service researchers, the federal government, and regulatory bodies. Increased interest in this area has been spurred by research on wide variations in medical practice and by the growing realization that traditional quality assurance methods have done little to ensure and improve quality and effectiveness of medical treatment.

Numerous health services researchers have contributed to the growing body of knowledge about ways to evaluate and improve the quality of medical care. As new approaches to measuring and managing medical quality continue to evolve, it is likely that techniques will be drawn from several different sources and integrated in a comprehensive approach. The developing fields of continuous quality improvement, clinical practice guidelines, and outcomes management will provide a solid basis for creating successful quality management programs.[5]

Continuous Quality Improvement

Continuous quality improvement (CQI), or total quality management (TQM) as it is sometimes referred to in health care, evolved from the manufacturing industry's experience with quality management. Industrial quality experts suggest that quality means "a continuous effort by all members of the organization to meet the needs and expectations of the customer."[7] Industrial quality management systems have adopted a number of CQI methods that increase the probability of improving quality. Central to these methods is use of multidisciplinary teams to identify problems, data collection and analysis to understand and correct underlying root causes of problems, and reductions in unwanted complexity and variation in systems through the use of statistical process control theory. Total quality management creates an open climate that fosters self-motivation and cooperation, where everyone in the organization shares responsibility for improving quality. Attempts are made to break down barriers between departments, to improve communication throughout the organization, and to drive out fear. CQI emphasizes that it is processes that should be the focus of quality improvement efforts, not individual workers. There is a belief that most workers are conscientious and are trying to do a good job, but that they face a multitude of system problems that can contribute to poor quality. By fully analyzing a process and understanding the root causes of variation, workers can develop and implement a plan to improve the process. CQI methods have been used successfully outside health care for a number of years and have resulted in significant improvements in the quality of products and services.

Evolution of CQI in Health Care

Application of continuous quality improvement techniques to health care has intrigued many health care providers and has been successful in a number of organizations. One of the initial success stories was the National Demonstration Project on Quality Improvement in Health Care.[8] In 1987, this ambitious one-year project matched 21 well-known health care organizations with experts in the field of industrial quality management. The nationwide experiment demonstrated that CQI techniques could be successfully used in the health care setting.

In the past few years, CQI has continued to gain considerable attention in health care, as is evidenced by the ever-increasing number of presentations at quality improvement conferences and by articles in the literature. A nationwide survey conducted by the American Hospital Association in 1990 reported that 44 percent of all respondents had adopted CQI methods to some degree.[9] In 1992, it was noted that some 1,500 hospitals and health care organizations, as well as the Health Care Financing Administration, had been actively involved in using continuous quality improvement techniques.[10]

CQI techniques differ greatly from traditional quality assurance approaches. Traditional techniques tend to focus primarily on physician decisions, underemphasizing the effects that nonphysicians can have on health care processes.[7] In reality, decisions are only one source of variability in processes. A significant amount of variation may be attributed to other causes, such as unclear policies and procedures, defective equipment, or variations in the work of other health care professionals. A program that encompasses CQI acknowledges the importance of teamwork and offers physicians an opportunity to participate in improving the entire workflow process. Because CQI focuses on improving processes, it does not single out individual employees as "bad apples" and is associated with fewer negative connotations than traditional QA programs. CQI allows the people who are intimately involved in the process to make changes in the system, resulting in significant improvements in the overall level of quality.

Some of the key concepts of CQI are:

- Poor quality usually stems from complex processes or variation within a system and not from individuals' lack of knowledge or skills.

- Because most work is accomplished through process, the focus of CQI is on evaluating and improving processes, not on identifying individuals with bad behavior and trying to change them.

- Quality needs to be built into processes so that poor quality is prevented upstream, not measured by inspection at the end of the line.

- Quality can always be improved. Just meeting the minimum established thresholds for acceptability or compliance does not ensure high quality.

- Quality is based on a thorough understanding of the needs and expectations of customers, both internal and external.

- Decisions are based on facts and scientific measurements, not on presumptions or anecdotal evidence.

- Poor quality is costly and results from unwanted variations and complexity in processes.

Although a number of different CQI models are used in health care, most models encompass the following general steps[8] to improve a process or fix a quality problem:

1. Clearly defined goals and objectives for the project are developed.

2. A multidisciplinary project team that knows the process is formed.

3. The team uses data to analyze a process and understand the key steps, variables, and root causes that contribute to quality problems.

4. A plan to improve the process is developed, implemented, and tested.

5. Data are collected and analyzed statistically to track the results of the improvement plan and to measure variation in the process.

Tools and Techniques of CQI

The cycle of continuously improving quality begins with identification of priority areas for improvements and then moves on to data collection and analysis. The remaining steps are better known as the "Plan-Do-Check-Act" cycle. Throughout this cycle, cross-functional teams trained in CQI techniques use a variety of data-driven tools to analyze process-related problems, reduce variations in the process, and monitor improvements in the process. One of the key factors in success is formation of a team with members who are intimately involved with the process being studied. If the team appropriately identifies the underlying root causes contributing to poor quality and makes the necessary changes, waste, rework, complexity, and the associated costs of poor quality can be reduced.[11]

Some of the tools that CQI teams use throughout the quality improvement cycle include[12]:

- Flowcharts are developed by the team to describe the sequence of steps that occur in a process. They provide a point of common agreement on what the process entails and help the group to focus on areas of redundancy and rework.

- Cause and effect diagrams are used to help identify and organize underlying root causes of problems or factors critical to the process.

- Pareto charts (bar graphs) illustrate the frequency and the impact of various problems in a process and help in the selection of improvement efforts. The Pareto chart is an extension of the Pareto Principle, which states that the majority of problems in a process can be attributed to relatively few factors.

- Histograms and scattergrams help in organizing and characterizing data and in looking for relationships among variables.

- Run charts are used to examine data for trends and patterns that occur over time.

- Control charts help to monitor a process for statistical control. Upper and lower statistical control limits are established to define the standard deviation from the mean. Points falling outside the control limits represent variations due to causes outside the usual process.

Two other techniques that have been used in health care to improve the quality and the efficiency of care are benchmarking and clinical pathway development.

- Benchmarking is used to compare the practices of an organization with the practices of leaders in the field. The goal is to identify and learn from the "best practices" and then to incorporate those practices into your own work.[13]

- Clinical (or critical) pathways are used to define the optimal sequence of events and timing for certain medical interventions. They are usually developed through the collaborative efforts of health care professionals in hospitals to reduce length of stay, delays, and variation in care. They also help to improve communication among physicians, nurses, and other health care professionals.[14]

A quality management program will also incorporate several managerial components: quality planning, quality measurement and control, and quality improvement activities.[15] Quality planning involves developing a thorough understanding of the wants and needs of the customer and linking them to the day-to-day activities of the organization. The organizational culture should foster pride, joy, collaboration, and scientific thinking. Quality measurement and control involves developing measures to reduce unintended, unwanted, or costly variations in work processes. Quality improvement consists of efforts to continuously improve overall performance through cross-functional teams that collect, analyze, and act on data.[16]

As CQI efforts have become more widespread, some health care professionals have wondered whether these efforts will replace quality assurance departments altogether. In practice, CQI is often developed and implemented with the help of existing QA programs and personnel. QA staff members often become a valuable resource for training and facilitating the work of cross-functional project teams. Other quality professionals may move into quality measurement and control functions within the organizational quality program. Each organization will likely develop its own approach within the context of its quality management program.

Barriers to CQI

Barriers to implementation of CQI in the health care sector have been described in detail by Ziegenfuss.[17] Most of these barriers relate to systems within health care organizations, such as technological, structural, psychosocial, managerial, or cultural subsystems. Within these systems, a number of organizational barriers may arise because of the complex nature of health care work, inadequate personnel, power conflicts, or concerns for authority over quality improvement programs. One of the most frequently mentioned challenges is that of involving physicians in CQI activities. Reasons cited by physicians for their lack of involvement include lack of time for or commitment to organizationwide activities.[8]

Additional barriers associated with planning, leading, and organizing quality improvement activities may prove to be difficult to overcome, but the existence of organizational barriers to quality improvement activities needs to be recognized and addressed before quality improvement initiatives can be fully adopted in health care settings.

CQI techniques offer the health care executive a structured approach to managing and improving the process and the outcomes of care.[15] It provides the tools necessary to reduce process variation, waste, inefficiencies, and complexity in health care processes. But, because CQI tends to focus on existing processes of care, it should be combined with an outcomes management program that focuses on the appropriateness and the outcomes of various medical interventions.[18]

Finally, Blumenthal and Kilo,[19] Nash,[20] and others have issued a "report card" on CQI. They noted that, regrettably, national CQI experts could not identify a health care organization that fundamantally improved its performance through CQI.

Practice Variations and Guidelines

There is significant interest in measuring patient outcomes to find out what works in medicine and what doesn't. A growing body of research has demonstrated the existence of wide variations in clinical practices. Research conducted by Wennberg[21-23] revealed the significance of variations in the rate of different medical and surgical procedures within small geographic areas. These variations could not be explained by differences in patients' medical conditions and did not correspond to differences in health outcome. They were attributable to differences in physician practice styles.[21] This research has suggested that patients in some areas may receive unnecessary care, while others may not receive needed care.

Additional studies conducted by researchers at the RAND Corporation revealed that as much as one-third of medical care provided to patients may be unnecessary or of little benefit.[24-25] These results have raised questions as to the "best" or "most effective" treatment for some medical conditions and have contributed to concerns about the value and the quality of medical interventions. Inappropriate care in the form of under- or overutilization of services for patients has indicated a great need to measure the appropriateness and the outcomes of various medical interventions.[26]

Outcomes Management

A third component of a comprehensive quality management program would include the use of outcomes management techniques. Outcomes management combines the use of clinical practice guidelines with the results of outcomes research and focuses on finding out what works from patients' points of view.

Outcomes management relies on the use of "standards and guidelines to assist physicians in selecting interventions; it routinely and systematically measures the functioning and well-being of patients; it pools clinical and outcome data on a massive scale; and it attempts to analyze and disseminate results from the segment of the database most appropriate to the concerns of each decision maker."[27] Outcome measures go beyond traditional measures of morbidity and mortality and consider patient satisfaction with the care received, changes in patients' functional abilities, and health-related quality of life. Outcomes management measures quality from patients' perspectives.

While the technical aspects of clinical quality may have been the primary focus of many quality assurance programs, increased attention is now being given to the dimension of quality associated with interpersonal aspects of care. This dimension considers patient preferences for treatment options, patient-practitioner relationships, and conveniences and courtesies of the medical service provided.[2] The attention given to this dimension of health care quality is becoming more evident as managed care organizations generate "report cards," with the results of patient ratings for satisfaction with physician office hours, waiting times, and friendliness of physicians and office staff.[28] As competition in health care increases and as providers seek to attract patients to particular health care facilities, this dimension will likely gain more attention and will be used to compare various health care programs.

Using patient satisfaction and outcomes as indicators of quality has led to questions about who should judge the quality of patient outcomes. Health economists suggest that "the ultimate judge of quality and value of a product or service should be the consumer. Thus medical quality can be defined by the nature of the medical outcome as perceived by the patient."[29] Outcomes research will provide information about the care that best reflects the needs and wants of health care consumers. This is entirely consistent with the new emphasis on measuring quality from patients' perspectives and reflects the customer-driven focus of CQI. It is no longer sufficient to measure quality by the traditional "assessment by inspection." Instead, quality must be built into health care processes, and outcomes of care must be measured in an ongoing fashion so that unwanted variation can be reduced and the overall quality of health care improved.

As leaders in health care, physician executives need to understand and address these issues if they are to participate in the debate on controlling costs and measuring quality. There is no doubt that quality can be improved by determining the best medical practices, adopting those practices, and continually measuring and improving the processes of care. Scientifically documented methods and tools to measure, analyze, and improve quality of care are already available and have been shown to be effective in the health care setting. We have entered an era of medical quality management that emphasizes the use of practice guidelines, embraces the concepts and techniques of continuous quality improvement, and incorporates new measures of patient health outcomes. The development of an integrated, comprehensive quality management program designed and run by clinicians will be the best approach to improving the quality of medical care.

References

1. Donabedian, A. "The Quality of Care: How Can It Be Assessed?" *JAMA* 260(12):1743-8, Sept. 23-30, 1988.

2. Donabedian, A. "Defining and Measuring the Quality of Health Care." *Assessing Quality Health Care: Perspectives for Clinicians,* Wenzel, R., Editor. Baltimore, Md.: Williams & Wilkins, 1992.

3. Nash, D., and Goldfield, N. "Information Needs of Purchasers." In *Providing Quality Care: The Challenge to Clinicians.* Nash, D., and Goldfield, N., Editors. Philadelphia, Pa.: American College of Physicians, 1989.

4. U.S. Congress, Office of Technology Assessment. *The Quality of Medical Care: Information for Consumers.* Washington, D.C.: U.S. Government Printing Office, June 1988, OTA-H-386.

5. Nash, D. *Buying Value in Health Care.* Washington, D.C.: National Association of Manufacturers, 1992.

6. Chassin, M., and others. *"The Urgent Need to Improve Health Care Quality."* JAMA 280(11):1000-5, Sept. 16, 1998.

7. Laffel, G., and Blumenthal, D. *"The Case for Using Industrial Quality Management Science in Health Care Organizations."* JAMA 262(20):2869-73, Nov. 24, 1989.

8. Berwick, D., and others. *Curing Health Care: New Strategies for Quality Improvement.* San Francisco, Calif.: Jossey-Bass Publishers, 1990.

9. "The Role of Hospital Leadership in the Continuous Improvement of Patient Care Quality." *Journal for Healthcare Quality* 14(5):8-14,22, Sept.-Oct. 1992.

10. Jencks, S., and Wilensky, G. "The Health Care Quality Improvement Initiative: A New Approach to Quality Assurance in Medicine." *JAMA* 268(7):900-3, Aug. 19, 1992.

11. Berwick, D. "Continuous Improvement as an Ideal in Health Care." *New England Journal of Medicine* 320(1):53-6, Jan. 5, 1989.

12. Plsek, P. "A Primer on Quality Improvement Tools." In *Curing Health Care: New Strategies for Quality Improvement,* Berwick, D., and others, Editors. San Francisco, Calif.: Jossey-Bass Publishers, 1990.

13. O'Rourke, L.. "Benchmarking: A New Tool for Quality Improvement in Healthcare." *Quality Letter for Healthcare Leaders* 4(7):1-9, Sept. 1992.

14. Coffey, R., and others. "An Introduction to Critical Paths." *Quality Management in Health Care* 1(1):45-54, Fall 1992.

15. Jennison, K. "Total Quality Management—Fad or Paradigmatic Shift?" In *Health Care Quality Management for the 21st Century,* Couch, J., Editor. Tampa, Fla.: American College of Physician Executives, 1991.

16. Berwick, D., "Controlling Variation in Health Care." *Medical Care* 29(12):1212-25, Dec. 1991.

17. Ziegenfuss, J. "Organizational Barriers to Quality Improvement in Medical and Healthcare Organizations." *American Journal of Medical Quality* 6(4):115-22, Winter 1991.

18. Reinertsen, J. "Outcomes Management and Continuous Quality Improvement: The Compass and the Rudder." *Quality Review Bulletin* 19(1):5-7, Jan. 1993.

19. Blumenthal, D., and Kilo, C. "A Report Card on Continuous Quality Improvement." *Milbank Quarterly* 76(4): 625-48, 1998.

20. Nash, D. "Trustees : Commit to Quality — Now." *Trustee* 52(5):20, May 1999.

21. Wennberg, J., and others. "Hospital Use and Mortality Among Medicare Beneficiaries in Boston and New Haven." *New England Journal of Medicine* 321(17):1168-73, Oct. 26, 1989.

22. Wennberg, J. "The Paradox of Appropriate Care." *JAMA* 258(18):2568-9, Nov. 13, 1987.

23. Wennberg, J. "Dealing with Medical Practice Variations: A Proposal for Action." *Health Affairs* 3(2):6-32, Summer 1984.

24. Brook, R., and others. *Appropriateness of Acute Medical Care for the Elderly: An Analysis of the Literature.* Santa Monica, Calif.: RAND Corporation, 1989.

25. Merrick, N., and others. "Use of Carotid Endarterectomy in Five California Veterans Administration Medical Centers." *JAMA* 256(18):2531-5, Nov. 14, 1986.

26. Chassin, M., and others. "Does Inappropriate Use Explain Geographic Variations in the Use of Health Care Services?" *JAMA* 258(18):2533-7, Nov. 13, 1987.

27. Ellwood, P. "Outcomes Management: A Technology of Patient Experiences." *New England Journal of Medicine* 318(23):1549-56, June 9, 1988.

28. Winslow, R. "Report Card on Quality and Efficiency of HMOs May Provide a Model for Others." *Wall Street Journal,* March 9, 1993, page B1.

29. Reinhardt, U. "The Importance of Quality in the Debate on National Health Policy." In *Health Care Quality Management for the 21st Century,* Couch, J., Editor. Tampa, Fla.: American College of Physician Executives, 1991.

David B. Nash, MD, MBA, FACPE is Director, Health Policy and Clinical Outcomes, Thomas Jefferson University Hospital,and Associate Dean for Health Policy, Jefferson Medical College, both in Philadelphia, Pa. This chapter is based on the author's chapter in New Leadership in Health Care Management: The Physician Executive, Second Edition, American College of Physician Executives, 1994. Dr. Nash wishes to acknowledge all of the help he received from Nelda Johnson, PharmD, in the preparation of the previous version of this chapter.

Chapter

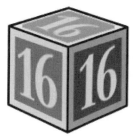

Introduction to Managed Care

by Mark A Bloomberg, MD,
MBA, CPE, FACPE

The parable is told of several blind men trying to describe the elephant they are each touching. Because each man touches the elephant in a different place and can describe only his part, their descriptions are very different. Managed care is like that elephant, except the blind men are the many observers trying to describe it from their individual perspectives. To make matters more complex, managed care itself is evolving. Not over the eons seen in natural evolution, but rather at the breakneck pace consistent with today's health care system. And with modern health care being increasingly represented and provided by managed care delivery systems, there is nowhere a physician can go and no setting in which a physician can practice in which an understanding of managed care is not required.

Therefore, it is critical for the physician executive to be knowledgeable of the world of managed care. Where did it come from? Why did it evolve? What is it evolving into? What are managed care's good points? What are its bad points? The purpose of this chapter is to provide the necessary background for the new physician executive to understand the whole picture. Like the elephant, managed care presents different looks to those not able to step back and view the entity in its entirety. Our purpose is to avoid the tunnel vision that hampers many in the field.

Managed care, as we know it today, began as a small number of "experiments" with prepaid group practice beginning nearly 100 years ago.[1] The earliest recorded prepaid practices were organized around major industrial efforts in the West, such as the Western Clinic in Tacoma, Washington (the lumber industry, 1910), the Ross-Loos Clinic (Los Angeles public utility workers, 1929), and Kaiser-Permanente (Colorado River aqueduct project, 1933, and the Grand Coulee Dam, 1937). Utilizing this prepaid model, an Oklahoma physician by the name of Michael Shadid sought to establish a prepaid hospital in his rural area in 1927 by selling shares to residents in return for hospital care. Following Dr. Shadid's example, some prepaid group practices were started by consumer activists, such as the Group Health Cooperative of Puget Sound (1947). These entities, while prospering regionally, remained a small part of the national health care system through the 1960s.

These early prepaid systems consistently faced strong opposition from organized medicine, a tradition that has generally continued throughout the century. Physician leaders of prepaid groups were routinely dismissed from county and state medical societies, were stripped of their hospital privileges, and had roadblocks erected to limit their ability to recruit other physicians to their systems. Numerous legal challenges were made to these punitive actions, all successful and upholding the right of physicians to enter into such prepaid arrangements without discrimination and/or interference from other physicians or their medical societies.

These prepaid models were in contrast to the predominant fee-for-service payment methodology, which would be maintained in the early indemnity health insurance vehicles, Blue Cross and later Blue Shield, for hospital and physician services respectively. While traditional health insurance developed "usual & customary (U&C)" payment schedules, the early prepaid groups reimbursed their clinicians on a salaried basis. The Great Depression, combined with the increasing cost of, and likelihood of surviving, an inpatient hospitalization, led to the development of hospitalization insurance, leading to the foundation and rapid deployment of Blue Cross plans across the country.

In areas in which there were successful and growing prepaid groups, such as Kaiser-Permanente in California, fee-for-service physicians would occasionally band together to offer an alternative system of care. These efforts led to the development of "foundations for medical care," in which fee-for-service physicians created loose networks that would then offer prepaid care to groups of patients. One of the first of these networks was started in 1954 in California's San Joaquin Valley. These foundations would gradually evolve into the independent practice associations (IPAs) common in the 1970s and 1980s. Despite all of this activity developing over a period of perhaps 60 years, by 1970 there were only about 30 prepaid group practices. There was still no such thing as "HMO" or "managed care," and the stage was merely being set for the rapid growth that would shortly ensue.

By the early 1960s, much of organized medicine's attention had been refocused on the federal government's effort to provide funding for the health care afforded to Medicare and Medicaid recipients. A bitter political battle was waged over this issue, with the federal government finally prevailing over the objections of the American Medical Association. Ironically, the provision of health insurance coverage for these populations in 1965-66 ushered in what would become the golden years of U&C physician reimbursement. Furthermore, the extensive lobbying surrounding the Medicare/Medicaid programs weakened the capability of organized medicine to subsequently block relatively liberal health care appointees in the new Nixon administration, allowing the health care reform movement of the early 1970s to take root and flourish.

HMOs Appear

Concurrent with these major changes in federally sponsored health insurance coverage, the medical profession was also experiencing an unprecedented amount of clinical specialization and rapid development and implementation of new medical technology. These developments led to a surge in health care costs as a percentage of Gross National Product and resulted in growing concern about the country's ability to fund these rising costs. The Nixon White House responded to these cost pressures by sending to Congress a bill to promote prepaid health plans as a more cost-effective way to provide services. It was at this time that the term "health maintenance organization (HMO)" was first used, credited to Dr. Paul Ellwood, a Minnesota physician prominent in prepaid care at that time.

The Health Maintenance Act of 1973 provided for federal funding to start HMOs and required large employers to offer their employees the option of HMOs within their geographic areas. The Act also established a federal office to regulate HMOs and certify them as "federally qualified," which then permitted the HMOs to approach large employers and to market their health plans to employees. Despite this federal inducement, overall HMO development and enrollment remained small, growing gradually through the 1970s.

This slow growth was in part related to the existing models of HMOs. The earliest plans developed from prepaid clinics or groups, in which the physicians were salaried, and this was by no means the predominant way in which physicians practiced in this era. Most physicians were based in solo or small practices, earning their income in the fee-for-service environment. Joining a clinic and being paid a salary was not attractive to the majority of new or experienced clinicians, limiting the attraction of the earliest HMOs. A review of the HMOs existing in the early 1970s reveals a preponderance of staff- or group-model HMOs. Many of these HMOs were descendants of those early prepaid plans, such as Kaiser-Permanente. There was also a number of staff-model HMOs that had started in the late 1960s or early 1970s and that were slowly growing in their respective communities.

The next iteration of HMOs, however, would spur a period of rapid growth as they attracted rank-and-file physician in private practice. These were the IPA-model HMOs mentioned earlier. Similar to the older "foundations," IPAs were a loose confederation of privately practicing physicians who came together for the purpose of providing a physician network that would take care of HMO members. By joining the IPA, physicians agreed to accept a set fee schedule and peer review and often assumed some degree of financial risk. IPA-model HMOs tended to develop whenever and wherever physicians felt threatened by staff- and/or group-model HMO growth in their local geographic areas. Because of local physician support and minimal capitalization requirements, i.e., no clinic facility to build or physician salaries to pay, IPAs could be started relatively easily. The growth that resulted from this new type of HMO was so dramatic that, by the end of the 1970s, there were more than 220 HMOs in 40 states with more than 8 million enrollees. This type of growth continued into the 1980s, with new HMOs developing in all major population centers.

The late 1980s also ushered in a period of significant consolidation, with smaller HMOs merging, being acquired, or failing financially and being shut down. By the end of the 1980s, there were more than 600 HMOs spread across all 50 states providing care to more than 40 million enrollees.

The Health Care Cost Crisis

The rapid growth in managed care seen in the 1980s was spurred not just by the federal HMO Act of the Nixon years. It was also stimulated by sharp rises in health care costs that, by the mid-1980s, were alarming both the federal government and the business community, the major payers of health care in the United States. The figure below depicts the rise in per capita health care costs through the 1980s and 1990s, from just over $1,000 to almost $4,000. The dotted line on the right side of the graph depicts the further rise that was predicted in 1990 if no steps were taken to control these costs. Note the sharp rise in HMO enrollments, as patients joined these managed care plans in record numbers. Whether the amelioration in the rise in health care costs was in fact due to increased managed care participation or not is a matter of opinion and probably depends on whether one is a supporter or a detractor of managed care in general. Nonetheless, some markets developed very successful HMOs with high percentages of their populations enrolled in HMOs. Foremost among these were the early sites of HMO development, California and Minnesota, each with approximately 40 percent of its population enrolled in HMO plans. Other states lag behind, with the national average being approximately 22 percent in 1997.

Common themes became recognizable as managed care grew in multiple geographic areas, leading to the description of a series of "stages" through which a typical metropolitan area would progress as it experienced local growth of managed care plans. Russ Coile[2] described these stages as:

Per Capita Health Care Costs and HMO Enrollment

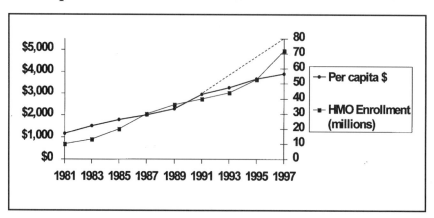

1. Can't Spell HMO.

2. Managed Care Gets Aggressive.

3. Managed Care Penetration.

4. Managed Competition.

5. Post Reform.

As an area progresses through these stages, there is greater HMO enrollment as a percentage of the insured population, more advanced provider risk sharing and contracting preferences, and more complex provider relationships. As with any artificial construct, specific metropolitan areas tend to represent a blend of these stages. We might see, for example, strong HMO enrollment consistent with Coile's Stage 3 coexisting with somewhat limited provider risk sharing arrangements consistent with Stage 2. Nonetheless, these stages form a very useful framework for understanding the many changes seen in the local health care environment as managed care grows and becomes the dominant form of health insurance. These stages also allow for some fairly reliable forecasting as to what trends are likely to develop in metropolitan areas as they become increasingly involved in managed care.

Managed Care Changes Physician Compensation

Coincident with the rise of managed care plans, changes developed in the manner in which physicians were being paid. Payment via a salary had long been a part of the prepaid group practices, of course, but fee-for-service (FFS) remained the trusted and preferred payment methodology for all other practice settings. As more independent practitioners joined IPA-model HMOs, payment under FFS continued, but risk-sharing arrangements became commonplace. The earliest of these entailed payment of an agreed-upon fee for each billed service, with a specified percentage, usually 10-30 percent, withheld and payable at year's end, depending on whether the HMO met its overall medical cost budget. If medical costs were over budget, practitioners would not be paid some or all of the withhold and therefore would be working for less than their hoped-for fees. Many HMOs also had upside arrangements, whereby practitioners would split some portion of the excess funds, if the year ended with medical costs under budget.

FFS reimbursement, however, was felt to promote unnecessary services, and risk withholds were limited in their ability to prevent them. This led to development of capitation as an alternative payment model. In capitation, a physician is paid a set monthly stipend for each member assigned under his or her care. Capitation models can be limited, paying a physician only for those services expected to be personally provided by that physician, or can be global, assigning all expected payments to that physician, regardless of who was expected to provide the service. The key requirements to drive a capitation model are knowing:

- What services are being covered in the capitation.

- Which physician is responsible for the overall management of each

- member's care.

- How much is being allotted to pay for each service.

Capitation has been used mostly as a means to pay primary care physicians (PCPs), but it is increasingly being used to pay specialty care physicians (SCPs) as well. Capitation models, a complete discussion of which is beyond the scope of this text, continue to evolve and be applied in more innovative ways. Capitation, however, is accused of promoting underutilization of services, creating concerns of poor quality of care. This has led to increasing scrutiny of capitation payment models and efforts to demonstrate that the quality of care remains high in HMOs using such payment methodology. An extensive review of capitation is available in a text edited by Howard Kirz.[3]

New Managed Care Alternatives Develop

The HMO enrollment figures noted above do not tell the entire story, however, because they fail to include the many people now enrolled in one of the non-HMO managed care alternatives that developed during the late 1980s and early 1990s. When traditional indemnity insurance companies saw the need to compete with the growing managed care plans, they developed a new managed care model known as the preferred provider organization (PPO). These approaches were characterized by a contracted network of providers with an agreed-upon fee schedule with no financial risk sharing but including inpatient utilization review. PPOs sought to capitalize on providers' willingness to accept the fee schedules and peer review that were typical of the IPA-model HMOs. The distinguishing factors of PPOs were their lack of an assigned PCP gatekeeper and their coverage of out-of-network services at a reduced rate, usually 70-80 percent of the covered fee schedule.

At the same time, HMOs were witnessing increasing resistance to the restrictions they placed on their members to receive all of their care within the network. Many HMOs responded to this pressure by forming an HMO variant known as a point-of-service (POS) plan. In the POS plan, members could typically receive full coverage by seeing an in-network contracted provider, but also receive 70-80 percent reimbursement if an out-of-network provider was seen. Many POS plans retained the primary care gatekeeper function common to most HMOs for any in-network care, but otherwise the consumer saw POS plans as being very similar to PPOs.

By the mid-1990s, the "managed care health care system" had come to encompass everything from the most restrictive HMO plans to the most permissive PPO plans, and it was becoming increasing difficult to define and differentiate the mix of restrictions and benefits being offered. Even in areas with a limited percentage of the insured population in HMOs, many more people were enrolled in POS and PPO plans, leading to managed care's dominance of the insurance market in all major geographic areas. By the late

1990s, indemnity health insurance, which at one time provided more than 95 percent of all health insurance, had diminished in scope to no more than 5-20 percent of the population, depending on the geographic region. All of the remaining consumers were covered by some form of managed care health insurance, whether HMO, POS, or PPO.

The Managed Care Backlash

By the mid-1990s, managed care's ascendance was met with the scrutiny that market dominance brings. Suddenly, every form of media outlet featured stories of excessive restrictions of care and resultant poor medical outcomes. Failure to diagnose and inappropriate treatment, long the predominant causes of medical malpractice suits, were presumed to be due to managed care's inherent restrictions to in-network care and/or utilization controls. In some of these cases, patients had been denied coverage for certain types of services, such as bone marrow transplants or similar new technologies that the HMO claimed to be unproved and experimental in nature. When terminally ill cancer patients subsequently died, their families would commonly ascribe death to HMOs' refusal to provide bone marrow transplants. Trial juries would sometimes agree and find for the plaintiffs, awarding sizable monetary damages that were newsworthy events. In reaction to these events, federal and state legislation was frequently proposed and often passed with the intention of ensuring patient rights and full disclosure by managed care plans of any restrictions they placed on access or services.

Were managed care plans acting recklessly without regard for appropriate medical standards? That usually depended on whom you asked. HMOs consistently argued that they were exercising sound clinical judgment and that any poor outcome was due to the underlying disease and not to their actions. Patients argued that that this was not the case, that they had been denied avenues of treatment that at least had a chance at success, however slight. Physicians were usually caught in the middle, properly advocating for their patients, even as they understood how slight the chances for success might have been. Making judgment all the more difficult was the reality that all of the facts rarely were made public. Press reports would be unlikely to have all of the details pertinent to a particular case, and the natural tendency was to find fault in the "system." It was often convenient to forget that medical malpractice was a crisis prior to managed care and was commonly alleged whenever outcomes were less than anticipated. Even as the trend has been to place the blame for poor outcomes on the managed care system, many managed care plans continue to benefit from exemptions of liability related to federal ERISA provisions, which has sparked new legislation to remove these exemptions and make all health plans liable for these cases.

The Outcomes Movement

Even before the backlash against managed care in the mid-1990s, there was a focus on demonstrating positive outcomes from the care provided within these systems of care. One of the earliest efforts to ensure quality in the industry was a move toward review and accreditation of managed care organizations by the

National Committee for Quality Assurance (NCQA).[4] Founded in 1979 as a private entity run by the managed care industry, it initially served to certify which HMOs were meeting federal qualification standards. After a period of dormancy in the late 1980s, NCQA was re-established as an independent, not-for-profit entity that has, since 1991, surveyed and accredited nearly 300 managed care organizations throughout the United States.

Another early response to the demand for useful outcomes data was the development of the Health Plan Employer Data and Information Set, commonly known as HEDIS. Developed in 1990 by a small number of HMOs and employers as a list of measures that managed care plans could measure and report, the responsibility for HEDIS was assumed in 1992 by NCQA. HEDIS measures focus on many areas, including clinical care, utilization rates, plan finances, and customer satisfaction. Over time, the number of measures has increased, and now many managed care plans report these measures annually to NCQA, permitting the development of national and regional performance benchmarks. The value of the HEDIS measures lies in the common measurement specifications that are explicitly stated and required of plans that submit data. Auditing of health plan results has been implemented to ensure that data are accurately reported and therefore reasonably comparable across health plans. NCQA publishes plans' HEDIS data, with the permission of each plan, annually in a format known as "Quality Compass."[4] An understandable but nonetheless disturbing recent trend has been the hesitancy of plans that perform poorly to permit release of their data by NCQA, diminishing the utility of Quality Compass for plan comparisons. Fortunately, NCQA has already announced a merging of its accreditation surveys with HEDIS reporting, such that some basic HEDIS data will now be a regular part of the normal NCQA accreditation reports. This new process, which began in July 1999, has a health plan's accreditation determination based 75 percent on how the plan complies with NCQA accreditation standards and 25 percent on how certain specific HEDIS data compare to regional and national benchmarks.

Central to the outcomes initiatives stimulated by NCQA accreditation and HEDIS reporting is application of continuous quality improvement principles to the delivery of health care.[5] Addressing both clinical care and service in the managed care environment, a number of national efforts have been undertaken to successfully implement quality improvement activities. One of these was the National Demonstration Project On Quality Improvement in Health Care. Spearheaded by a consortium of managed care plans and hospitals, with strong support from industry QI experts, the project sought to describe how such efforts could be initiated and successfully managed.[6] Another quality initiative was the Foundation for Accountability (FACCT), started by Dr. Paul Ellwood and other researchers from the Jackson Hole Group. FACCT was initiated in an attempt to foster a more vigorous look at true clinical outcomes, as opposed to the process measures that had been the predominant focus of the HEDIS clinical measures.

Another result of managed care attention to outcomes is the development of programs designed to address the health care needs of specific defined populations. When the population is otherwise healthy, these programs address preventive health care services and beneficial lifestyle education. When the population has a chronic illness, disease management programs seek to maximize effective treatment according to recognized clinical guidelines, reducing disease exacerbations and morbidity and improving the patient's quality of life. Disease management programs are now becoming common and address conditions such as diabetes, asthma, and heart disease.

Regardless of how one decides to approach the issue of quality improvement in health care, there is a fairly uniform belief that current efforts have just scratched the surface of what can and must be done to improve clinical care and service in the delivery of health care in this country. Much is made of how expensive our system of care is when compared to other industrialized countries, without a concomitant superiority in simple measures such as life expectancy, infant mortality, and percentage of population covered. While our wide access to care (for those with health insurance) and the quality of our practitioners and facilities is envied worldwide, there have been open calls to address the need to improve on what we currently have.[7] These efforts will likely accelerate in the years ahead, stimulated by the inevitable pressure to demonstrate quality of care in the face of continuously rising costs and the resulting restrictive management of health care delivery systems.

The Role of Physician Executives in Our Managed Care System

Now that you have been able to absorb this brief history of managed care and the key issues driving the industry, it is much easier to envision the central role that physician executives are playing in managed care today. For those working in managed care plans, some of the areas requiring their attention are the relationship between managed care plans and their associated provider networks, support of both individual practitioners and health care facilities, quality improvement programming, and both patient and provider education. Senior physician executives will also be involved in shaping MCOs' strategic direction and the selection and development of new business ventures and will take a role in shaping the future of the overall managed care industry. A key role for all physician executives is safeguarding the professionalism and the ethics of medicine and ensuring a continuing central role for physicians over the complete spectrum of the health care delivery system. This will involve balancing the needs of the larger system with preservation of the patient-doctor relationship, a crucial issue that can only be fully appreciated and managed by physician executives.

For physician executives involved in other areas of the health care delivery system, understanding the managed care environment is key to their successful interaction with this increasingly important and powerful component of the overall system. The physician executive responsible for a medical group, for example, will need to negotiate contracts, promote quality improvement efforts, support provider education, and deal with increasingly critical issues of resource allocation. The physician executive with responsibility for a hospital system will have largely similar issues to deal with, including resource allocation, contract negotiation, and quality improvement initiatives. In health care, as in any other discipline, the ability to understand the pressures and motivations of those on the other side of the table can only help in dealing with the normal business issues that arise. Physician executives in any field will benefit from an in-depth understanding of the managed care system.

The Future

How will the managed care system evolve in the years ahead? Recognizing my predictions to be as suspect as any on the subject, there do appear to be a number of trends that will characterize the industry's future. The first of these is the move toward freer access to care, with open access plans permitting self-referral to specialty care. The second trend is the shift of fiscal responsibility onto the shoulders of the provider network, whether primary care or specialty care. This recognizes the central role of the provider in guiding the patient through the health care system and determining or at least influencing the actual services provided. The third trend is the effort to measure and improve customer service and health care quality, especially in defined populations. Demonstrated improvements will be seen in many areas and will be increasingly publicized and touted as evidence of excellence among competing health care systems. The fourth trend is expansion of managed care across all populations. We are already seeing this in the Medicaid and Medicare populations and will likely see managed care applied to the uninsured population as well, possibly through a federal voucher system.

Conclusion

Managed care has assumed responsibility for the majority of the population because of its ability to provide excellent care at lower cost. It has done many things well, including reducing obvious waste in the health care system, addressing issues of quality of care and service, and promoting preventive care and systematic treatment of chronic illnesses. Managed care has also raised fears in a number of areas, including limited access to specialty care and the denial of care on financial grounds. Despite the current backlash, however, which was probably predictable and inevitable, the inexorable pressure of national health care economics will continue to drive patients into managed care systems at an increasing rate in the years ahead.

References

1. Mayer, T. "HMOs: Origins and Development." *New England Journal of Medicine* 312(9):590-4, Feb. 28, 1985.

2. Coile, R. *The Five Stages of Managed Care.* Chicago, Ill.: Health Administration Press, 1997.

3. Kirz, H., Editor. *Thriving in Capitation: A Practical Guide for the Medical Leader.* Tampa, Fla.: American College of Physician Executives, 1999.

4. National Committee for Quality Assurance, http://www.ncqa.org

5. Berwick, D. "Continuous Improvement as an Ideal in Health Care." *New England Journal of Medicine* 320(1):53-6, Jan. 5, 1989.

6. Berwick, D, *Curing Health Care.* San Francisco, Calif.: Jossey-Bass, Inc., 1990.

7. Chassin, M. "The Urgent Need to Improve Health Care Quality." *JAMA* 280(11):1000-8, Sept. 16, 1998.

Mark A. Bloomberg, MD, MBA, CPE, FACPE, is President, The Bloomberg Healthcare Group, Sudbury, Massachusetts.

Chapter

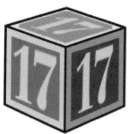

Integrated Delivery Systems

by Jerry Royer, MD, MBA

When physician/hospital organizations fail, they fail for one (or both) of two reasons: incongruent cultures and values, and/or a rush to organizational integration before economic integration.—Curt Pelley, Consultant

Embarking on the path of creating an integrated health care organization from a matrix of private practice is a little like driving a truck loaded with nitroglycerin along a bumpy road. Leaders without the political skills to sense the bumps in the road before they hit them will never know what happened. They will be steak tartare.—from "Driving the Nitroglycerin Truck,"—Jeff Goldsmith.[1]

Case #1

Mercy Hospital receives fixed reimbursement for more than two-thirds of its admissions: 46 percent from Medicare (DRGs) and 21 percent from capitated contracts. The physicians have no capitated contracts; they are reimbursed on the basis of discounted fee for service. The hospital improves its bottom line by decreasing days/1000—by decreasing length of stay and reducing inappropriate admissions. However, physicians, especially specialists whose practices are primarily inpatient, increase their revenue through increased days/1000; there is no incentive—indeed there is even a disincentive—to decrease days/1000.

Case #2

The physicians in Centerville, both those in the multispecialty group and those in a wraparound IPA, are capitated for more than 80 percent of their practice. The Centerville Hospital System, on the other hand, has not been able to secure global capitation from any of the payers in the market; the opportunity for capitation arbitrage eludes the four-hospital system.

The physicians have developed a congestive-heart-failure clinic. This successful chronic disease management program has improved the health status of patients, decreased CHF admissions, improved the physicians' bottom line, and decreased the overall health costs of the community. The hospital, however, lost revenue as a result of the decreased CHF admissions.

Case #3

At Kaiser-Permanente, the division between hospital and physicians differs from that in other health systems. Permanente physicians have fiscal responsibility for many hospital-based services (emergency department, laboratory, radiology, anesthesiology, cardiac cath lab, physical therapy, occupational therapy, and outpatient clinics)—all of which are cost centers. The hospital has only nursing and hotel services.

When a Kaiser hospital temporarily closes a nursing unit, as a cost-cutting measure during low census, patients may back up in the emergency department, thereby increasing the cost for Permanente Medical Group. Even at Kaiser-Permanente, incentives are not always aligned.

Integration remains elusive. The path to integration is fraught with political, economic, legal, and cultural land mines.

Background and Core Concepts

The United States continues to experience the largest industry reorganization since the 19th Century—the corporatization of American health care.[2,3] Hospitals and health plans continue to consolidate through a steady parade of mergers and acquisitions. Wall Street has become a player. Physicians increasingly practice in groups.

Perhaps the greatest transition, however, is that providers now reduce (rather than boost) their profit with every additional inpatient day, procedure, office visit, and test. In this new world, the traditional measures of success, such as high occupancy rates and more procedures, are no longer valid. In the past, more volume meant more profit. Now, more volume means less profit.

Many hospitals formed multihospital systems during the 1980s. Considerable research and literature of the late 1980s focused on multihospital systems that had formed during that decade.[4,5] There was little evidence that these systems added significantly more value than did independent hospitals.[6,7] The first generation of multihospital systems did not demonstrate superior cost, quality, or access performance compared to independent hospitals. These systems achieved some economies of scale (such as group purchasing), but little was known about their impact on clinical performance—that is, the extent to which they provided an integrated continuum of coordinated services to meet patient needs.[8]

During the 1990s and now, the primary driver behind the formation of integrated delivery systems has been the new economics of managed care. In response to managed care pressures and imminent legislative health care reform, provider organizations across the United States have come together to form integrated delivery systems as a means to offer better coordinated, more cost-effective care.

The year 1998 was not a good year for national-scale, Wall Street-funded health care companies—Columbia, MedPartners, Oxford, FPA, and Foundation Health Systems. The CEOs of these companies are gone, each having left behind a troubled enterprise. The common theme: Largely for-profit, national companies suffered from overly aggressive expansion plans to the detriment of day-to-day operations. They had "trouble managing care, trouble managing physicians, and trouble managing hospitals."[8] The real news, however, has been the strength and prosperity of a much larger number of integrated delivery systems, e.g., Presbyterian in New Mexico and Alliant Health System in Kentucky. The Advisory Board found, for the first time, "real evidence of significant health system price leverage and scale advantage."[9]

Based on an ongoing national study of nine integrated delivery systems, Stephen Shortell and his colleagues have examined what is known about the performance of such systems, the barriers they face, and the likely key success factors.[10] They define an integrated delivery system as "a network of organizations that provides or arranges to provide a coordinated continuum of services to a defined population and is willing to be held clinically and fiscally accountable for the outcomes and the health status of the population served."[11]

The core concept of an integrated delivery system is that it is an organization that can effectively coordinate services to patients across the range of care required to maintain, restore, or enhance a patient's health status. Gillis *et al.* define three types of integration[8]:

> *"Clinical integration—the extent to which patient care services are coordinated across the various functions, activities, and operating units of a system.*
>
> *"Physician-system integration—the extent to which physicians are economically linked to a system; use its facilities and services; and actively participate in its planning, management, and governance.*
>
> *"Functional integration—the extent to which key support functions and activities (such as financial management, human resources, strategic planning, information management, marketing, and quality improvement) are coordinated across operating units so as to add the greatest overall value to the system."*

The relationships among the different forms of integration are shown in the figure on page 292. Clinical integration includes both horizontal and vertical integration. Horizontal integration refers to "the coordination of functions, activities, or operating units that are at the same stage in the process of delivering care."[8] Hospitals, for example, have consolidated and merged across geographic regions. Vertical integration, by contrast, refers to "the coordination of functions, activities, or operating units that are at different stages of the process involved in delivering patient services."[8] Examples include hospital linkages with physician groups, ambulatory

Framework* for Examining Integration8

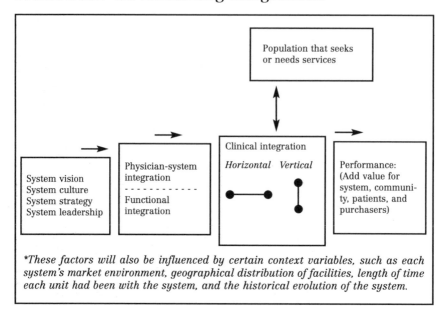

These factors will also be influenced by certain context variables, such as each system's market environment, geographical distribution of facilities, length of time each unit had been with the system, and the historical evolution of the system.

surgery centers, home health, long-term care, retirement centers, hospice care, etc. (Perhaps the ultimate vertical integration would include funeral homes and cemeteries.)

Clinical integration is the most important integration, in that it focuses on the patient. The extent to which a patient's care needs to be coordinated depends on the patient's illness and on decisions made by the patient's physician. The extent to which physicians are integrated into the system and the extent to which certain functional activities (e.g., information management, financial management, and marketing) are integrated will promote clinical integration.

Barriers to System Integration

Shortell *et al.* discuss nine major barriers to system integration.[10,11]

1. **Failure to Understand the New Core Business.** An ever-increasing volume of health care is being provided in non-acute settings. Acute inpatient care is no longer the core business. The shift to outpatient settings, cost containment pressures for lower-cost settings, and patient preferences have contributed to the shift toward an integrated continuum of care as the new core business. The more interesting developments in patient care for the foreseeable future are beyond the hospital walls—ambulatory care, prevention and wellness, early diagnosis, and after-care recovery. We have the opportunity to become what we have not been in the recent past—a provider in the higher-growth segments of the health care industry.

2. **Inability to Overcome the Hospital Paradigm.** As a corollary to barrier #1, the hospital may no longer be the starting point or center of integration efforts. Shortell et al. ask, "What multidivisional organization in corporate America would attempt to organize its efforts around the unit that is not only least in demand but declining in demand?"[11] Inpatient care is the sole non-growth market in all of health care. Defending inpatient beds is a disheartening journey into the wind.

3. **Embryonic Development of Clinical Information Systems.** Information technology must link patients and providers across all care settings: physician offices, acute inpatient care, home care, etc.

4. **Inability to Convince the "Cash Cow" to Accept System Strategy.** "Cash cow" refers to an operating unit—e.g., a hospital in a good payer market—that generates the most revenue for the system. Historically, a "cash cow," because of its prime cash-flow source, has had the autonomy to pursue its own priorities. There is often an unwillingness to reallocate funds away from the "cash cow" to support emerging system priorities.

5. **Inability of Board to Understand New Health Care Environment.** Traditional hospital board members bring a hospital mindset to system governance, reinforcing the above barriers.

6. **Ambiguous Roles and Responsibilities.** Operating unit managers, fearful that their power and influence will be reduced, fail to understand their role in the evolving system. This barrier is heightened when there is a regional level of management operating between the system office and the individual operating units.

7. **Inability to "Manage" Managed Care.** Learning to manage care is a daunting undertaking. For managed care to operate effectively, certain building blocks must be in place: "sufficient numbers of physician leaders who understand the new realities of health care, a sufficient number of physicians organized in group practices, a sufficient number of primary care physicians, case manager roles, and information systems in place that can provide clinical and financial data that both improve internal processes of care and provide external information for purchasers' decision making."[11]

8. **Inability to Execute Strategy.** CEOs and operating unit managers, satisfied with the status quo and fearful of loss of autonomy, are unwilling and may lack the new competencies required to focus on a new core strategy.

9. **Lack of Strategic Alignment.** Various components of the system may lack alignment, "particularly in regard to its orientation toward the market versus its administrative or managerial control of the strategy."[11] Accounting and financial controls may be overemphasized, as opposed to customer satisfaction, market research, and community health status needs assessment.

I would suggest a tenth barrier:

Lack of a Management Culture of Collegiality. As Paul Starr and others remind us, the relationship between physicians and hospitals has been one of conflict for the past century. One system CEO lamented, "There continues to be a breech of trust between our hospitals and physicians." (See below, Critical Success Factor #3.)

Critical Success Factors

Since 1993, Advisory Board staff members have reviewed the literature and conducted interviews to obtain detailed information on integration strategies being pursued by North America's most successful health care systems. Their initial research report, Grand Alliance: Vertical Integration Strategies for Physicians and Health Systems, sought to define the qualities of a stable, successful integrated system. Ongoing research (both the Advisory Board and Stephen Shortell's group) and discussions with health care leaders (both providers and payers) suggest the following critical success factors:

1. **A thriving medical group environment is the single most critical factor.**

   - The core enterprise of many integrated delivery systems—Mayo, Henry Ford, Kaiser—is a large multispecialty group practice.

   - The medical group must have its own governance structure and business plan—a separate board that includes elected and full-time physician managers.

   - The Advisory Board evaluated eight organizational models, concluding that only three models are sustainable[3]:

Transitional Models	Sustainable Models
Management Service Bureau	Foundation Model
Group Practice without Walls	Staff Model
Open PHO	Equity Model
Closed PHO	
Comprehensive MSO	

     Follow-up research with physicians, however, indicates that there is only limited allure of equity; most physicians view equity as (at best) moderately desirable, and clearly subsidiary to a host of other facility attributes.[12]

     ❑ Physicians will require new skill sets, such as assembling and managing a large medical group, managing risk, and allocating resources. Inexperienced physician managers will require mentoring by experienced physician leaders. (Nonphysician managers are less effective mentors for physicians.)

     ❑ Physician income must be tied to proceeds.

     ❑ Any health system investment must be identified and isolated.

2. **The health system leadership must be committed to overcoming the barriers to system integration.** (See above, "Barriers to System Integration.")

3. **Closer alignment of physicians and hospitals is a requisite for prosperity if not survival.**

"The key feature of the new integrated health care enterprise is not a balance of power, but the emergence of collegiality as the fundamental organizing principle. The essence of collegiality is tolerance and a sharing of common professional values. This trust and sharing of values is, in turn, the central precondition of the ability to share and successfully manage the economic risk of health costs.

There are not many truly integrated health care organizations in America, and those that come to mind, such as Kaiser Permanente or Mayo, are not only unambiguously physician-run but are anchored in a long tradition of collegiality. This collegiality—not who owns what, how physicians are compensated, or who works for whom—is literally what integrates them."[1]

In a collegial system, physicians are full partners, privy to all information. The system CEO works his or her relationships with physicians daily; there is no decision he or she does not discuss with the physicians. (Also see the Advisory Group's study, The Physician Perspective: Key Drivers of Physician Loyalty.[12])

4. **A rich primary care base is essential for any viable system.** The system must create a structure to support the practice of primary care, one in which physicians are not merely employees but participants who share and exercise real power.

5. **The system must be committed to clinical practice/process improvement (CPI).** CPI refers to the application of continuous quality improvement (CQI) principles in the health care setting. Variation in clinical practice may be the single greatest challenge we face.[13] Edwards Deming 101: Decreasing variation improves quality and decreases cost.

6. **Strong information systems are required for improving quality and cost performance and for generating data for external stakeholders.** Credible data are essential for an electronic medical record, evidence-based practice, guideline/pathway development, and outcomes measurement.

7. **Patient care management systems and technology management systems are critical for efficacious, cost-effective care.** These systems include case management for chronic disease, demand management, health status assessment, integration of clinical and financial data, and assessment of the relative cost/benefit ratios of alternative technologies.

Coda

The behaviors one should observe in more integrated health systems include downsizing of acute care capacity; consolidation of programs and services;

development of regionwide clinical service lines (such as cardiovascular care, women's and children care, and neuromuscular care); expansion of the primary care base and growth of primary care and multispecialty group practices; identification of best practices, leading to clinical guidelines and pathways; care management systems; commitment to clinical practice improvement; and development of outcome measures.

The ultimate measure will be the extent to which integrated delivery systems improve the health and welfare of our patients and communities.

References

1. Goldsmith, J. "Building Integrated Systems—Driving the Nitroglycerin Truck." *Healthcare Forum Journal* 36(2):36-8,40,44, March/April 1993.

2. Starr, P. *The Social Transformation of American Medicine.* New York, N.Y.: Basic Books, 1982.

3. The Governance Committee. *The Grand Alliance: Vertical Integration Strategies for Physicians and Health Systems.* Washington, D.C.: Advisory Board Company, 1993.

4. Zuckerman, H., and Kaluzny, A. "Strategic Alliances in Health Services: The Challenges of Cooperation." *Frontiers of Health Services Management* 7(3):3-23,35, Spring 1991.

5. Zuckerman, H., and D'Aunno, T. "Hospital Alliances: Cooperative Strategy in a Competitive Environment." *Health Care Management Review* 15(2):21-30, Spring 1990.

6. Shortell, S. "The Evolution of Hospital Systems: Unfulfilled Promises and Self-Fulfilling Prophesies." *Medical Care Review* 45(2):177-214, Fall 1988.

7. Shortell, S., and others. *Strategic Choices for America's Hospitals: Managing Change in Turbulent Times.* San Francisco, Calif.: Jossey-Bass, 1990.

8. Gillies, R., and others. "Conceptualizing and Measuring Integration: Findings from the Health Systems Integration Study." *Hospital and Health Services Administration* 38(4):467-89, Winter 1993.

9. Health Care Advisory Board. *The Chief Executive's Agenda: Physician Defection, Physician Retention, and Long-Term Physician Relationships.* Washington, D.C.: Advisory Board Company, 1998, p. 11.

10. Shortell, S., and others. "The New World of Managed Care: Creating Organized Delivery Systems." *Health Affairs* 13(5):46-64, Winter 1994.

11. Shortell, S., and others. "Creating Organized Systems: The Barriers and Facilitators." *Hospital and Health Services Administration* 38(4):447-66, Winter 1993

12. Health Care Advisory Board. *The Physician Perspective: Key Drivers of Physician Loyalty.* Washington, D.C.: Advisory Board Company, 1999.

13. Wennberg, J., Editor. *The Dartmouth Atlas of Health Care in the United States.* Chicago, Ill.: American Hospital Publishing, Inc., 1996.

Jerry Royer, MD, MBA, is Senior Vice President and Chief Medical Officer, Mercy Health Plans, Chesterfield, Missouri.

Chapter

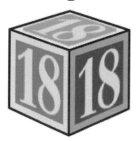

A Multidisciplinary Approach to Clinical Resource Management

by Alan H. Rosenstein, MD, MBA

As health care organizations face increasing pressures to manage financial risk, the demands to provide and demonstrate cost-effective, high-quality patient care will steadily increase. Successful strategies designed to improve efficiencies in care come from a multidisciplinary commitment to developing and implementing both operational and clinical programs focused on effective resource management based on sound information systems and clinical decision support. The Clinical Resource Management Program described in this chapter has proved to be an effective vehicle for managing one organization's resources by developing a structured program that integrated the efforts of individuals who have control over processes involved in patient care. Experience has shown that, if you provide clinicians with accurate and meaningful information and give them adequate support, they will enthusiastically participate in development and use of the tools that will provide optimal, efficient patient care. The process will benefit the organization, physicians, and the populations they serve.

By now, we are all well aware of changes affecting almost every aspect of the health care delivery system. With one trillion dollars estimated to have been spent on health care services in 2000, concerns continue to mount about the availability and value of the health care dollar. Nowhere is this concern felt more intensely than by health care payers. With more than 40 percent of health care spending coming from government-sponsored programs such as Medicare and Medicaid, federal and state governments are extremely concerned about the future ability to continue to fund these programs. Business, the second largest payer category, accounting for nearly 35 percent of health care spending, is concerned about the $4,800 average annual cost of providing health care benefits for covered employees. The remainder of the spending falls into the category of self-pay or, in many cases, of no pay because of the nearly 20 percent of the population not covered by health care insurance. Needless to say, most of the efforts geared at reducing health care spending have come from the payer sector. Starting in the mid-1980s and continuing through today, payers began to initiate a series of programs and initiatives designed to reduce their health care financial burden. Using a combination of legislative mandates and market force dynamics, their goal was to reduce health care spending by directly limiting dollar outflow and/or placing more of the financial risk for services rendered onto the shoulders of health care providers. These initiatives can be consolidated into three main areas of concentration:

• The first attempt to limit health care spending came though the implementation of a series of direct utilization controls. Recognizing the high percentage of inappropriate and/or ineffective services being provided in patient care (which in some estimates ranged from 15 to 40 percent), payers recognized that they needed to exert some control over these services. Starting with the TEFRA legislation in 1983, affecting inpatient services for Medicare beneficiaries, the government initiated the first major set of utilization guidelines tying financial reimbursement to appropriateness and necessity of care. Using a set of severity of illness and intensity of service criteria, hospitals treating patients who did not meet these necessity criteria would run the risk of having payments denied. The utilization control program was so effective that it quickly spread across the entire health service system. Some studies suggest that utilization review by itself was successful in taking 20 percent of unnecessary care out of the system. Others suggest that the costs were merely transferred to a different level of care.

• The second major change occurred in reimbursement restructuring. Recognizing the financial misincentives of the fee-for-service system, payers quickly realized that they needed to change the nature of the reimbursement incentives. The new vehicles for reimbursement included fee-for-service at a percentage discount, payment by diagnosis (DRG) and other types of global payments, payment per diem, and capitation. As illustrated in table 1, page 295, this set up a different set of financial incentives based on insurance category and type of payment. Looking at the hospital sector, if you're lucky enough to still have true fee-for-service or modified fee-for-service patients, the economic incentive is to encourage the hospital admission, prolong the length of stay, and consume multiple resources. The more you do, the more you get reimbursed. Under per-case reimbursement, you want the hospital admission (if it's clinically justified and meets the established severity of illness/intensity of service criteria discussed earlier), but you want to shorten the length of stay and reduce resource consumption, because you accrue no additional revenues for these services under per case reimbursement. For per-diem coverage, you want the hospital admission (if it's clinically justified), and you want a longer length of stay because it's only during the latter, less intensive part of the hospitalization that the per-diem rate exceeds the actual costs of providing care.

Unfortunately, if the patient does not continue to meet acute care criteria, you run the risk of having these less acute days denied if services could have been safely provided at a lower level of care. As with the per-case

Table 1. Hospital Payment Incentives

Payment Method	Admission	LOS	Services per Case
Charge Based	↑	↑	↑
Diagnosis Based	↑	↓	↓
Per Diem Based	↑	↑	↓
Capitation	↓	↓	↓

patient, with a fixed amount of dollars per day, the economic goal is to reduce resource consumption. Under capitation, where you have the money up front, the economic incentive is to avoid unnecessary hospital admissions, reduce lengths of stay, and be conservative in resource utilization. In one philosopher's view, the goal is to lock the front doors and provide only bread and water and an uncomfortable bed, if they ever make it into the building. Note that, in the latter three payment categories, the emphasis is on resource management. From the attending physician's perspective, the only time hospital and physician incentives are truly aligned for inpatient services is through either a fee-for-service or a capitation arrangement. I'll leave it to your imagination as to which way the payers would like it to go.

- The third major influence is managed care. The conceptual intent of managed care, or managed competition as it was once called, is to encourage providers (hospitals and clinicians) to organize together into integrated groups in an effort to more effectively contract with a host of intermediary organizations (HMOs or PPOs) that are able to sign up large groups of patients. Employers began to shuffle their employees into these managed care organizations in hopes of lowering their health care premiums. Following suit, the government began to encourage Medicare and Medicaid enrollees to join these plans in an effort to get control of health care costs. Providers, while resentful of the external interference exercised by these organizations, were forced to join them because of the rules of supply and demand. With an excess of hospital beds and an excess of physicians, providers who did not join these plans were left out in the cold. Being left out in the cold meant that you would not have access to the growing number of patients enrolling in these plans. It was a Catch 22. But managed care has not turned out to be the salvation that people were looking for. In fact, a new crisis has arisen, with the growing perception that managed care plans have cut revenues and services to the point that they compromise direct patient care. The patient's bill of rights is now a hot ticket item in Congress and is currently going through bipartisan review.

On the delivery side of the equation, these changes have had a profound impact on the practice of medicine. Providers, whose core business is to provide the best and highest possible quality of care, are now faced with a situation of providing more for less. Significant restrictions in reimbursement have forced providers to restructure their entire line of business and develop new modalities and processes for delivering patient care. The following sections will focus on the various strategies and techniques used by providers in an effort to more effectively manage utilization of health care resources and supply appropriate, cost-effective, high-quality care.

Resource Management

Before we begin to discuss the merits of effective resource management, we need to come to an understanding of what we mean by health care resources. For the purposes of this discussion, we will assume that the term "resources" refers to all the manpower, supply and materials, technology services, and physical and organization infrastructure involved either directly or indirectly in patient care. These components can be grouped into three distinct categories.

- Operational resources, which includes all the labor and structural overhead.

- Material and supplies, which includes all the resources related to consumables.

- Clinical resources, which refers to all diagnostic and treatment resources directly related to patient care.

The next question is, Why is resource management so important? Basically in comes down to pure economics. If you think of the fundamental economic equation, Net Income = Net Revenues – Net Expenses, providers in today's health care environment are struggling to make ends meet and to maintain a positive net balance. Net income can be affected by price and volume. But with less reimbursement, there is limited opportunity to increase the net revenues side of the equation. You can charge whatever you like, but, for most payments, the price has already been fixed through up-front negotiations. You can try to increase quantity, but profit and loss for each additional patient depend on reimbursement structure and how effectively the patient is managed. Therefore, most attention has been directed to the expense side of the equation, attempting to increase net income by lowering the costs of care.

Going back to the definition of resource management presented above, there are several different areas that can be affected by efficiencies gained in effective resource management. Using a 350-bed acute care hospital as an example, figure 1, page 297, provides a graphic overview of the potential dollars that could be saved in one year if the hospital were to achieve benchmark performance in each of the categories discussed above. The greatest opportunity lies in the area of improving operational efficiency, where $16.5 million could be saved by achieving benchmark performance in labor management and another $7.6 million could be saved by maximizing efficiencies in overhead control.[1] Figures 2 and 3, pages 300 and 301, present an example of the type of analysis that can be used to identify key operational indicators in an effort to uncover potential opportunities for improvement by achieving benchmark performance results.[2] In this analysis, benchmark performance is measured by averaging the results from the top 25 percent of hospitals in each hospital class. In each sector, further drill-down analysis will discover cost centers with the greatest opportunity for savings. This type of comparative analysis allows the institution to select and monitor key indicators of operational performance related to labor and productivity and expense control reflected by staffing ratios and costs per discharge. Improvements are gained by implementing an action plan geared to improve operational function.

In another area, we have the costs associated with materials and supplies. Again using the example of a 350-bed acute care hospital, a projected $5.5 billion could be saved by achieving efficiencies in the cost of material and

Figure 1. Cost Savings Potential

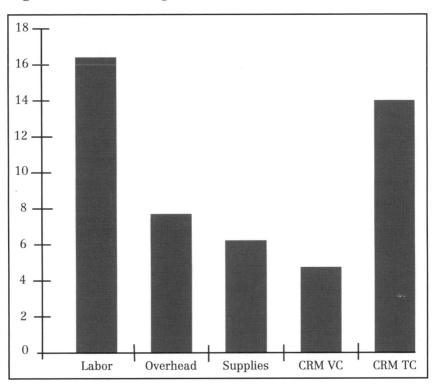

supply acquisition and by improving resource utilization through standardization and waste reduction programs. While each institution can try on its own to negotiate lower price contracts, many institutions have turned to large group purchasing organizations (GPOs) that are able to exercise more clout in the contracting process by virtue of the large number of hospitals affiliated with the organization. VHA and Premier are two examples of this type of organization.

In the clinical area, we have resources related to direct patient care. Again following the example of the 350-bed acute care hospital discussed above and using a variable cost per day of $300, the hospital might be able to save $3.75 million in direct costs of care by providing benchmark care maximizing efficiencies in length of stay and resource utilization. Using a total cost of care of $1,000 per day, potential savings could reach $12.5 million per year. (Actual cost savings will be discussed later in the section on return on investment.) While the direct dollar savings from clinical resource management is far less than potential total dollar savings related to efficiencies in labor, operational control, and materials management, efficiencies in resource management will eventually influence each of these sectors accordingly (see figure 4, page 302). As illustrated in figure 5, page 302, a critical point is eventually reached when the cumulative reduction in clinical unit consumption allows a corresponding reduction in labor and supplies. Timeliness, appropriateness, and efficiency of care are the hallmarks of clinical resource management, and this topic will be discussed in greater detail in the following section.

Tools for Improvement
Resource Management/Information Sharing/Physician Education

Table 2, page 299, gives a listing of 10 different tools for improvement designed to inject efficiencies into the clinical resource management piece of the pie. You'll note that none of the tools are mutually exclusive. In fact, most are complementary in their goal to improve process efficiencies and outcomes of care. Table 3, page 299, takes the same approach and extends the tools to cover the materials and supplies and the labor and operations sectors discussed previously.

Tool number one relates to organizational structure. In order to be effective in its resource management efforts, the institution must have the proper vehicle for assimilating and distributing all the information necessary to develop and implement an effective clinical resource management program. While many institutions attempt to solve this problem by redefining the roles of one of the already existing performance improvement and/or cost and quality management programs, to really be successful there needs to be an integrated multidimensional approach to resource management. One way to accomplish this objective is to use a model similar to the Clinical Resource Management Steering Committee illustrated in figure 6, page 304.[3] In this model a multidisciplinary committee consisting of representatives from administration, medical staff, nursing, case management, quality improvement, finance, ancillary services, information systems, and decision support was formed as a steering committee that was given responsibility

Table 2. Ten Tools For Improvement

1. Resource Management - Organizational Structure

2. Information Sharing/Physician Education

3. "Hawthorne Effect"/Accountability

4. Case Management/Disease Management

5. Guidelines/Protocols/Policies & Procedures

6. Clinical Pathways

7. Computer Assists

8. Benchmarking/Best Practice Performance

9. Aligning Provider Incentives/Gainsharing

10. Outcome Management

Table 3. Sector Based Tools for Improvement

Materials and Supplies	Labor and Operations	Clinical Resource Management
1. Information Management • Supply cost • Supply consumption • Automation	1. Information Management • Staffing/Overhead • Productivity/Flow • Benchmark standards	1. Information Management • Variations in care • Practice standards • Cost/Quality outcomes
2. Enduser Education • Materials Management • Integrated care	2. Enduser Education • Operational Management • Integrated care	2. Enduser Education • Clinical Management • Integrated care
3. Utilization Management • Standardization	3. Utilization Management • Productivity	3. Utilization Management • Disease Management
4. Care Redesign • Product Assessment	4. Care Redesign • Process Re-engineering	4. Care Redesign • CQI/Process Improvement
5. Benchmarking • Pricing/Consumption	5. Benchmarking • Productivity/Staffing Ratios	5. Benchmarking • Clinical Markers
6. Best Practice	6. Best Practice	6. Best Practice
7. Critical Pathway • Supply Flow	7. Critical Pathway • Labor Flow	7. Critical Pathway • Patient/Resource Flow
8. Guidelines/Protocols • Supply Efficiency	8. Guidelines/Protocols • Labor Efficiency	8. Guidelines Protocols • Patient Care Efficiencies
9. Incentive Alignment	9. Incentive Alignment	9. Incentive Alignment
10. Outcome Management • Price • Efficacy • Employee Satisfaction	10. Outcome Management • Labor Supply • Labor Demand • Employee Satisfaction	10. Outcome Management • Cost • Quality • Staff/Patient Satisfaction

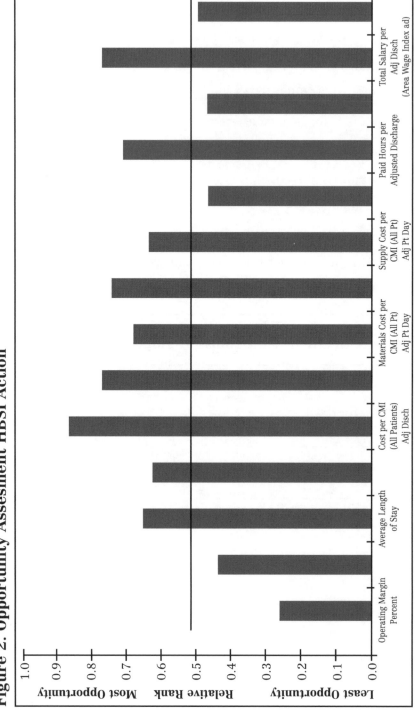

Figure 2. Opportunity Assesment HBSI Action

Figure 3. HBSI Action Performance Report

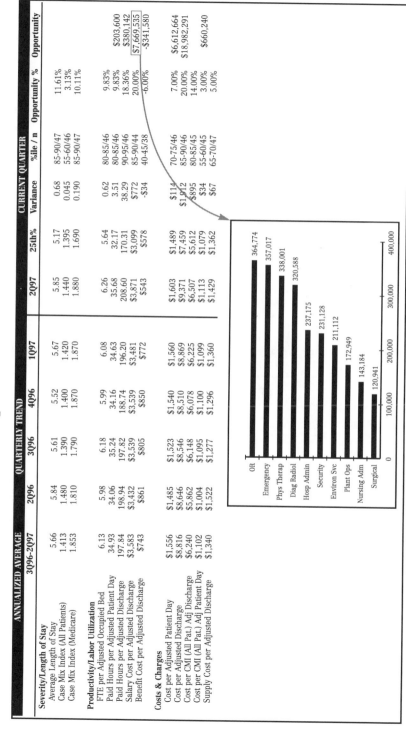

	ANNUALIZED AVERAGE	QUARTERLY TREND					CURRENT QUARTER				
	3Q96-2Q97	2Q96	3Q96	4Q96	1Q97	2Q97	25th%	Variance	%ile / n	Opportunity %	Opportunity
Severity/Length of Stay											
Average Length of Stay	5.66	5.84	5.61	5.52	5.67	5.85	5.17	0.68	85-90/47	11.61%	
Case Mix Index (All Patients)	1.413	1.480	1.390	1.400	1.420	1.440	1.395	0.045	55-60/46	3.13%	
Case Mix Index (Medicare)	1.853	1.810	1.790	1.870	1.870	1.880	1.690	0.190	85-90/47	10.11%	
Productivity/Labor Utilization											
FTE per Adjusted Occupied Bed	6.13	5.98	6.18	5.99	6.08	6.26	5.64	0.62	80-85/46	9.83%	$203,600
Paid Hours per Adjusted Patient Day	34.93	34.06	35.24	34.16	34.63	35.68	32.17	3.51	80-85/46	9.83%	$380,142
Paid Hours per Adjusted Discharge	197.84	198.94	197.82	188.74	196.20	208.60	170.31	38.29	90-95/46	18.36%	$7,669,535
Salary Cost per Adjusted Discharge	$3,583	$3,432	$3,539	$3,539	$3,481	$3,871	$3,099	$772	85-90/44	20.00%	
Benefit Cost per Adjusted Discharge	$743	$861	$805	$850	$772	$543	$578	-$34	40-45/38	-6.00%	-$341,580
Costs & Charges											
Cost per Adjusted Patient Day	$1,556	$1,485	$1,523	$1,540	$1,560	$1,603	$1,489	$114	70-75/46	7.00%	$6,612,664
Cost per Adjusted Discharge	$8,816	$8,646	$8,546	$8,510	$8,869	$9,371	$7,459	$1,912	85-90/46	20.00%	$18,982,291
Cost per CMI (All Pat.) Adj Discharge	$6,240	$5,862	$6,148	$6,078	$6,225	$6,507	$5,612	$895	80-85/45	14.00%	
Cost per CMI (All Pat.) Adj Patient Day	$1,102	$1,004	$1,095	$1,100	$1,099	$1,113	$1,079	$34	55-60/45	3.00%	$660,240
Supply Cost per Adjusted Discharge	$1,340	$1,522	$1,277	$1,296	$1,360	$1,429	$1,362	$67	65-70/47	5.00%	

Bar chart values:

Department	Value
OR	364,774
Emergency	357,017
Phys Therap	338,001
Diag Radiol	320,588
Hosp Admin	237,175
Security	231,128
Environ Svc	211,112
Plant Ops	172,949
Nursing Adm	143,184
Surgical	120,941

Figure 4. Cost Control Opportunities

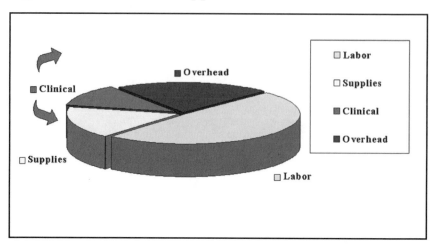

Figure 5. Consumption Based Staffing Requirements

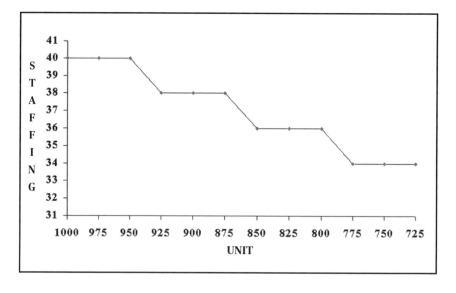

for developing and overseeing the entire clinical resource management program at the institution. The first objective of the committee was to centralize all the current, often independent, performance improvement activities in the institution. By setting clearly defined goals and objectives, the committee developed an action plan that coordinated all the performance improvement efforts into a consistent unified approach to information gathering and dissemination that was then presented to the appropriate clinical teams to be used in their individual department performance improvement projects. The results of these efforts were reported back to the committee on a regular basis.

Tool number two is information management and staff education. Having access to the right information provides the backbone to any successful clinical resource management program. Information is needed to identify and prioritize efforts, to compare and analyze performance outputs, and to measure and monitor the impact of resource management efforts. In order to be influential, the information must be accurate, timely, and presented in a meaningful, well-constructed format. The next step is to deliver the information to all those who need to know. Because physician are most responsible for directing care, educational efforts need to be targeted directly to the physician audience, but other groups intimately involved in the patient care process should be included. The information should be presented in an educational, constructive, non-threatening manner, designed to influence positive behavioral change. The full scope of the process of information gathering and sharing will be discussed in the case examples presented below.

Tool number three is the Hawthorne Effect. The principle behind the Hawthorne Effect is the fact that we all tend to perform better when we know that someone is looking over our shoulder. To say it another way, what gets measured is what gets managed. Performance tends to improve when you know you're being monitored. While both physician education and the threat of external monitoring do have some value, their ability to consistently influence change diminishes over time unless these efforts are continually reinforced.

Tool number four is case management. Unlike the relatively passive and often short-lived impact of education and performance overview, case management has the potential to provide a real-time opportunity to influence change at the point of care. Besides performing customary preadmission review and concurrent review, which focus on appropriateness and length of stay of the hospital admission, case managers can provide a vital service to the overall resource management effort through timely intervention. The hallmark of an effective case management effort is to prevent a less satisfactory alternative from occurring by making a recommendation for a more effective alternative before the order is actually transcribed. In many institutions, case managers have assumed more responsibility for monitoring compliance with recommended treatment standards, pathways, and protocols discussed below. In order to be successful, the case management program must have a clear vision of its goals, objectives, and priorities; be supported by adequate staffing and assignment of appropriate responsibilities; and have access to all the

Figure 6. Clinical Resource Management Model

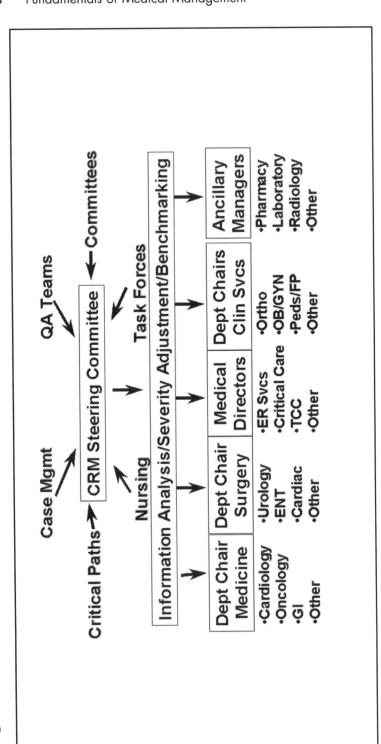

information necessary to monitor and affect care.[4] True disease management occurs when the case management process is extended across the entire continuum of care.

Tool number five is the development of guidelines, protocols, policies, and procedures. Guidelines should be tied to a specific outcome, designed as a framework to reduce unwanted variations in care, and focused on a specific circumstance or event. While many guidelines can be based on already established external criteria, success is more readily assured if they are built with consensus internal input that reflects local community standards of care.

Tool number six is clinical pathways. Whereas guidelines reinforce efficiencies for a single event, clinical pathways are designed to reinforce efficiencies for a confluent episode of care. As with guidelines, there are many prefabricated external pathways available for implementation, but results are better if the framework is built internally from a well-focused multidisciplinary perspective supported by well-accepted, evidence-based, best practice patterns of care. Many institutions have had a huge amount of success with guidelines and pathways, but much of the success depends on the individual institution's level of commitment and resource management maturity. Clinical pathways are often time and resource intensive and inherently have their own set of potential benefits and disadvantages. The first benefit is just getting the right people to the table. The pathway development process provides a unique opportunity to facilitate a multidisciplinary approach geared to identifying the important aspects of care and to begin the value-added component of discussing, developing, and implementing the essential ingredients of an effective process improvement plan. A second advantage is the benefit to the casual admitter. Cardiologist are well aware of the latest trends in effective management of the patient with CHF, but the internist or family practitioner who admits only one or two patients a year with this diagnosis has the greatest potential for improving efficiencies in care when following the pathway protocols. On the disadvantage side, while many hospitals have 20 or 30 different pathways, many of them are having problems with compliance and adherence. If the pathways aren't used or don't cover the right diagnoses, there's no added value. Similarly, someone has to take on the responsibility for active pathway management. Retrospective variance analysis does little to improve real-time treatment. Another problem with pathways is the time to implementation. Full pathway development can involve a two-year commitment. Short-term rewards can be gained by focusing on the two or three key elements of care that are unique to each diagnosis and that drive the entire process of care.

Tool number seven is the interactive computer. If you can get physicians to go to the computer for order entry, you have a wonderful real-time opportunity to make recommendations for a more appropriate alternative. Physicians will find the computer useful if it saves them time or provides information that will enable them to make better decisions. Computers that provide cost information, quality information, guidelines, algorithms, drug dosing regimens, standing orders, pathways, alerts and reminders, and Web site compatibility have proved to be a remarkable force in improving efficiencies in physician behavior.

Tool number eight is benchmarking. Benchmarking is a term used to describe individual comparison to a like group of peers who seem to obtain more favorable results for selected outcomes of care. Internal benchmarking refers to identifying optimal peer group performers within your institution and using this group as an example of benchmark performance. The advantage of internal benchmarking is consistency in measurement and analysis. External benchmarking infers comparisons to like groups of external peers. An example of external analysis for operational efficiency was presented in figure 3, page 301. Figure 7, page 307, gives an example of clinical benchmarking. Notice that, in Hospital #3, CHF patients appear to consume an unusually large amount of time and resources in the CCU setting. The hospital might not have recognized this from its internal analysis, but the point becomes obvious when performing external comparisons. The problem with external benchmarking is peer group homogeneity and lack of consistent measurement definitions and applications. Benchmarking's strength is its ability to compare results and identify potential opportunities for improvement. The real value occurs after process review and implementation of the appropriate improvement strategies.

Tool number nine is incentive alignment. Having physicians and the hospital financially motivated to supply the most efficient care along the health care continuum is one of the strongest motivators of behavioral change. As we evolve into a more integrated health care delivery system with more equal sharing of financial risks and rewards, we will see many efficiencies not otherwise gained through the improvement strategies discussed previously.

The final tool is outcome management. Being able to provide cost-effective, high-quality care with positive perceptual and functional patient satisfaction is the hallmark of medical care. Being able to measure and monitor critical indicators for each of these disciplines and to aggregate all the results into a meaningful overview across the entire spectrum of care is the ultimate direction in which we all need to go. Figures 8 and 9, pages 308 and 309, illustrate a display format for integrated outcome assessment. Figure 10, page 310, links utilization, cost, quality, functional, and perceptual improvement into a working format designed to integrate outcomes into a framework in which those in charge can gain a greater appreciation for the overall impact of care.

Case Example—Congestive Heart Failure

Following the process described above, after team organization and setting of objectives, the next step in the resource management process is to use information to identify opportunities for improvement. As illustrated in table 1, page 295, the economic incentives for resource management are different for different payer categories. While we don't recommend differences in management based on payer class, we do recommend promoting the most appropriate, expedient, cost-effective, high-quality care for all patients admitted to the institution. Using the case example of the 350-bed acute care

Figure 7. CHF Service Line Costs By Hospital HBSI Explore Report

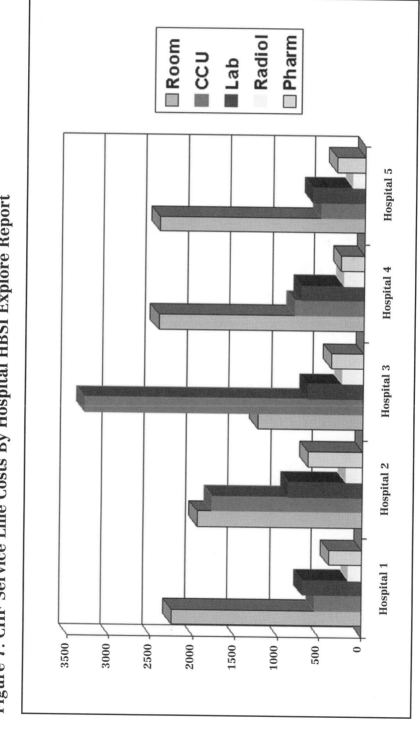

Figure 8. Outcomes Comparisons DRG 209 HBSI Integrated Outcomes Report

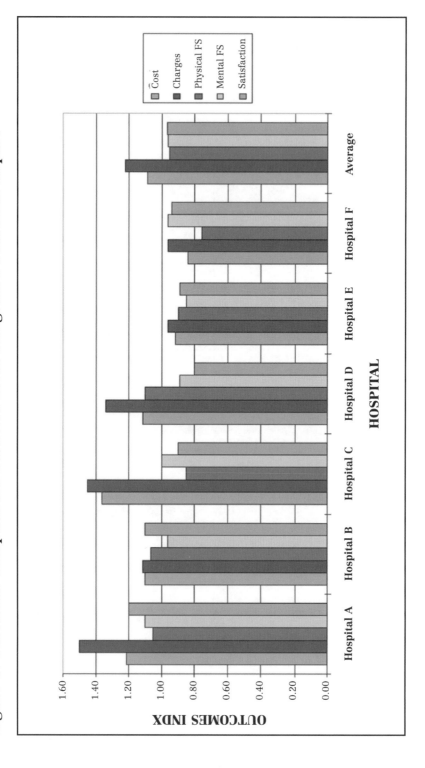

Figure 9. Variations In Care CHF > 5 Discharges

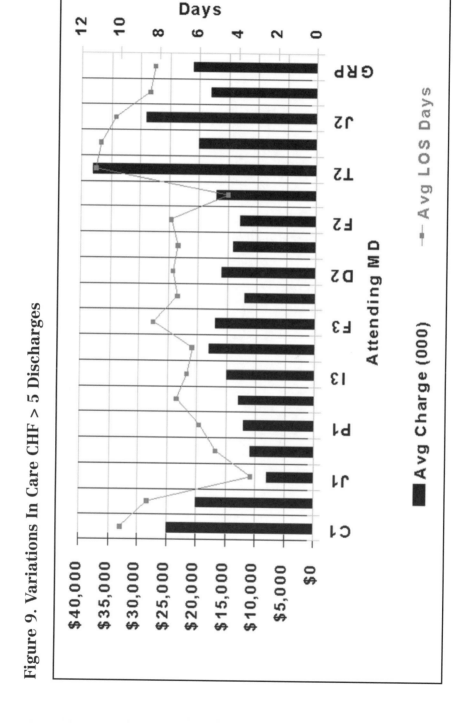

Figure 10. Aggregate Outcome Management

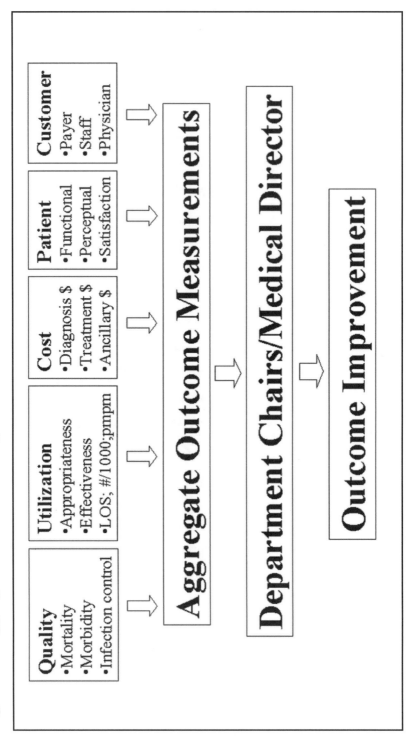

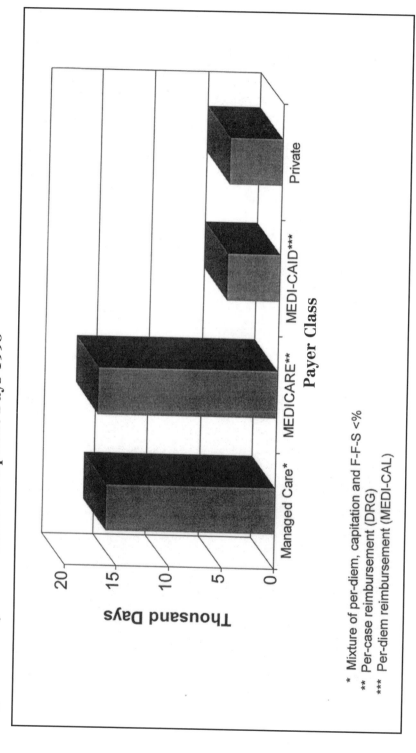

Figure 11. Payer Mix based on Inptient Days 1998

*   Mixture of per-diem, capitation and F-F-S <%
**   Per-case reimbursement (DRG)
*** Per-diem reimbursement (MEDI-CAL)

Table 4. Top Ten Admissions By Volume Profit/Loss

DRG	Cases	ALOS	Charges	Payment	T. Costs	P/(Loss)
112 PTCA	272	3.0d	$28,867	$11,989	$9,210	$2,779
127 CHF	205	5.3d	$21,012	$5,296	$7,680	($1,984)
14 CVA	170	4.9d	$22,891	$6,904	$7,856	($952)
89 PNEU	159	5.3d	23,645	$9,366	$11,565	($2,199)
209 JOINT	157	5.1d	$31,985	$14,323	$12,987	$1,336
359 TAH	116	2.5d	$16,134	$4,204	$6,189	($1,985)
88 COPD	112	5.0d	$18,443	$5,589	$6,524	($935)
106 CABG	105	8.7d	$92,154	$38,787	$31,969	$6,818
79 RESP	70	7.1d	$35,380	$9,587	$11,832	($2,345)
148 Bowel	69	10.2d	$53,679	$17,689	$19,632	($1,963)

Table 5. Projected Ancillary Charges 1998

SERVICE	CHARGES
Pharmacy	$41,077,528
Laboratory	$21,377,316
Respiratory	$13,439,218
Imaging	$3,146,880
EKG	$2,193,864
Other	$619,638
Total	$81,854,444

hospital discussed previously, figure 11, page 311, describes the hospital's patient mix based on inpatient days. You'll notice that, in an area of high managed care penetration, the bulk of the payments come from fixed dollar reimbursements. While there are mixed financial incentives in regards to length of stay, in all three of the fixed dollar categories the goal is to provide effective resource management.

The first step in the information assessment phase is to look at the top diagnoses admitted to the hospital. Table 4, page 312, sorts the top 10 diagnoses by volume, with categories for hospital charges (gross revenues), payments received (net revenues), and operating costs (fully allocated costs). Profit or loss is based on the difference between net revenues and operational costs. Figure 12, page 315, gives a graphic display of these same data plotted by profit and loss. From an institutional perspective, seven of the top 10 admissions were financial losers, in that the total costs of care exceeded total reimbursement. Congestive heart failure (CHF) was the number two diagnosis by volume, with 205 cases and an average loss per case of $1,984.

The next step is to look at the same type of information by individual department. As indicated in figure 6, page 304, both clinical and ancillary departments were targeted for study. Let's consider the ancillary departments first.

Why would you bother doing a separate analysis for ancillary services? If you refer back to figure 11, page 311, 75 percent of the hospital's payer mix falls into Medicare, Medicare Risk, Medicaid, Medicaid Risk, per-diem, or capitation payments. In all of these payer categories, there is a fixed dollar reimbursement, with no additional revenues earned for additional services rendered. Table 5, page 312, provides a listing of 1999 inpatient charges for the major ancillary departments. At year's end, there was a total of more than $81 million in charges, less than 25 percent of which would earn revenue. With this in mind, each ancillary department director was instructed to consider his or her department as a cost center rather than a revenue center and was asked to come up with strategies to improve utilization of services in the department. Each department manager was given an individual top 10 list similar to the list provided in table 6, page 314. Using respiratory services as an example, there were over $13 million in charges. The number one charge item was measurement of oxygen saturation, at $2.37 million. The number two item was delivery of oxygen, at $2.35 million. By establishing guidelines for appropriate administration and discontinuation of oxygen therapy and protocols for oxygen saturation measurement, the hospital was able to save more than $200,000 in this area alone. A similar savings was gained by developing guidelines for use of meter-dose inhaler treatments rather than the more intensive therapist-applied aerosol therapy treatments.

A similar type of process was followed for the clinical departments. Each department chair was given a listing of the top 10 diagnoses for his or her clinical department and was asked to review the data and select an appropriate

Table 6. Respiratory Care Services

Charge Code	Service Item	Charges Total (1)	Charges % of Total (2)	Charges Cum. % (3)	Units Total (4)	Units % of Total (5)	Units Cum. % (6)
183784	SAO2-Monitor-Hourly	2,378,873.20	17.70%	17.70%	102118	18.63%	18.63%
183204	Oxygen-Hourly	2,356,212.20	17.53%	35.23%	177006	32.29%	50.91%
183306	Ventilator-Continous	1,616,448.50	12.03%	47.26%	44296	8.08%	58.99%
183705	Aerosol-Treatment	1,504,259.30	11.19%	58.45%	30884	5.63%	64.62%
183785	SAO2-Measurement	1,262,136.20	9.39%	67.85%	33621	6.13%	70.76%
183206	Isolette-Oxygen	580,598.00	4.32%	72.17%	21910	4.00%	74.75%
183400	Posit-Drainage-with-	504,142.50	3.75%	75.92%	11194	2.04%	76.79%
183769	TCPO2-Hourly-Rate	397,559.00	2.96%	78.88%	18175	3.32%	80.11%
183716	Metered Dose Inhaler Trtmnt	372,183.70	2.77%	81.64%	9248	1.69%	81.80%
	80% Cutoff Total	10,972,412.60	81.64%		448452	81.81%	
	All Others	2,466,805.70	18.36%		99802	18.20%	
	Department 27 Total	13,439,218.30			548254		

Figure 12. Top 10 Admissions By Volume Profit/Loss

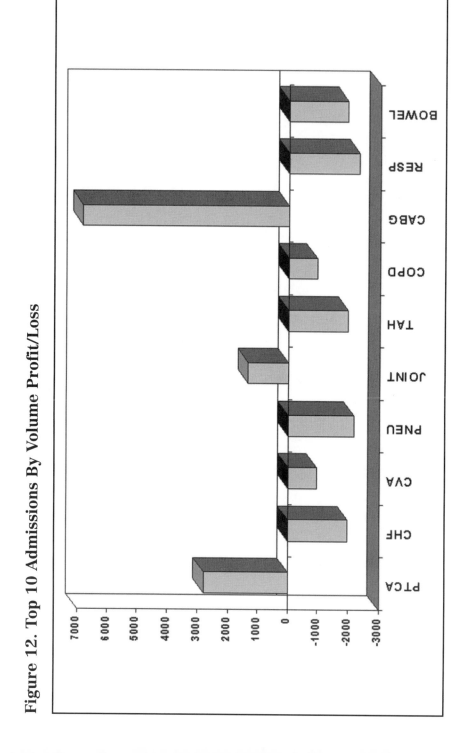

Figure 13. Distribution of Charges DRG 127

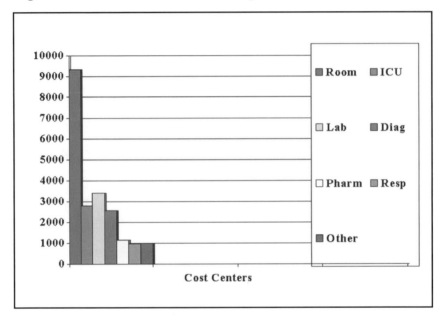

Figure 14. CHG: Break-Even Analysis

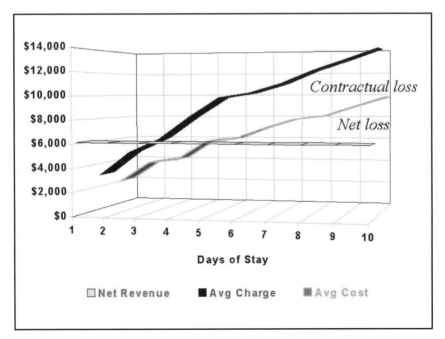

Figure 15. Variations In Care>5 Discharges

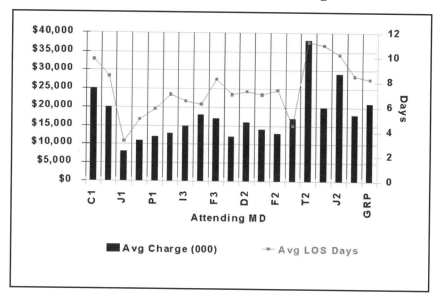

Figure 16. LOS/Cost Variance Analysis DRG127 HBSI Explore Report

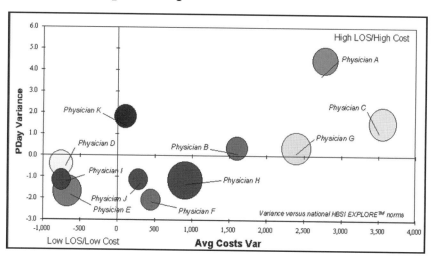

Figure 17. Distribution of Charges DRG 209

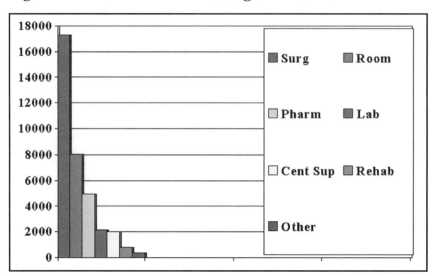

diagnosis for further study. The chairs were encouraged to select diagnoses based on volume, costs of care, and potential opportunity for improvement. Table 7, page 319, gives a listing of the top 10 diagnoses for the department of medicine. Congestive heart failure was selected as the diagnosis for further study.

With the help of the Clinical Resource Management Team (a subset of the Clinical Resource Management Steering Committee), a multidisciplinary task force was put together to study congestive heart failure. Included in the group were representatives from nursing, case management, quality assurance, decision support, and ancillary services and medical staff physicians from cardiology, the emergency department, and the department of medicine. Other members were added as the efforts became more focused. The next step in the process was to go into more depth, analyzing actual inputs and outputs of care.

As in most resource management efforts, the primary targets were services that consumed the greatest dollar outlay and had the greatest variability in care. Figure 13, page 316, gives an overview of the comparative costs of care for each of the major ancillary categories in CHF. When indicated, more detailed costing information was provided for each ancillary service, as described previously. The next step was to look for potential opportunities for improvement in each of these categories (table 8, page 320).

One of the first areas of focus was treatment in the emergency department (ED). For non-elective admissions, the bulk of the patients admitted to the hospital came in through the emergency department. Recognizing the significance of the emergency department as the major portal of entry, concentrate

Table 7. Top 10 Admissions Department Medicine

DRG	Cases	ALOS	Charges	Payment	T. Costs	P/(Loss)
127 CHF	205	5.3d	$21,012	$5,296	$7,680	($1,984)
14 CVA	170	4.9d	$22,891	$6,904	$7,856	($952)
89 PNEU	159	5.3d	$23,645	$9,366	$11,565	($2,199)
88 COPD	112	5.0d	$18,443	$5,589	$6,524	($935)
79 RESP	70	7.1d	$35,380	$9,587	$11,832	($2,345)
121 AMI	57	5.3d	$31,981	$9,524	$10,098	($574)
174 GI Hem	55	5.4d	$24,324	$6,676	$8,402	($1,726)
182 Esoph	52	5.3d	$18,520	$5,672	$6,567	($895)
296 Nutrit	50	3.7d	$11,876	$4,433	$4,256	$177
143 Chest p	48	1.8d	$6,921	$2,292	$2,391	($99)

ed efforts were made to focus on ED treatment and patient disposition.[6] With an ED physician and several cardiologist on the task force, efforts were begun to maximize treatment in the ED setting. With prompt and effective diuresis as the primary objective, a set of standardized ED orders that emphasized rapid and effective diuresis through the initiation of a progressive diuretic dosing schedule directly linked to patient response was developed. The orders also reinforced appropriate patient disposition with criteria developed for ED discharge, protracted treatment in the ED setting, admission to "observation status," and/or admission to the hospital or coronary care unit. The emergency department became such an integral part of the resource management program that a dedicated task force was formed to analyze overall performance in the ED setting, using the same type of data modeling and consensus group input described previously.

As evidenced by the graphic, the biggest dollar spending for CHF was for room and board. Room and board rates are a reflection of total days in the hospital (length of stay) and of the intensity level of the bed being occupied. It is obviously more costly to treat the patient in the CCU setting than it is to treat the patient on the medical floor. Remember, most of the patients with CHF are elderly, and, under the Medicare DRG case rate reimbursement schedule, you get a fixed dollar reimbursement regardless of how long the patient is in the hospital and the services supplied while they're there. Because room and board charges accounted for more than 50 percent of the patient's bill, strategies designed to promote transfer to the most appropriate level of care and expediency in discharge will have a significant dollar impact for patients reimbursed under traditional Medicare (per-case) or Medicare Risk (capitation) contracts.

Table 8. CHF Cost Center Analysis

ER Services	Portal of entry
Room Charge	CCU VS Telemetry*
Board & Care	Medical Surgery/ SNF
Nursing	Discharge Status
Laboratory	Isoenzymes?
	Blood Gas VS Oximetry
Pharmacy	Diuretic Therapy
	Ace Inhibitors?
	Other?
Respiratory	Oxygen therapy
	Aerosol treatments
Diagnostics	Echocardiogram?
	Tread Mill/ Thallium scan?
	Cardiac Catheterization?

As is true for most medical diagnoses, the remainder of the costs are more or less evenly spread across the other ancillary services. Efficiencies can still be gained through proper use of the pharmacy, laboratory, and respiratory services as discussed previously. When looking at additional diagnostics, you must always ask yourself if the additional testing is really going to change the way you manage the patient. This is particularly true if you have a teaching program. Residents love to order the latest and greatest in technological assessment, yet rarely use the information to change their patient management regimen. Using this rationale, the group discussed what it felt represented optimal patterns of care based on best demonstrated practice patterns and developed a set of preprinted admission orders and appropriateness criteria for admission to the CCU. In conjunction with the appropriateness criteria and guidelines, a clinical pathway that focused on managing the key critical elements of care appropriate for this group of patients was developed. Effective diuresis, use of ACE inhibitors, home health consultation, and assessment of readmission rates were the key elements used to monitor patient response and outcomes of care.

After the group decided on the best course of care, the information was presented to members of the department of medicine. Two weeks prior to the meeting, each physician received a letter from the department chair stating that there would be an information-sharing educational session on CHF at the next meeting. As part of the letter, each physician also received a copy of his or her practice profile, as indicated in Table 9, below. At the department meeting, findings and recommendations of the task force committee were presented to the physicians. In order to stress the importance of financial risk, the physicians were presented with a series of additional graphics that emphasized the need for providing more cost-effective patient management. Figure 14, page 316, shows the average break-even point for all patients admitted to the hospital with CHF. The top line represents the daily accrual of patient charges. The straight line is the average net payment. When total charges exceed the average payment, there is a contractual loss. The lower line represents the average costs of care as they accrued per day. The break-even point is 3.4 days. In order to illustrate significant variations in care, several graphics were used to highlight the notable physician differences in care.

Figure 15, page 317, shows the differences in lengths of stay and charges among a selection of physicians with at least five admissions for CHF. Figure 16, page 317, was used to highlight individual differences in performance outcomes. Benchmark performers achieving optimal results are highlighted in the lower left quadrant of the bubble graph.

The basic assumption for process and outcome improvement is that, for several reasons, there are significant variations in overall patient management. First and foremost, some patients are sicker than others and require more resources. In order to more fairly interpret these data, one must account for differences in patient severity through some form of severity, risk, or case-mix adjustment. A second reason for variation is in clinical management. Decisions when to admit; recommendations for a procedure or special testing; the use of consultants; and other differences in overall diagnosis, treatment, and patient disposition account for a significant degree of variation in patient processing and outcomes of care. A third important source of variations is related to system issues. Are you able to get the patient on the operating room schedule? Is the patient waiting for a test result? Are lower level of care beds available? Do you have utilization management and discharge

Table 9. DRG 127 Physician Profile

MD	Cases	LOS	G Rev	Room	Pharm	Lab	X-Ray
C	11	9.7	24123	10870	1019	4126	1060
H	8	8.4	20246	9555	706	2770	820
Klein	12	11.1	20057	11264	1183	3803	595
JJ	11	10.2	29466	11500	925	3772	1044
VV	9	4.4	8619	4092	258	2240	265
JJJ	23	6.9	12645	6973	741	2428	349
...	...	...	...	...	...	...	...
Total	280	8.3	21012	9349	1154	3427	705

planning working on the weekends? Reducing unnecessary variations in care will go a long way in improving efficiencies in care.

It took about nine months to generate and have accepted a set of preprinted ED and inpatient orders for treatment of patients presenting with congestive heart failure. It took another three months to get the key indicators of the clinical pathway up and running. One year later, there was a 15 percent reduction in overall costs of care and a 0.5 day reduction in average length of stay.

Case Example: Total Hip Procedures

A similar type of process was followed for the department of orthopedics. A task force was convened, with physicians, nursing, and administrative representatives from the departments of surgery and orthopedic surgery, pharmacy, physical therapy, case management, quality management, and central supply in an effort to provide multidisciplinary input to important aspects of care that could potentially benefit from targeted process improvement activities. As with the process used for congestive heart failure, information was aggregated into specific performance templates designed to present an overview of utilization and resource consumption patterns for patients undergoing total hip procedures. Table 10, page 323, gives an example of Dr. Casey's performance profile compared to his peers for total joint procedures. Figure 17, page 318, gives an overview of the comparative costs of care for each of the major resource centers affected by these procedures. Unlike a medical diagnosis, where most of the costs are more or less evenly distributed across all ancillary departments, surgery accounts for most of the costs in a pure surgical admission. Under the surgery cost center is included time in surgery, anesthesia, supplies, and recovery room. The biggest item under central supply is the cost of the hip prosthesis and associated nuts and bolts reinforcements.

Through the efforts of a designated sub-task force, a group was convened to address opportunities for improving efficiencies in scheduling, staffing, patient flow, and overall supply management and utilization. A dedicated program of orthopedic supply-demand matching that significantly improved costs and efficiencies in prosthesis utilization was also implemented. Unlike with the complicated acute emergency medical admission in the case of congestive heart failure, the task force found it easier to develop, implement, administer, and monitor the key elements of care for a relatively straightforward surgical diagnosis through a multidiscipline-supported clinical pathway. The pathway focused on the key elements of care related to the hospital admission and procedure and included a preoperative education and assessment phase as well as a post hospitalization rehabilitation phase as part of its structure. Studies one year later showed significant reductions in lengths of stay and total costs of care.

Return on Investment

As we move through the realm of performance improvement and resource management, it is essential to be able to document the impact and benefits of

Table 10. DRG 209 Physician Profile

MD	LOS	Surg	Room	Phar	Lab	PT
A	4.9	14087	7736	4888	1642	721
B	6.0	11621	9176	4233	2186	1023
Casey	4.8	14873	7925	4724	2316	714
D	5.5	12454	8088	5623	2359	778
......	......	......	......	......	......	......
Avg.	5.1	13339	8016	4963	2147	767

what we do. Despite the fact that our core business is to provide high-quality care, with the overall concern about managing financial risk, providers have

been forced to focus on the cost-savings impact of their process improvement activities. In the inpatient sector, the traditional way of assessing the cost-savings impact of resource management activities is to assess the impact on LOS and costs of care. Unfortunately, the financial impact is often misrepresented, as indicated in the examples presented below.

The traditional interpretation in reducing length of stay is that, for every day's reduction, the hospital saves x dollars. If we assume an average variable cost per day of $300 in a hospital with 10,000 admissions per year, and a reduction in LOS from 4.5 days to 4.0 days, the hospital will have reduced its total inpatient days by 5,000. One might assume that the hospital has just saved $1,500,000 (5,000 days x $300) in hospital-related costs. But reducing LOS only benefits the hospital for those patients reimbursed on either a per-case or capitation arrangement. Reducing LOS actually works against you financially for patients reimbursed under a fee-for-service (FFS) or per-diem payment schedule. A more realistic approach would be to factor in the impact on all payment categories. If 60 percent of the inpatient population is reimbursed under either per-case or capitation arrangements, the hospital will save $900,000 in daily costs. However, for the 40 percent of the patients covered under FFS or per-diem contracts, shortening the LOS would actually reduce revenues by $600,000. The savings is only $300,000. These assumptions are illustrated in table 11, page 324.

Another traditional method used to assess costs of care is to analyze the financial impact of clinical pathways. As illustrated in table 12, page 325, if we assume that the hospital had 10,000 admissions per year with an the

Table 11. Lengths of Stay and Payer Mix

- Average variable cost/ day $300
- 10,000 admissions/ yr. ALOS 4.5 days (Non OB)
- $10,000 \times 4.5 = 45,000$ days
- $10,000 \times 4.0 = 40,000$ days
- $5,000 \times 300 = \$1,500,000$?
- $5,000 \times \$300 = 900,000^1 - 600,000^2 = \$300,000$

1 60% per-case/ capitation

2 40% FFS/ per diem

average cost per case of $6,000 and that 30 percent of the admissions are covered by critical paths with an average cost savings of 10 percent, the initial assumption might be that the hospital saved $1,800,000. In this case, the cost savings are attributable to a reduction in both length of stay and resource consumption. Reducing resource consumption is of financial benefit for per-case, per-diem, and capitation coverage, but it works against you in FFS. If we consider a hospital with a 25 percent FFS mix and the fact that there is an financial tradeoff between length of stay and cost reduction for the 15 percent per-diem mix, the actual savings is $630,000. Note that neither of these analyses takes into account the cost of decision-support services provided.

A third aspect to consider is the financial impact of quality of care. Quality is often difficult to measure, and incorporating measurement of quality into the cost accounting methodology often adds an additional level of complexity to the analysis. In fact, most quality measurements in health care focus on unwanted quality outcomes. Mortality rates, morbidity rates, infection rates, and readmission rates are examples of traditional quality assessment indicators, and each of these unwanted events comes at a price. Prevention of adverse events not only will improve the likelihood of positive patient outcomes but also will prevent accumulation of unnecessary additional costs of care attributable to these conditions. One of the most frequently studied quality indicators is adverse drug events (ADEs). According to expert sources, potentially preventable ADEs can add $2,000 to $4,000 in increased cost and two to four additional days to the length of stay of a hospitalization.[5] Other quality indicators with equally important financial implications are nosocomial infections, surgical wound infections, decubitus ulcers, and patient falls.

Table 12. Lengths of Stay and Payer Mix

- Top 25 DRGs 30 - 50% of hospital business
- Average cost $6,000.
- Average number of admissions 10,000
- Cost savings CP 10%
- 10,000 x 30% x $600 = $1,800.000?
- 10,000 admits x 30%[1] x 35%[2] x $600[3] = $630,000

1   30% admissions covered by CPs
2   60% at per-case/ capitation - 25% FFS
3   6000 cost x 10% cost savings CP

Table 13, page 326, provides a listing of the average frequency and the cost implications of potentially preventable adverse events. Given the relatively frequent

occurrence of these adverse events, any cost analysis should be able to assess the impact of pharmacy support, quality control, and risk manage

ment programs designed to reduce the likelihood of their occurrence.

A more accurate measure of financial impact falls under the umbrella of return on investment (ROI). Measuring ROI in health care is a tricky business. As illustrated in table 14, page 326, there are intricacies in health care measurement that are different from the usual expense and revenue determinations afforded by traditional ROI methodologies. First is the issue of revenues. Whereas, in the retail marketplace, revenues are measured as monies earned, under fixed dollar reimbursement incentives in health care, the economic benefits are gained from cost reduction. Second is the lack of proficiency and consistency in cost analysis. Many hospitals still do not have accurate cost accounting systems, and, for those that do, there is no consensus on cost accounting methodologies. Another confounding factor is the multiple divergent financial incentives for inpatient care. As alluded to earlier, the same action may have different economic consequences because of the financial implications of different insurance categories. Payer mix must be considered in order to provide a more reliable assessment of revenue activity. A fourth aspect is the cause and effect attribution. Just because a program was implemented doesn't necessarily mean that, by itself, caused the noted effect.

Table 13. Average Cost Implications of Adverse Events

Incident	Occurrence	Cost per episode
ADEs	5%	$3,000
Falls	2%	$2,000
Decubitis ulcers	5%	$9,000
Nosocomial	1%	$2,000

Table 14. Intricacies in ROI Assessment

- Traditional ROI maximizes revenue return
  PI ROI maximizes cost reduction

- Financial/ system % allocation to clinical PI?

- Cost measurement/Methodology/Interpretation?

- Divergent payment incentives*

- Quantitative vs. qualitative cost-benefits

- Short-term vs. long-term benefits

- Cause and effect? Multidisciplinary efforts

- Cost-quality impact

- Cost shifting?

Despite these shortcomings, it is still possible to perform an accurate ROI analysis for resource management activities. The two crucial components are the ability to capture all the underlying costs of decision-support/resource management activities and then to be able to document in financial terms all the related outputs of these efforts.

Decision support is a catchall term used to describe the various performance improvement/resource management activities needed to support the delivery of cost-effective, high-quality care. Included in decision-support activities are programs related to case management, quality management, infection control, risk management, and any other specialized programs geared to improve efficiencies in the management of ancillary or special services. Much of this activity is supported by a heavy investment in information technology.

Because clinical pathways have had such a vital impact on patient outcomes, let's go back to the clinical pathways scenario presented previously. In order to perform a more appropriate ROI evaluation of critical pathway activities, you need to assess the overall costs and benefits of the entire program. Table 15, page 328, illustrates a straightforward analysis of the labor costs involved in building a clinical pathway. On the average, we estimate that it takes three nurses, each contributing 40 hours of work; two (paid) physicians, each contributing a 20 hours work; and three other support staff, each contributing 40 hours, to create a single pathway. Other personnel may be involved in pathway design, and the appropriate costs, either direct or indirect opportunity costs, should be accounted for in the process. We then estimate that it takes about 26 weeks to build a pathway and that five pathways could be produced in one year. After the process is learned, subsequent pathways should cost less and be produced in a more productive fashion. If the institution has implemented an automated process for pathway development wherein data are collected and assimilated through a software program designed to provide computerized assistance for pathway building, the labor costs and the speed of implementation would be reduced. Also important to consider are the after-pathway construction costs involved in monitoring, variance tracking, and pathway maintenance. Various studies have estimated that the cost savings of clinical pathways can average between 10 and 40 percent per pathway case. Success rates will vary, depending on the magnitude of influence of the external environment and the internal culture and commitment of the individual institution. Using a conservative estimate of 10 percent, table 16, page 328, presents a listing of the projected cost savings attainable through implementation of clinical paths. For a hospital averaging 150 admissions per year for the top five diagnoses (excluding OB) and having an average cost of $6,000 per case, the hospital would accumulate a projected cumulative cost savings of $450,000, payer mix not considered. The projected cumulative cost savings for the next five DRGs averaging 100 admissions per year would be $300,000. The total projected cost savings for all 25 DRGs would be $1,305,000.

For a more comprehensive decision-support perspective, table 17, page 331, presents an overview of the cost appreciation of all the components necessary for building, implementing, and monitoring a decision-support/clinical

Table 15. Costs of Pathway Development

```
LABOR            Manual                          Automated*
3 RNs 40hrs 35.00 =   4,200.00   3 RNs 30hrs 35.00 =   3,150.00
2 MDs 20hrs 150.00 = 6,000.00    2 MDs 15hrs 150.00 = 4,500.00
3 other 40hrs 25.00 = 3,000.00   3 other 20hrs 25.00 = 2,250.00
TOTAL LABOR      13,200.00                         9,900.00


TIME TO DEVELOPMENT
Weeks to complete        26      Weeks to complete  15
Paths year one            5      Paths year one      6


* Time, labor, compliance monitoring, variance tracking, erosion
```

Table 16. Clinical Paths: Cost Savings

TOP 25 DRGs	Cases/DRG	Total cases	Total cost[1]	Proj. savings[2]
1-5	150	750	4,500,000	450,000
6-10	100	500	3,000,000	300,000
11-15	75	375	2,250,000	225,000
16-20	60	300	1,800,000	180,000
21-25	50	250	1,500,000	150,000
Total		2175	13,050,000	1,305,000

[1]Average cost per DRG 6,000.00
[2]Average cost reduction CP 10%

pathway program. The various components and dollar attributes will differ from institution to institution; the model should be construed merely as a template for documenting appropriate variables. In year one, we allocate the cost of the base information system devoted for decision support as a percentage of the utility of system use in that area. If the core information system cost was $2,000,000 and 25 percent of its utility was used for decision support, $500,000 would be applied as the cost of the system. Factored into the cost in year one is $20,000 for maintenance, $50,000 for other technical support, $5,000 for annual license fees, $50,000 for training fees, and $100,000 to cover the costs of additional FTEs dedicated to the program. The subtotal information technology cost is $725,000. Although not included in the present analysis, systems specializing in severity of illness or risk assessment; benchmarking systems; software products that support case management, quality management, infection control, or risk management; point of care systems; specialty software systems designed to provide analytical services for special units or services such as the intensive care unit, cardiology, perinatal care, surgery, or pharmacy services; and any other computer application used in the decision-support process would be applicable to the analysis.

Following the example depicted in table 15, we assumed an average labor cost per pathway of $10,000 and attributed a total of $50,000 to the first year labor costs necessary to generate five clinical pathways. An additional $75,000 was allocated for the labor costs required for pathway monitoring. This amounted to a subtotal of $125,000 for pathway labor costs, with a cumulative year one cost of $850,000. The same approach was used for years two to five. Obviously, hardware and software costs would be less in subsequent years, unless the institution purchased additional decision-support information technology. After the one-year learning curve, the institution would be able to implement and monitor more pathways (an additional 10 per year for at least the next two years) at a lower total cost per pathway. The cumulative costs after five years amounted to $2,325,000.

On the revenue side, one must look at cost savings rather than earned revenue because of the payment incentives discussed previously. We not only must account for the direct cost impact related to room and board and resource consumption, but also must be able to account for the benefits of appropriate cost avoidance programs. For example, one of the advantages of an effective case management program is to expedite process flow and timely treatment and disposition, thereby avoiding potential delays in service. Another advantage of real-time case management is to make recommendations for ordering a more effective treatment alternative, thereby avoiding the additional cost of a nonessential or less effective service alternative. Other examples of cost avoidance programs include quality management, infection control, risk management, and pharmacy intervention programs. Unfortunately, the value of many of these services is rarely appreciated because no one has gone to the trouble of documenting the impact of these interventions and bringing it into the cost avoidance revenue stream.

As hard as it is to quantify the direct cost impact on patient services, quantifying the impact on quality of care poses an even more difficult problem. While we were able to attach a dollar value related to adverse events, how do you attach a dollar value to high-quality care and patient improvement, particularly when the benefits may not show up for years?

Table 18, page 331, combines all the expense and cost saving figures into a ROI table. In year one, there is no direct cost savings to the institution, as it takes awhile to realize the savings from pathway implementation. However, it is assumed $75,000 is gained through the Hawthorne Effect described previously. Experience has shown that, once a program has been targeted for study, improvement occurs almost instantaneously, as the perception of performance monitoring produces notable changes in behavior well before actual implementation of the completed action plan. In a similar vein, based on the cost-saving values presented earlier, newly instituted decision-support activities from case management, resource management, pharmacy intervention programs, risk management programs, and computer-assisted artificial intelligence were estimated to save an additional $75,000 in the first year, for a total decision-support savings in year one of $150,000. In year two, most of the programs will have been well on their way, and the savings should increase substantially. Assuming that five clinical pathways were implemented in year two, based on the previous assumptions, a total of $450,000 would be saved. However, taking into account the economics of payer mix, in the first two years the cost savings would only be realized for that portion of the patients covered by risk contracts. For years two and three, we'll assume that 50 percent of the patients were at risk through either per-case or capitation contracts. In year two, the adjusted savings from clinical pathways would add $300,000 and the total savings from decision support activities would add up to $500,000. In year three, the projected savings from clinical pathways, now 15 in number, would save an adjusted total of $450,000 and decision-support activities would generate another $500,000 in cost reductions. Cumulative cost savings at the end of year three would be $1,900.000. Applying the costs of operation depicted in table 17, the total cumulative costs at the end of year three amounted to $1,695,000. In years four and five, we make an assumption that 75 percent of the patients will migrate into financial risk contracts, and the pathway costs have been adjusted accordingly. At the end of year five, there is a projected cumulative critical pathway savings of $2,684,000 and a total cumulative clinical pathway/decision-support savings of $4,759,000. The cumulative costs of information systems and personnel is $2,325,000. As illustrated in the bottom of the table and in figure 18, page 332, the break-even point for clinical pathway implementation is in year five. The break-even point for combined clinical pathway and decision support efforts is in year three.

Conclusion

As health care organizations face increasing pressures to manage financial risk, the demands to provide and demonstrate cost-effective, high-quality patient care will steadily increase. Successful strategies designed to improve efficiencies in care come from a multidisciplinary commitment to developing

Table 17. Decision Support/Pathway Costs

Expense Category	Year 1	Year 2	Year 3	Year 4	Year 5
Hardware/software[1]	500,000	35,000	15,000	15,000	15,000
Annual maintenance	20,000	20,000	20,000	25,000	25,000
Decision support (1.5 FTE)	100,000	100,000	110,000	110,000	110,000
Other technical support	50,000	25,000	30,000	25,000	25,000
Annual license fees	5,000	5,000	5,000	5,000	5,000
Training (opportunity costs)	50,000	30,000	10,000	10,000	5,000
Subtotal direct IT costs	**725,000**	**215,000**	**190,000**	**190,000**	**185,000**
Labor costs (development)[2]	50,000(5)	75,000(10)	65,000(10)	15.000	10,000
Monitoring[3]	75,000	150,000	150,000	125,000	100,000
Subtotal indirect labor costs	**125,000**	**225,000**	**215,000**	**140,000**	**115,000**
Cumulative total costs	**850,000**	**1,290,000**	**1,695,000**	**2,025.000**	**2,325,000**

[1]Dollar allocation of information system to decision support (25%)
[2]10,000.00 labor costs per critical pathway (5)
[3]CM/ CNS % time CP 0.25 FTE ($40,000) Pathway monitoring

Table 18. Cost Reductions Clinical Path/Decision Support

	Year 1 (0)	Year 2 (5)	Year 3 (15)	Year 4 (25)	Year 5 (25)
Cost reduction all payors[1]		450,000	750,000	975,000	1,305,000
Cost savings 50%[2]	75,000a	300,000	450,000	.....	.....
Cost savings 75%[3]	.....	.....	.....	806,000	1,053,000
Cumulative CP cost savings	**75,000**	**375,000**	**825,000**	**1,631,000**	**2,684,000**
Additional DS savings[4]	*75,000*	*500,000*	*500,000*	*500,000*	*500,000*
Cumulative DS savings	**75,000**	**575,000**	**1,075,000**	**1,575,000**	**2,075,000**
Cumulative total savings	**150,000**	**950,000**	**1,900,000**	**3,206,000**	**4.759,000**
Information system costs	725,000	215,000	190,000	190,000	185.000
Labor support costs	125,000	225,000	215,000	140,000	115,000
Cumulative total costs	**850,000**	**1,290,000**	**1,695,000**	**2,025,000**	**2,325,000**
Projected savings CP5	775,000)	(915,000)	(870,000)	(394,000)	359,000
Projected savings CP & DS	(700,000)	(340,000)	205,000	1,181,000	2,434,000

aHawthorne effect
[1]CP projected savings assume 10% reductions in costs via implementation/ CPs savings: a payor mix
[2]50% Medicare/ capitation/ global payments
[3]75% Medicare/ capitation/ global payments
[4]Additional Decision Support Interventions: Case management, Alerts & reminders, Resource management, Supply and materials management, Operational efficiencies, Pharmacy intervention, Risk management, Reduction in adverse events, other (50% cost benefit years 1-3; 75% cost benefit years 4-5)
[5]Cumulative costs - CP savings

Figure 18. ROI Break—Even Analysis

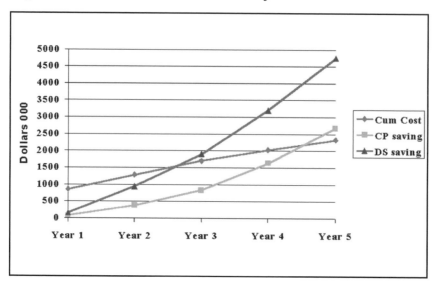

and implementing both operational and clinical programs focused on effective resource management based on sound information systems and clinical decision support. The Clinical Resource Management Program described here proved to be an effective vehicle for managing one organization's resources by developing a structured program that integrated the efforts of the individuals who have control over the processes involved in patient care. Experience has shown us that, if you provide clinicians with accurate and meaningful information and give them adequate support, they will enthusiastically participate in the development and use of tools that will provide optimal, efficient patient care. The process will benefit the organization, physicians, and the populations they serve.

With the growing need to document outcomes and to demonstrate the value of services, hospitals and physicians need to develop a template for outcome measurement and outcome management. In order to provide cost-effective, high-quality care, institutions need to invest heavily in human and technical support services. In an effort to assess the impact of this commitment, institutions need to be able to develop a methodology for measuring the quantitative and the qualitative costs and benefits of services rendered. Using an ROI model that considers the financial impact of both cost and quality care will help institutions in this process.

References

1. Rosenstein, A. "Healthcare Resource Management: Integrating Apples and Oranges." *Journal of Healthcare Resource Management* 15(10):10-7, Dec. 1997.

2. HBSI Action Module, Operational Benchmarking Performance Analysis software, Bellevue, Wash.

3. Rosenstein, A. "Using Information Management to Implement a Clinical Resource Management Program." *Joint Commission Journal on Quality Improvement* 23(12):653-66, Dec. 1997.

4. Rosenstein, A., and Proptnik, T. "Case Management." *Journal of HealthCare Management* 15(2):11-6, March 1997.

5. Rosenstein, A. "Measuring the Benefits of Clinical Decision Support: Return on Investment." *Health Care Management Review* 24(2):32-43, Spring 1999.

6. Rosenstein, A. and others. "Timing Is Everything: Impact of Emergency Department Care on Hospital Length of Stay." *Journal of Clinical Outcomes Management.* 7(8):31-6, Aug. 2000.

Alan H. Rosenstein, MD, MBA, is Vice President/Medical Director, VHA West Coast, Pleasanton, California, and Medical Director, Clinical Decision Support, HBSI, Bellevue, Washington.

Chapter

A Personal View of the Growth of the Medical Management Profession

by James E. Hartfield, MD, CPE, FACPE

In a rather evangelistic speech to assembled medical directors almost 15 years ago, I proclaimed that "physicians have only themselves to blame if we let government and politicians, insurance companies and actuaries, or hospitals and administrators determine the future of our profession. We are capable of learning and managing." Shortly thereafter, I was approached by a health care organization and asked basically "to put my money where my mouth was," and I left clinical practice to do just that. Actually, I never left practice—I shifted my patient base to the corporate millions of plan members and, through a variety of management venues, have never regretted that shift. It has certainly not been a "success story" in the storybook fashion, but the ride has been as thrilling as any roller coaster.

The evolution of medical management as a certifiable specialty within medicine and of an individual physician as a certified physician executive has been a remarkable progression of stunning leadership, stupefying serendipity, and classic hard work. Although perhaps not as dramatic as the theoretical rise from amphibian to astronaut, the emergence of this proud professional niche is almost as unnatural in concept.

In a classic booklet, *Doctor in the Making,* published in 1943 by Drs. A.W. Ham and M.D. Salter, the first chapter, entitled, "You and the Medical Course," contains this opening paragraph: "Embarking on a medical course bears certain similarities to embarking on a polar expedition. Both are arduous adventures. Anyone who sets off on either without a true appreciation of the hardships involved is not likely to reach his goal. And, even if a person thinks the goal is worth the hardship, he is not likely to succeed unless he has enough and the right sort of equipment. So, before you take the final step and register in medical school, you should satisfy yourself that you neither underestimate the hardships nor overestimate your desire to reach your goal, and that you have enough and the right sort of equipment to finish the journey."[1]

It is clear from the admonitions to prospective students of medicine that the authors never entertained the scope of scientific challenge faced by contemporary physicians. It is ever more apparent that the insertion of business and management in that learning curriculum was inconceivable and, perhaps, unconscionable, as some of our senior colleagues affirm even today. The wisdom of their initial warnings and the comparison to a "polar expedition" are certainly current and relevant.

Successful physicians have always been "creative scientists," whether as a surgeon manipulating through an unexpected operative finding or as an internist paring away unrelated complaints to determine an accurate diagnosis. It was within this creative mode that medical management as a formally defined course of study arose. Generations of physicians had served as managing leaders and had made business decisions that had sustained practical impact, but it was not until the late 1960s that political and economic realities demanded a more structured approach to curriculum development. Rising health care costs, post-Vietnam unrest, and evolving managed care mechanisms placed physicians in the unaccustomed role of defending the integrity of the medical profession. Most agreed that seeking a workable solution, i.e., "going on the offense," was more desirable than reactionary rhetoric, but physicians were not adequately prepared to deal with issues of contracting, marketing, financing, or time and conflict management.

Against this challenging backdrop, the American Group Practice Association convened in Washington, D.C., during an annual meeting in 1974, a collection of group practice medical directors. The focus was educational, and potential target audiences of physicians were listed: group practice, hospitals, managed care, insurance, military, academic, etc. The American Academy of Medical Directors was born, and a new specialty was described with a defined basic curriculum. The response from physicians who had customarily been "appointed to serve" as medical directors was dramatic, and, even through an organization name change to the American College of Physician Executives, growth and recognition of the specialty of medical management continues on an unprecedented curve.

It is particularly appropriate in this concluding chapter of a book that takes a continuing and updated look at the "Fundamentals" of this specialty to recognize some of the things that have been learned thus far in the "expedition"; to reflect upon the personal impact of the travels; and to postulate briefly, and conservatively, on the road ahead.

Choices

The warning that "you have to kiss a lot of frogs before you find a real prince" was undoubtedly issued to mid-level managers concerning their CEOs, whether corporate executives, commanding officers, or hospital administrators. As physicians assume management responsibilities, they are more likely today to enter at a middle management position until some track record of experience can be accumulated. The process of management progress is filled with a wide array of choices, with no guarantee about the outcome of a right or wrong selection or even that such options exist. It is clear that what might be a successful venture for one physician manager may prove to be a disaster for another because of differences in personality compatibilities, mastered skills, and available opportunities. More often than not, the disappointments are related to "things beyond my control," such as organizational restructuring or failure, unrealistic expectations, or personnel changes. The "toady" CEO is a significant force, depending on how he or she intends to use the physician's talents. Perhaps it reflects some latent hostility toward a personal doc in the past, but, whatever the cause, many nonphysician executives seem to enjoy emphasizing their positional superiority or authority over staff physicians. It rarely helps to point out their personality disorders or to offer to prescribe medications.

So some choices must be made: Does the end of this employment justify the means? Is this an inherent company/organizational problem, or it is mine? Should I even be in this job? The often too-late and personally painful realization surfaces that those questions are in the wrong order. It is of primary importance that physicians interested in becoming "executives" address honestly the basic question: "Is this the job for me? Should I even be in this job?"

Examine carefully your motives for electing the specialty of medical management. Honest answers to the following questions might be of some help in your evaluation:

- *Is this job decision in line with my reasons for entering Medicine?*

- *Will my becoming a successful physician executive be as satisfying to me as becoming a respected clinician?*

- *In which frame of reference do I currently find myself:*

Defensive:

> "I cannot stand any more paperwork in my practice!"
> "If you can't beat 'em, join 'em!"
> "I'll never make enough money to survive in this practice!"
> "I won't have nurses or actuaries telling me how to practice medicine!"

Offensive:

> "I have the ability to make a significant contribution to management!"
> "Something must be done to help control the cost of medical care!"
> "I can work productively in a non-clinical office to improve clinical care!"
> "I can work cooperatively with non-physicians to enhance health care delivery!"

It is fair to acknowledge that a mixture of some of these offensive and defensive reference questions will exist in many satisfied physician executives, but unless a personal future offers some enlightening challenge or stimulating anticipation, it is rarely worth the effort to make a major change in professional activity. Look around at your colleagues and you will find adequate examples:

- "Burned out" practitioners who are increasingly confrontational with patients, late or absent from work, or sour with associates and employees.

- Over-involved physicians whose involvements are in any area other than medicine. Note in passing the number of lawyers who practice anything other than law.

Sometimes I worry a bit about the sustained volume of physicians from every specialty who are joining the American College of Physician Executives. Not everyone who joins is leaving medical practice totally, probably just the converse, but if medical management is just another "involvement," I have doubts about that physician's success or satisfaction in this very different arena of service. I heartily applaud learning efforts if they are directed toward improving personal business knowledge or skills for any professional application.

Full- or Part-Time Management

One of the choices encountered early after deciding to pursue a management focus is the question of full- or part-time commitment. Essentially, this is a question of whether to try staying current in my field of clinical expertise or not. That "not" is a knotty consideration. In this era of rapid technological advances and pharmaceutical developments, maintaining a current state of clinical awareness in any single field is a major challenge. It is not made particularly easier by keeping a part-time foot in the clinical office, but admittedly it is probably somewhat enhanced. Often, the choice is made by the job description of the prospective management position; however, the more senior the position or the greater the management responsibility, the more likely that full-time commitment is required.

This issue of part- or full-time management has been reviewed repeatedly[2] and has been frequently associated with maintaining credibility among one's peers. While I doubt that my continuing to practice pediatrics made my management decisions any more acceptable to neurosurgeons or radiologists, I do agree that my having practiced for many years was significant. My part-time practice was probably of greater concern to me during those hours when I knew my colleagues were being overwhelmed in the outpatient clinic while I sat reeling with management imponderables in my other office. One of my most cherished comments came from a dear friend and pediatric associate who stopped by my office one morning "to take a break from the crying crowds in the clinic." When I apologized for not being there to help, he shook his head and stated pointedly, "Hey, don't give it another thought. We need you here to do for us what we cannot do for ourselves. We will take care of the kids—you take care of us!" I will quit managing when I find I am no longer needed.

The Entry Point

The next major choice confronting a physician entering management involves the entry point—that is, where and how to enter management.

While the subject of career choices has been effectively reviewed elsewhere,[3-5] one look at the number of opportunities currently available to medical managers should emphasize several considerations:

- What am I best prepared to do? Academic leadership appointments require a vastly different résumé than a managed care medical director opening. Hospital administrative officers demand different experiences than medical underwriters for insurance companies.

- Am I willing to move my home? Geographic relocation is a basic component of a military career or of most managed care positions. This question is a family consideration and relates to spouse employment, children's education, and health requirements.

- Do I need to enhance or supplement my education for this position? An MBA or MPH may not be required, but adequate educational time allotment may be necessary to attend ACPE courses or to develop required computer skills.

- Am I willing to adopt this organization's "corporate culture?" Everyone understands uniforms and saluting within a military position, but not everyone is prepared for the dress codes or environmental restrictions that are common in large corporations.

Some of the answers to these and other cautious considerations may require only a simple and honest self-assessment. Without a doubt, if you are not honest with your own personal appraisal, someone else eventually will be—and your job, or at least your bonus, may depend on it. Other answers should be sought with the assistance of a search firm representative utilized by the employer or your own contracted organization. Many job conflicts that occur after employment might have been avoided with an up-front understanding of job expectations and performance objectives, both for you personally and for the company. For some unexplained reason, physicians seem reluctant to seek such advance job clarification, yet it can provide important insight into the critical choice of accepting a job offer.

Time To Move On

After devoting substantial energies in one medical management position, whether successful or not, the question of changing positions usually arises. To most physicians, the decision on where to practice after completing residency training is projected to be a life-long commitment, and indeed, for generations of practitioners, such was the case. The opposite is more likely to be found in medical management. Job changing is often dictated by the availability of advancement potential, corporate stability, or performance evaluations. Some employers even prefer a broad and varied background of employment experiences. The decision to move, if the choice is yours, should be based on a careful review of several additional considerations, plus those identified previously at "The Entry Point":

- Do I have another solid job option? Storming into the CEO's office and resigning on the spot may have dramatic appeal or induce personal satisfaction, but it is best to have Plan B well in hand first. The success of the development of medical managers and CPEs has produced serious competition in all management fields. Much of the groundwork for identifying and investigating a new position can be done, and should be done, on your own time before the march on authority.

- Can I resign from this position and remain on good terms with office personnel? Notwithstanding the impact on your current job or the possibilities of a new position, it is always preferable to leave in glory rather than gloom. Avoid revealing your relocation plans with close work associates before the resignation discussion with your supervisor. Agree with the supervisor on how the announcement will be made and allow that agreement to proceed before other in-office discussions. Many companies are now requesting references from someone who directly reported to you or was a peer associate. Trying to maintain a good exit relationship is worth the effort and should begin with an assessment of how your leaving will affect the jobs of others. A discussion of your concerns for those impacts is a good leading-off point for a farewell announcement and will be appreciated much more highly than a glowing description of your new job or reflections upon your misery in the current position.

- Do I have existing contractual considerations about termination? In an era in which health care activities are coalescing into nationwide conglomerates, be certain that your employment contract contains no restrictive covenant language that would prevent your planned job move. A review of your current contract by a trusted attorney is wise. It is also important to know if the new company has any job advertising requirements that must be fulfilled before you can be hired or other employment conditions that interject some time lapse (such as state medical licensure). Understand clearly what your current contract requires about notification of termination.

- Will the new position actually satisfy your reasons for leaving this company? To leave over job dissatisfaction only to accept a different format for the same dissatisfactions is rarely considered progress. Sometimes changes in personnel will suffice, but be careful to analyze your reasons for leaving before resigning. Often a frank discussion with a supervisor or someone in an authority position may effect resolution of the problems. Such a "frank discussion" includes constructive suggestions, avoiding personnel finger-pointing if possible, and offers descriptions of how the concerns affect your ability to perform in the job.

Involuntary Termination

Rarely is a physician executive told bluntly, "You're fired!" However well phrased or regardless of the circumstances, the effect is just about the same. Physicians do not cope well with a perception of failure. We are trained to succeed, to cure, to remedy, and we usually have difficulty saying, "I'm sorry," even to loved ones when it is appropriate, because confidence bordering on omnipotence is drummed into our psyche early during training. In the 1970s and 1980s, when malpractice claims became fashionable, among the most devastating blows with which I, as a medical director, had to deal were allegations of negligence against litigation virgins in my group practice. The road through all stages of dealing with death and dying, from denial to acceptance, was experienced as a staggering, emotional struggle for most physicians.

When a physician manager loses a job for whatever reason, the effect can be almost as devastating. In spite of the smug comfort contained in "Golden Parachutes," the message comes through loud and clear that his or her services are no longer necessary. The pain of job loss is more acutely exacerbated when the more senior executive attempts to re-enter the job market. Jobs are there, to be sure, but qualified competitors are everywhere in increasing numbers.

This is the time when another personal appraisal is appropriate and mandatory. Often this honest evaluation is best accomplished by a career counselor with special focus on medical managers. Résumés need to be updated and, usually, refined. Accomplishments should be clearly enumerated and extraneous involvements eliminated. Only relevant and recent publications or presentations have any interest. Most significant, serious preparation for a job interview must be defined and focused. The personal image must be sharp and suited to the role being sought.

When a job offer comes and is accepted, the physician manager takes a long stride toward re-establishing professional confidence, personal acceptance, and productive resilience. Rejection, on the other hand and for whatever reason, has just the opposite effect and can be progressively defeating and personally demeaning. Unfortunately (although in all probability, fortunately), there is rarely a fallback position, i.e., returning to a clinical practice that will sustain a comparable lifestyle. The best choice, and most secure hope, lies in a personal regrouping and in pressing ahead. Again, career advice from a reliable source may prove an enlightening and encouraging experience. The job choice may involve accepting a less substantial position to begin again or another household move, but the jobs are available. Learn from the rejection—make late-course corrections—and move forward.

Moving Forward

For physicians in management, the direction ahead means:

- Believing that medicine is still a "Lifelong Obsession," to paraphrase Lloyd C. Douglas.[6]

- Committing to be a part of the changes taking place in our profession.

- Encouraging the best of our younger colleagues to pick up the mantle of responsibility as physician executives.

Regardless of the system of payment for health care services, the role of the physician executive has been clearly defined and, in my view, will remain of increasing necessity through decades of changes to come. There has never been a period in history with more demands on medical management to sustain the miraculous disease interventions of the recent years, to distribute those interventions to citizens of our nation and the world, and to confront the ethical issues that those interventions have spawned and that cannot be abrogated to nonmedical professionals. The certified physician executive designation should be carefully guarded and reserved for physician managers who are willing to accept these New Century challenges.

In the End

The summary of all of these writings lies in the appropriate preparation of the physician manager to accept these challenges. I am eternally grateful to the physician colleagues, the corporate executives, the academic faculties, the supporting co-workers, and the long-suffering patients who gave me opportunity. Of all the experiences within my years of maturing, the most significant, then and now, is the day I was declared a doctor of medicine. The MD or DO degree provides the most effective access to productive involvement in health care. While I might not have controlled everything that transpired during my professional career, I have retained ultimate control over my personal integrity and that control will never be relinquished. It remains my challenge, and that for physician executives everywhere, to maintain the integrity of our profession. Studious application of the fundamentals within this guide will enable successful pursuit of that challenge.

References

1. Ham, A., and Salter, M. *Doctor in the Making.* London, England: J.B. Lippincott Company, 1943, p. 1.

2. Weiner, L. "Part-Time Medical Director: Way Station or End of the Line?" *Physician Executive* 20(3):12-5, March 1994.

3. Many of the issues of career management are addressed in a one-day course, "Career Choices," conducted in various locations throughout the year by the American College of Physician Executives.

4. Linney, B. *Hope for the Future: A Career Development Guide for Physician Executives.* Tampa, Fla.: American College of Physician Executives, 1996.

5. Linney, G., and Linney, B. *Medical Directors: What, Why, How?* Tampa, Fla.: American College of Physician Executives, 1993.

6. Douglas, L. *Magnificent Obsession.* Boston, Mass.: Houghton Mifflin Company, 1929.

James E. Hartfield, MD, CPE, FACPE, is Medical Director, Quality Management, CIGNA Healthplans, Tampa, Florida. He is a Distinguished Fellow and Past President of the American College of Physician Executives.

Index

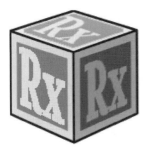

You May Have Paid Too Much for This Book

Members of the American College of Physician Executives receive discounts and special prices on all of our educational and informational products.

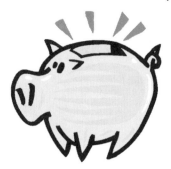

On a single item, that may not seem like much, but a few books and attendance at an educational program can sometimes recover an entire year's membership dues.

That is only one of many reasons for joining the College, of course. Many of our programs are offered only to members. The Graduate Program in Medical Management, whereby completion of College educational programs in the first step to a master's degree in medical management from a prestigious university, is a prime example.

The best reason for joining the College is the many opportunities to network with other physicians who have opted for management careers. In a variety of formal and informal programs, the College encourages and promotes the concept of networking and group discussion. The addition of Internet services has made networking an easy and compelling method of growing a management career.

Give us a call at **800/562-8088**
or drop by our Web site **(www.acpe.org)**
to learn more about the advantages of membership in ACPE.